Introduction to Clinical Neurology

22/4/79

Introduction to Clinical Neurology
Second Edition

Douglas J. Gelb, M.D., Ph.D.
Clinical Associate Professor of Neurology,
University of Michigan Medical School, Ann Arbor

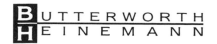
BUTTERWORTH
HEINEMANN

Boston•Oxford•Auckland•Johannesburg•Melbourne•New Delhi

Butterworth–Heinemann supports the efforts of American Forests and the Global ReLeaf program in its campaign for the betterment of trees, forests, and our environment.

Library of Congress Cataloging-in-Publication Data
Gelb, Douglas James, 1957-
  Introduction to clinical neurology / Douglas J. Gelb.--2nd ed.
    p. ; cm.
  Includes bibliographical references and index.
  ISBN 0-7506-7202-1
    1. Neurology. 2. Nervous system--Diseases. I. Title.
  [DNLM: 1. Nervous System Diseases. WL 140 G314i 2000]
  RC346 .G45 2000
  616.8--dc21
                                                              99-044004

British Library Cataloguing-in-Publication Data
A catalogue record for this book is available from the British Library.

The publisher offers special discounts on bulk orders of this book.
For information, please contact:
Manager of Special Sales
Butterworth–Heinemann
225 Wildwood Avenue
Woburn, MA 01801-2041

Tel: 781-904-2500
Fax: 781-904-2620

For information on all Butterworth–Heinemann publications available, contact our World Wide Web home page at: http://www.bh.com

10 9 8 7 6 5 4 3 2 1

Printed in the United States of America

To my father, the best teacher I know

Contents

Contributing Authors

James W. Albers, M.D., Ph.D.
Professor of Neurology and Director, Neuromuscular Program, Department of Neurology, University of Michigan Medical School, Ann Arbor

Mark B. Bromberg, M.D., Ph.D.
Associate Professor, Department of Neurology, University of Utah School of Medicine, Salt Lake City

Marc I. Chimowitz, M.B., Ch.B.
Professor and Director, Stroke Program, Department of Neurology, Emory University School of Medicine, Atlanta

Ivo J. Drury, M.B., B.Ch.
Chairman, Department of Neurology, Henry Ford Health System, Detroit; Adjunct Professor, Department of Neurology, University of Michigan Medical School, Ann Arbor

Linda M. Selwa, M.D.
Clinical Associate Professor, Department of Neurology, University of Michigan Medical School, Ann Arbor

Preface

I am writing these words at the twilight of one millennium; you are reading them at the dawn of another. How did that Y2K thing turn out, by the way?

In the 5 years since the first edition of this book appeared, new drugs have been released for stroke, seizures, amyotrophic lateral sclerosis, Alzheimer's disease, Parkinson's disease, narcolepsy, multiple sclerosis, and migraine. New surgical and endovascular treatments have been developed for stroke, epilepsy, Parkinson's disease, and tremor. The genetic mutations responsible for dozens of neurologic diseases have been identified, and the pathophysiologic mechanisms of many neurologic disorders have been clarified. My co-authors and I have attempted to incorporate these advances into this edition. At the same time, we have retained our focus on practical issues of diagnosis and management. The purpose of this book remains unchanged: to present a systematic approach to the neurologic problems likely to be encountered in general medical practice.

Although the first edition of this book included an extensive discussion of the neurologic examination and its interpretation, it did not contain step-by-step instructions for performing the examination. This was intentional, because I thought that such material was readily available elsewhere. Apparently I was wrong. In response to suggestions from readers, I have included a systematic discussion of the basic techniques of the neurologic examination in the present edition.

My thanks to Roger Albin, Mike Aldrich, Judy Heidebrink, Suzy Hickenbottom, Karen Kluin, Lori Schuh, and Jonathan Trobe for reading selected chapters and providing helpful suggestions. I remain grateful to my wife, Karen, for her encouragement and understanding, and for cutting me some slack while I tried to get this book done. Thank you to our daughters, Elizabeth and Molly, for sharing the computer with me, and so much more.

D.J.G.

Preface to the First Edition

Is neurology obsolete? Two current trends prompt this question. First, dramatic biologic and technologic advances have resulted in increasingly accurate diagnostic tests. It is hard to believe that CT scans have only been widely available since the 1970s; MRI scans, PET scans, and SPECT scans are even more recent, and they are constantly being refined. While chess-playing computers have not quite reached world champion status yet, neurodiagnostic imaging studies have long since achieved a degree of sensitivity that neurologists cannot hope to match. There is more than a little truth to the joke that "one MRI scan is worth a roomful of neurologists." Moreover, advances in molecular genetics and immunochemistry now permit more accurate diagnosis of many conditions than could have been imagined 25 years ago. Some conditions can even be diagnosed before any clinical manifestations are evident. With tests this good, what is the point of learning the traditional approach to neurologic diagnosis, in which lesion localization is deduced from patients' symptoms and signs?

The second major trend challenging the current status of neurology is health care reform. As of this writing, the first great national legislative debate concerning health care reform has ended, not with a bang but a whimper. Yet the problem itself has not disappeared. The already unacceptable costs of health care will continue to escalate if the current system remains unchanged. While the various reform plans that have been proposed differ in many fundamental respects, there appears to be a consensus that there should be more primary care physicians and fewer specialists. Indeed, several forces are already pushing the medical profession in that direction even in the absence of a comprehensive national legislative plan. As a concrete example, it is anticipated that the number of residency training positions in neurology will drop, perhaps to only half of the current level. With so much nationwide emphasis on primary care, what is the point of studying neurology?

Ironically, these two trends together provide a compelling reason to study neurology. In coming years, there will be increasing pressures on primary care physicians to avoid referring patients to specialists (and there will be fewer specialists in the first place). One response of primary care physicians might be to order more diagnostic tests. Unfortunately, the only thing more impressive than the sensitivity of the new tests is their price tag. Just at the time when diagnostic tests are reaching unprecedented levels of accuracy, the funds to pay for the tests are disappearing. Rather than replacing neurologists with MRI scans and genetic testing, primary care physicians will have to become neurologists (to some degree) themselves.

In short, the role currently played by neurologists may well be obsolete, but neurology itself is not. All physicians, regardless of specialty, must become familiar with the general principles of neurologic diagnosis and management. That is the rationale for this book.

The purpose of this book is to present a systematic approach to the neurologic problems likely to be encountered in general medical practice. The focus throughout the book is on practical issues of patient management. This is a departure from the traditional view of neurologic diseases as fascinating but untreatable. Neurologists are often caricatured as pedants who will pontificate interminably on the precise localization of a lesion, produce an obscure diagnosis with an unpronounceable eponym, and smugly declare the case closed. In years past, this stereotype was not wholly inaccurate. Even when therapeutic options existed, there were few controlled studies of efficacy, so it was easy to take a nihilistic approach to therapy. "First do no harm" could often be legitimately interpreted to mean "Do nothing." This was obviously a frustrating position for physicians, and even more so for patients, but at least it kept things simple. All this has changed. Controlled trials of both new and traditional therapies are being conducted with increasing frequency. In the two years since the original versions of some of the current chapters were first prepared, sumatriptan has been approved for treatment of headache, beta interferon for use in multiple sclerosis, ticlopidine for stroke, and tacrine for Alzheimer's disease. Felbamate has appeared and (practically) disappeared. Gabapentin and lamotrigine have been approved for use in epilepsy. The long-term results of a large cooperative study of optic neuritis have challenged traditional practices involving the use of steroids for that condition and for multiple sclerosis. Preliminary reports have appeared concerning the value of endarterectomy for asymptomatic carotid stenosis, a new preparation of beta interferon for MS, and Copolymer I for MS. These are exciting developments, but many of the studies raise as many questions as they answer. They certainly change the way physicians have traditionally approached many neurologic diseases. This book reflects that change. Esoteric diagnostic distinctions with little practical relevance are avoided. Distinctions that affect treatment are emphasized. In most chapters, the available treatment options and general approach to management are presented first, to clarify which diagnostic distinctions are important and why.

For many physicians and medical students, the most difficult aspect of neurology is deciding where to start. It is relatively straightforward to manage a patient who has had a stroke; it is often harder to determine whether the patient had a stroke in the first place. When does hand weakness indicate carpal tunnel syndrome, and when is it a manifestation of multiple sclerosis? When does back pain signify metastatic cancer or a herniated disk? These general issues are addressed in the three chapters of Part I. In Part II, common neurologic disease categories are discussed. Part III concerns common symptoms and issues that cross disease categories. Features that distinguish neurologic problems in the pediatric and geriatric populations are discussed in Part IV.

This book is not meant to be comprehensive. Certain topics are omitted, notably specialized management issues that primary care physicians will probably not need to address and other conditions for which treatment is a matter of standard medical care. For example, most patients with primary brain cancer will probably be referred to specialists even in an age of health care reform, so the different types of brain cancer and their treatment are not addressed in this book. Diabetes, chronic alcohol abuse, vitamin B_{12} deficiency, and other metabolic disturbances can affect many parts of the nervous system. These conditions are mentioned in the relevant sections of this book, but there is no chapter devoted specifically to metabolic problems and their management because these topics are covered in standard medical textbooks. Even for the topics that are included in the book, much detail has been omitted. Again, detailed discussions are available in standard reference books. Use of those books requires some sophistication about neurology, however. A physician trying to figure out why a patient's hand is weak may be overwhelmed by a one or two thousand page textbook. Even when the patient's diagnosis is known, the standard references often fail to distinguish the forest from the trees, making it difficult to glean the main principles governing patient management. Those principles are the focus of this book.

Each chapter in this book begins with a set of clinical vignettes and associated questions. These are intended to help the reader focus on practical clinical questions while reading the chapter. Readers should try to answer the questions before reading the rest of the chapter. After finishing the chapter (but before reading the discussion of the clinical vignettes) readers should return to the questions and revise their answers as necessary. Readers can then compare their answers with those given in the discussion at the end of the chapter.

The vignettes are also intended to convey the message that neurology is fun. Many students who used the original version of this book reported that they enjoyed working through the vignettes, and they even suggested that more be included. This response is gratifying. Still, the best "clinical vignettes" come from patients themselves, not from books. Ideally, readers of this book will be inspired to seek out patients with neurologic problems, and will approach them not only with confidence, but with enthusiasm.

D.J.G.

Introduction to Clinical Neurology

The Basic Approach

I

1

Where's the Lesion?

I. Sample Localization Problems

Example 1. A patient is found to have the following:

   1. weakness of abduction of the little finger on the right hand

   2. reduced pinprick sensation on the palmar surface of the little finger of the right hand

Where's the lesion?

Example 2. A patient is found to have the following:

   1. reduced pinprick sensation on the left forehead

   2. reduced pinprick sensation on the palmar surface of the little finger of the right hand

Where's the lesion?

Example 3.   A patient is found to have the following:

1.   reduced joint position sense in the left foot

2.   reduced pinprick sensation on the palmar surface of the little finger of the right hand

Where's the lesion?

Example 4.   A patient is found to have the following:

1.   reduced joint position sense in the left foot

2.   reduced pinprick sensation on the palmar surface of the little finger of the right hand

3.   weakness of left ankle dorsiflexion

4.   hyperreflexia at the left knee

Where's the lesion?

Example 5.   A patient is found to have the following:

1.   reduced joint position sense in the left foot

2.   reduced joint position sense in the right foot

3.   reduced joint position sense in the left hand

4.   reduced joint position sense in the right hand

Where's the lesion?

Example 6.   A patient is found to have the following:

1.   reduced joint position sense in the left foot

2. reduced pinprick sensation on the palmar surface of the little finger of the right hand

3. reduced visual acuity in the left eye

Where's the lesion?

Example 7. A patient is found to have the following:

1. reduced joint position and pinprick sensation in the left foot

2. reduced joint position and pinprick sensation in the right foot

3. reduced joint position and pinprick sensation in the left hand

4. reduced joint position and pinprick sensation in the right hand

5. normal strength and sensation proximally in all four limbs

Where's the lesion?

II. The Game

"Where's the lesion?" Generations of medical students and house officers have learned to dread being asked this question. Having just presented an eloquent summary of a patient's history and physical examination, they are determined to proceed to an elegant differential diagnosis, when they are interrupted by those three pesky little words. Why do neurologists become so obsessed about localization? Is it just an intellectual game they like to play, a form of mental gymnastics?

As a matter of fact, it is. Neurologists tend to view each diagnostic challenge as a logical exercise and approach localization as a kind of puzzle or game. It is by no means frivolous, however. It is an essential step in the generation of a differential diagnosis. Once the site of the problem is identified, certain diseases become prime suspects, while others can be rejected out of hand. If this step is omitted, diagnosis becomes purely a process of pattern recognition, which is an unwieldy approach when there are hundreds of diseases to consider. Localization of the lesion can help to focus and prioritize the evaluation, an important goal in an age of health care cost containment.

The principle of localization is not unique to neurology. For example, a patient with hematemesis is evaluated not for cardiac or pulmonary diseases, but for diseases of the gastrointestinal tract, and specifically the upper gastrointestinal tract; diseases of the jejunum and below can be ignored. The main reason neurologic localization is distinctive is that the nervous system has so many different functions, each one mediated by anatomic structures that overlap or abut structures responsible for many other functions. Moreover, most of the anatomic structures are inaccessible to direct examination. Neurologic localization is thus analogous to the problem of debugging a miniature integrated circuit (although some might argue that a more appropriate analogy would be the problem of finding the site of obstruction in an underground sewer system—without swimming in it!).

Fortunately, most of the functions of the nervous system can be assessed even without examining the anatomic structures that mediate them. The nervous system is primarily responsible for coordinating an organism's interactions with its environment, so it must process sensory information from the outside world and generate some form of motor response. Whether the motor response involves highly coordinated patterns of muscle activity (such as those necessary for speaking or hitting a baseball) or simply the reflex contraction of a single muscle, it can be directly observed by an examiner. The sensory input is also subject to the examiner's observation. By knowing the way the nervous system is organized, and by observing the "output" that results from a known sensory "input," the examiner attempts to deduce the site of nervous system dysfunction. This is the localization game played by neurologists.

The rules of the game are presented in the following section. For practicing neurologists, the reasoning involved in localization is so instinctive that explicit rules are unnecessary, but most would agree that localization ultimately depends on the kind of logical, stepwise approach summarized in these rules.

III. The Rules

1. Each symptom or abnormal physical finding can be thought of as a line segment connecting the central nervous system to the periphery (a muscle or sensory receptor).

2. If all of these line segments intersect at a single point, that point is the site of the lesion.

3. There may be two or more points where all the line segments intersect, and hence, two or more potential lesion sites. If so, each potential site must be evaluated further by determining whether the patient has the other symptoms or signs that would be expected with a lesion in that location.

4. There may be no points that fall on all of the line segments. If so, the goal is to explain all of the patient's symptoms and physical findings on the basis of just two lesions (i.e., to find two points such that every line segment passes through one or the other point).

5. If even two lesion sites are not sufficient to explain all the symptoms and findings, the process is considered to be multifocal. The goal then becomes one of detecting a unifying property that applies to all the lesion sites. For example, they may all be located at the neuromuscular junction, or they may all be in the white matter of the central nervous system.

When stated in this way, the rules appear abstract and somewhat obscure, but they are actually quite straightforward to apply. This is demonstrated in the following three sections by considering specific examples. It might seem that detailed knowledge of neuroanatomy would be required. Certainly, more precise neuroanatomic knowledge permits more refined localization, but for most purposes some fairly rough neuroanatomic approximations are adequate. To show this, several examples of careful neuroanatomic analysis are presented in Part IV, and simpler analyses of the same clinical scenarios are presented in Part V. In Part VI, the kind of reasoning applied in Parts IV and V is used to derive some useful general localization rules.

IV. The Play—The Long Version

Note: Some readers may choose to proceed directly to Part V if the following discussion seems too complicated. In fact, some may wish to focus on the simple rules presented in Part VI, which can be used to localize the majority of neurologic lesions. At some point, however, the reader should return to Part IV to understand the detailed reasoning process that underlies the more simplified approaches.

Example 1.   A patient is found to have the following:

1. weakness of abduction of the little finger on the right hand

2. reduced pinprick sensation on the palmar surface of the little finger of the right hand

Where's the lesion?

Item 1 could be caused by a lesion anywhere in the line segment shown in Figure 1-1. The pathway begins in the precentral gyrus of the left cerebral cortex (i.e., the motor strip). The representation of the hand in this strip is midway between the leg representation medially and the face representation laterally. From this point of origin, the segment passes through the corona radiata and the internal capsule, then through the cerebral peduncle in the midbrain and the basis pontis to the pyramid in the medulla. At this point, the pathway crosses to the right side, proceeds downward in the lateral white matter of the spinal cord, and exits the spinal cord via the right C8 and T1 roots. It proceeds through the lower trunk and then the medial cord of the brachial plexus, exits in the ulnar nerve, passes through the neuromuscular junction, and terminates in the abductor digiti minimi muscle.

The line segment corresponding to item 2 is shown in Figure 1-2. It starts in sensory receptors in the little finger of the right hand, continues in the ulnar nerve, proceeds proximally through the medial cord and lower trunk of the brachial plexus, and enters the spinal cord via the right C8 nerve root. It ascends one or two segments in the cord, then crosses to the left spinothalamic tract, ascending in this tract through the medulla, pons, and midbrain. After synapsing in the ventral posterolateral nucleus of the thalamus, the pathway continues through the internal capsule and corona radiata, terminating in the parietal cortex (just posterior to the region of the motor strip where the line segment for item 1 originates).

Figure 1-3 illustrates both of these line segments together. One obvious point of intersection is in the frontoparietal cortex, where one segment lies directly behind the other. In addition, there is a whole set of possible intersection sites falling between the ulnar nerve distally and the C8/T1 nerve roots proximally. To decide which of these potential localization sites is the true focus of pathology, the next step is to consider what other signs and symptoms might be expected from a lesion at each site. For example, a lesion in the C8/T1 nerve roots or the lower trunk of the brachial plexus would be likely to affect fibers des-

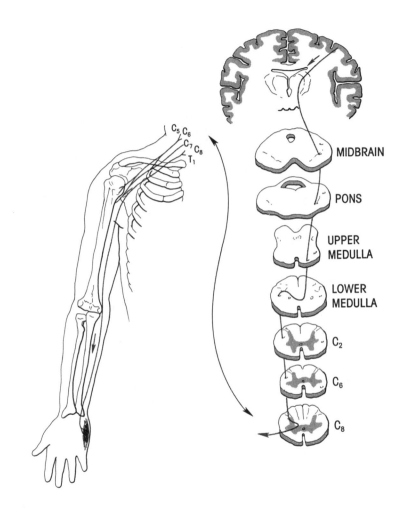

Figure 1-1. *The solid red line shows the pathway corresponding to weakness of abduction of the little finger on the right hand.*

C₅ C₆
C₇ C₈
T₁

MIDBRAIN

PONS

UPPER MEDULLA

LOWER MEDULLA

C₂

C₆

C₈

9

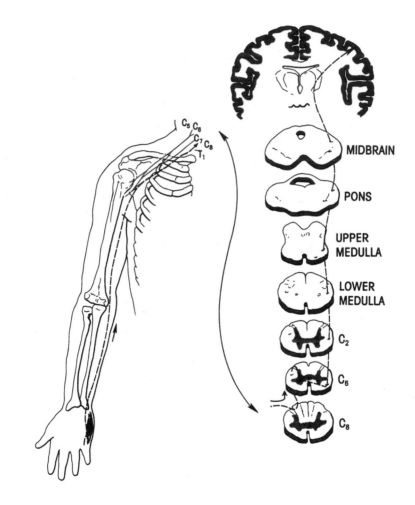

Figure 1-2. *The dashed black line depicts the pathway corresponding to reduced pinprick sensation on the palmar surface of the little finger on the right hand.*

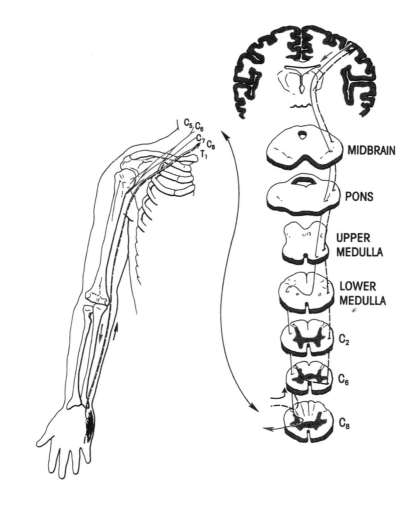

MIDBRAIN

PONS

UPPER
MEDULLA

LOWER
MEDULLA

C_2

C_6

C_8

C_5, C_6

$C_7 C_8$

T_1

Figure 1-3. *Diagram illustrating both the pathway corresponding to weak abduction of the right little finger (solid red line) and reduced pinprick sensation (dashed black line) in that finger (i.e., the pathways of both Figure 1-1 and Figure 1-2). The regions common to both pathways are in the frontoparietal cortex and in the peripheral nervous system (from the C8/ T1 nerve roots to the ulnar nerve).*

tined for the median nerve, affecting muscles innervated by that nerve, whereas these muscles would clearly be spared by a lesion in the ulnar nerve itself. In contrast, a cortical lesion affecting the arm could extend far enough laterally or medially to affect the cortical representation of the right face or leg, whereas a nerve, plexus, or root lesion clearly would not affect anything outside the right upper extremity. Abnormalities of vision or language function would also imply a cortical localization and would be inconsistent with a lesion in the peripheral nervous system.

Example 2.   A patient is found to have the following:

1.   reduced pinprick sensation on the left forehead

2.   reduced pinprick sensation on the palmar surface of the little finger of the right hand

Where's the lesion?

The line segment corresponding to item 2 was already discussed in the previous example (see Figure 1-2). The pathway for item 1 is shown in Figure 1-4. It starts in sensory receptors in the left forehead and continues in the first division (the ophthalmic division) of the trigeminal nerve (cranial nerve V). This nerve travels through the superior orbital fissure and enters the lateral wall of the cavernous sinus. It then emerges to join the other two divisions of the trigeminal nerve in the trigeminal (gasserian) ganglion. From here, the pathway enters the pons, descends in the left spinal tract of the trigeminal nucleus, and synapses in the nucleus of that tract at about the C2 spinal level. At this point, the pathway crosses to the right side of the spinal cord and ascends in the ventral trigeminothalamic tract to synapse in the ventral posteromedial nucleus of the right thalamus. The final section of the line segment runs from the ventral posteromedial nucleus through the internal capsule and corona radiata to terminate in the lateral aspect of the postcentral gyrus of the parietal lobe.

   Figure 1-5 combines Figures 1-2 and 1-4. Potential intersection sites lie between the mid-pons and the high spinal cord (C2) on the left. At all other points, the line segments are nowhere near each other. In fact, they are generally on opposite sides of the nervous system! Again, the localization can be made even more precise by determining whether the patient has other abnormalities that might result from a lesion at each potential site. For example, facial nerve involvement could occur

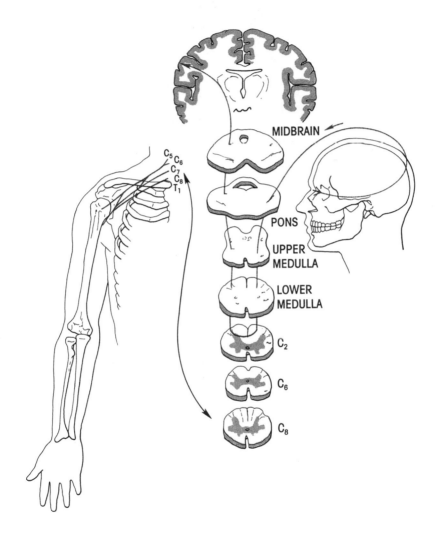

Figure 1-4. *The solid red line shows the pathway corresponding to reduced pinprick sensation on the left forehead.*

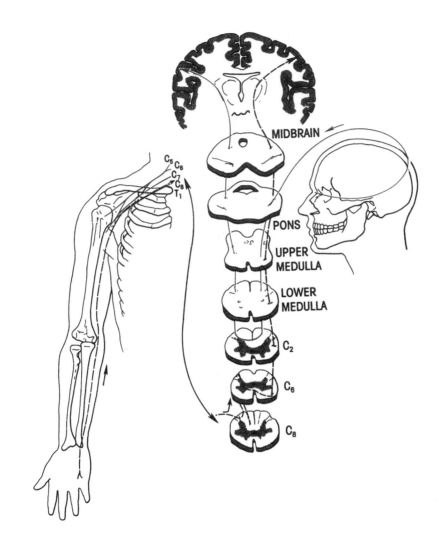

Figure 1-5. *Diagram illustrating both the pathway corresponding to (dashed black line) reduced pinprick sensation in the right little finger and (solid red line) reduced pinprick sensation on the left forehead (i.e., the pathways of both Figure 1-2 and Figure 1-4). The regions common to both pathways lie between the mid-pons and the C2 level of the spinal cord on the left.*

with a lesion in the mid-pons, but not at any of the lower sites, whereas hypoglossal nerve involvement would indicate a lesion at the level of the medulla.

For all the neuroanatomic detail presented in Figures 1-1 through 1-5, these are still only simplifications. For example, Figure 1-1 reflects a tacit assumption that the lateral corticospinal tract is the principal descending pathway affecting limb muscles. The ventral corticospinal tract and other descending motor pathways (such as the vestibulospinal, tectospinal, rubrospinal, reticulospinal, and ceruleus-spinal projections) are not included in the figure. The importance of these other descending pathways is best appreciated by recognizing that a selective lesion of the corticospinal tract (e.g., in the medullary pyramid, one of the few locations where it is physically isolated from other descending tracts) results in minimal long-term weakness. Even so, the pathway presented in Figure 1-1 proves to be very useful in clinical localization. Presumably, the contributions of all the descending tracts sum up in such a way that the net effect is something similar to the pathway shown in the figure.

V. The Play—The Abbreviated Version

The best way to identify all plausible lesion localization sites (and only those sites) is to follow the approach outlined in Part IV. In many cases, however, much coarser analysis of the symptoms and signs will give nearly the same results. In particular, the lesion can often be localized with surprising precision simply by considering where the relevant nervous system pathways cross the midline.

Example 1 Revisited

Figure 1-6 shows a schematic diagram of the pathway portrayed in Figure 1-1, corresponding to weakness of the right abductor digiti minimi muscle. Much of the detail has been eliminated. In fact, the same diagram would apply to any muscle in the right upper extremity. Figure 1-7 shows a schematic diagram for the right hand numbness represented in Figure 1-2. Figure 1-8 combines Figures 1-6 and 1-7. It is clear even from this simplified diagram that the lesion could not possibly be located within the spinal cord: The two pathways are on opposite sides! Instead, the lesion must either be in the periphery (i.e., at the level of nerve roots, plexus, or peripheral nerves) or rostral to the level at which the motor pathway crosses in the medulla. Although

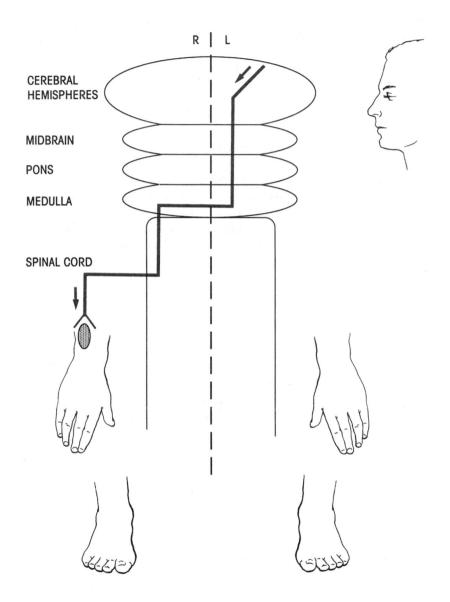

Figure 1-6. *Schematic drawing of the pathway shown in Figure 1-1, representing weakness of right little finger abduction. The same diagram would be used to represent weakness in any muscle of the right upper extremity.*

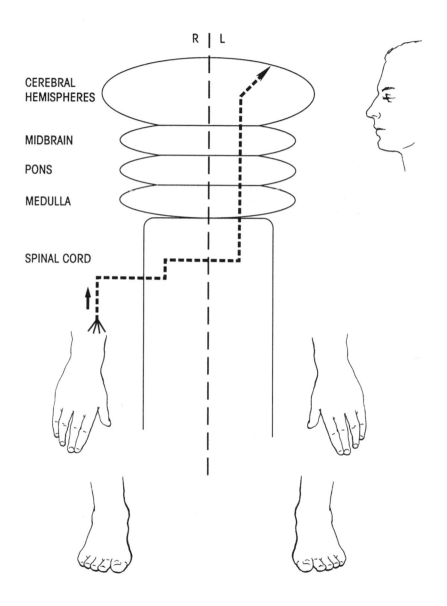

Figure 1-7. *Schematic drawing of the pathway shown in Figure 1-2, representing reduced pinprick sensation in the right upper extremity.*

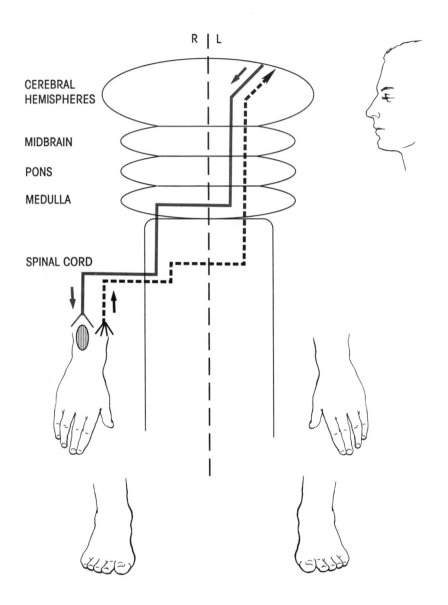

Figure 1-8. *Schematic representation of Figure 1-3, combining Figures 1-6 and 1-7. The only regions common to both pathways are at the level of the mid-medulla or above, or in the periphery.*

the more detailed analysis presented in Part IV results in a more refined final localization (ruling out all of the rostral structures except the cortex), this additional refinement may not have much practical consequence. The entire region from the medulla to the cortex is visualized on magnetic resonance imaging (MRI) of the brain, so as long as the lesion can be localized to somewhere within this region the appropriate diagnostic study will be obtained. In contrast, elimination of the cervical spinal cord from consideration does have a significant practical result, because it makes an MRI scan of the cervical spine unnecessary.

Example 2 Revisited

Figure 1-9 presents a schematic diagram for the pathway shown in Figure 1-4, representing left forehead numbness. Again, Figure 1-7 represents a schematic diagram for right hand numbness. Both pathways are shown together in Figure 1-10. It is clear from the diagram that the only potential intersection points lie in the region extending from the left mid-pons down to the left side of the spinal cord at the C2 level. This is exactly the same localization deduced earlier from the more detailed analysis.

This simplified approach to localization involves only a small number of schematic diagram templates. Weakness in any limb is represented by Figure 1-6 or an analogous pathway in another limb. A diagram analogous to Figure 1-7 can be drawn to represent a deficit in pain or temperature sensation in any limb. A deficit in proprioception or vibration sense is represented by Figure 1-11 (or something analogous in another limb). Figure 1-9 portrays the pathway for impaired pain and temperature sensation in the face. The pathway for facial weakness is represented in Figure 1-12, and analogous figures can be drawn for the motor components of other cranial nerves. These pathways are complicated because there is bilateral cortical input to many of these cranial nerve nuclei, making interpretation difficult at times. Analogously, the auditory and vestibular pathways project bilaterally once they enter the central nervous system, making peripheral lesions much more straightforward to localize than central lesions. For example, unilateral hearing loss implies a lesion in the ipsilateral eighth nerve, cochlea, or inner ear. Bilateral hearing loss is of much less localizing value.

The distinction between the central and peripheral portions of a pathway is often very powerful. When considered schematically, the peripheral portion of a pathway (connecting a muscle or sensory

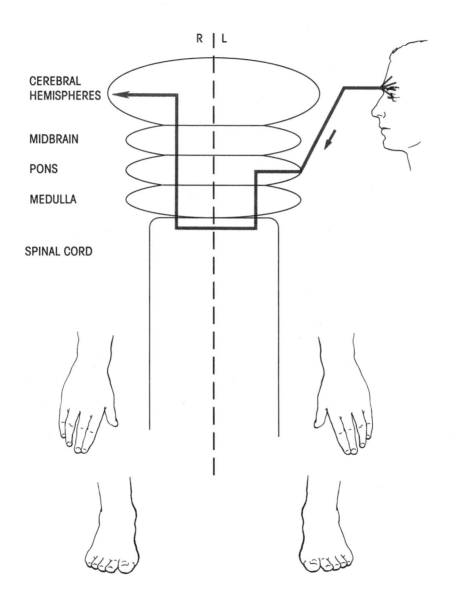

Figure 1-9. *Schematic drawing of the pathway shown in Figure 1-4, representing left facial numbness.*

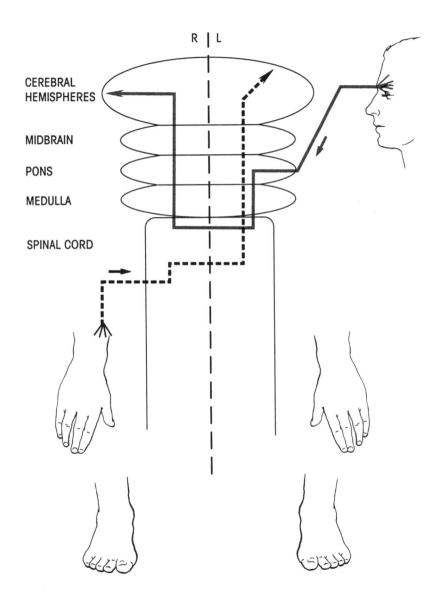

R | L

CEREBRAL
HEMISPHERES

MIDBRAIN

PONS

MEDULLA

SPINAL CORD

Figure 1-10. *Schematic representation of Figure 1-5, combining Figures 1-7 and 1-9. The only regions common to both pathways lie between the mid-pons and the C2 level of the spinal cord on the left.*

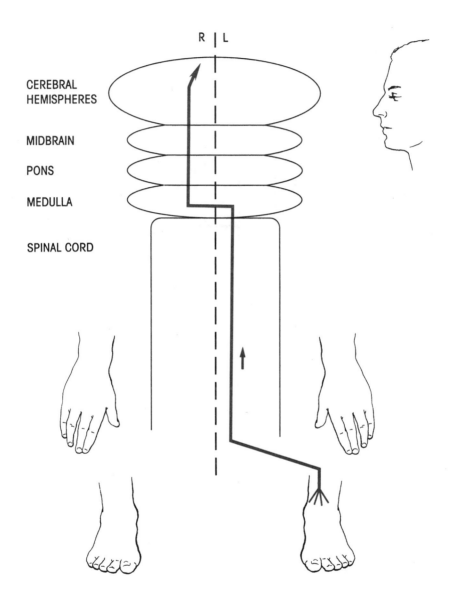

Figure 1-11. *Schematic drawing of the pathway corresponding to reduced position or vibration sense in the left lower extremity.*

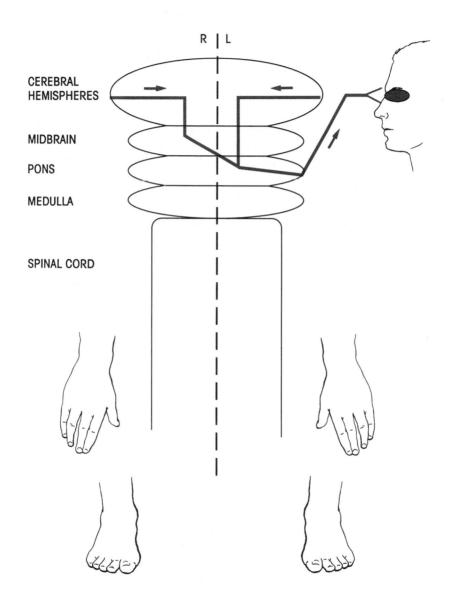

Figure 1-12. *Schematic drawing of the pathway corresponding to left facial weakness.*

receptor organ to the spinal cord or brainstem) is perpendicular to the "long axis" of the nervous system (the neuraxis), which runs from the cortex to the base of the spinal cord. A lesion that can be localized to the peripheral limb of one pathway and the central limb of another is thus "caught in the cross-hairs," permitting very precise localization.

For example, a patient who has a lesion compressing the spinal cord typically has hypoactive deep tendon reflexes at the level of the lesion and hyperactive reflexes below that level. **Hypoactive reflexes indicate dysfunction in the peripheral portion of the reflex pathway, the reflex arc.** The reflex arc begins in a sensory receptor, travels along sensory nerve fibers to the spinal cord, then synapses with a motor neuron in the anterior horn at the same level, proceeding out along motor nerve fibers to the muscle. In essence, this pathway is formed by joining the peripheral components of Figures 1-6 and 1-11. In normal individuals, the deep tendon reflexes are continually suppressed by descending motor tracts. These tracts constitute the central, or "upper motor neuron," portion of the reflex pathway. **When there is a lesion in this central pathway, the peripheral reflex arc is no longer suppressed, and a hyperactive reflex results.** A variety of different descending tracts are involved, but as already discussed with regard to weakness, the net effect is approximated by the central limb of the pathway shown in Figure 1-6. Both the peripheral and the central portions of the pathway for the right biceps reflex are represented schematically in Figure 1-13. A compressive lesion at the C5 level of the spinal cord interrupts the peripheral portion of the biceps reflex pathway and at the same time interrupts the central portion of the pathways mediating the triceps and lower-extremity reflexes. Other examination findings useful in distinguishing central (e.g., upper motor neuron or supranuclear) from peripheral (e.g., lower motor neuron or nuclear) lesions are discussed in Chapter 2.

Visual information is transmitted from the eyes to the brain by another pathway that is perpendicular to the neuraxis (Figure 1-14). Some very elegant principles of localization can be deduced from a detailed understanding of this pathway, but at the most basic level it suffices to know that the optic nerves from each eye merge at the optic chiasm. Anterior to the chiasm, a structural lesion will affect vision from only one eye, whereas a lesion at the chiasm or posterior to it will produce visual problems in both eyes. Moreover, when the fibers merge at the chiasm, they sort themselves so that all the fibers on one side of the brain correspond to visual input from the opposite side of the visual world. To be specific, the fibers passing through the left side of the brain to reach the left occipital cortex originate in retinal cells

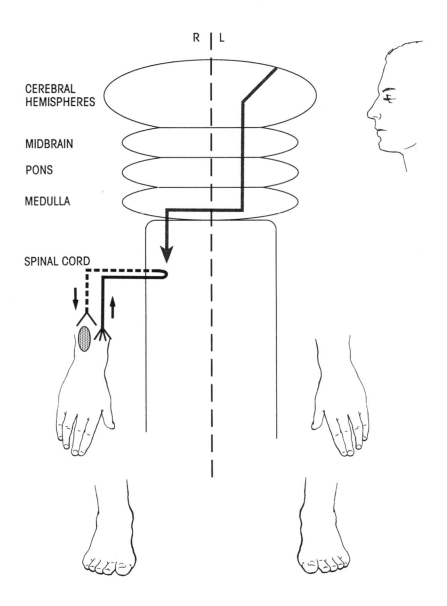

Figure 1-13. *Schematic drawing of a reflex arc in the right upper extremity, together with the central pathway providing descending input to the reflex arc.*

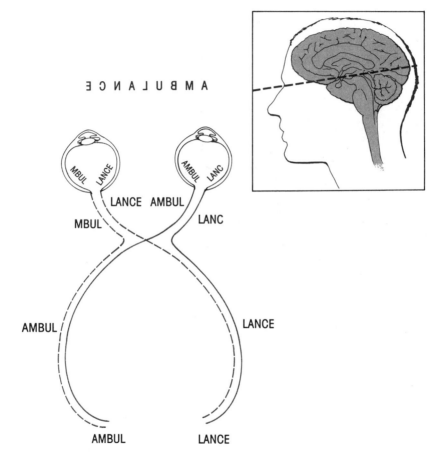

Figure 1-14. *Schematic drawing representing the visual pathways.*

that respond to stimuli in the right half of the world. By the rules of optics, this is the left half of each retina (i.e., the temporal half of the left retina and the nasal half of the right retina). In order to achieve this organization, the fibers from the nasal half of each retina must cross at the chiasm. A single large lesion at the chiasm can damage all the crossing and uncrossing fibers, resulting in total blindness. A smaller, centrally placed lesion may damage only the crossing fibers. Since these fibers originate in the nasal retina of each eye, the result is impaired vision in the temporal field of each eye (a bitemporal hemianopia).

The pupillary light reflex is mediated by yet another pathway that is perpendicular to the neuraxis (Figure 1-15). The pathway runs from the eye through the optic chiasm, just as in Figure 1-14, but soon after leaving the chiasm some fibers diverge from the rest of the visual fibers to synapse in the dorsal midbrain on parasympathetic nerve fibers that run with the oculomotor nerve (cranial nerve III) and terminate in the pupillary constrictor muscles. Note that even with input to just one eye, the bilateral projections in the optic chiasm and again in the midbrain result in bilateral output—that is, both pupils constrict. The net output is actually a function of the input to both eyes. In most natural circumstances, the overall illumination is the same in both eyes, so the input to each eye is the same. When the input to each eye is different (e.g., when an examiner holds a bright flashlight up to one eye, or when one optic nerve is defective), the midbrain essentially averages the illumination from the two eyes to produce a single net output signal that is the same for the two pupils.

Pupillary size is determined not only by the parasympathetic pathway but also by the sympathetic pathway, represented in Figure 1-16. This pathway begins in the hypothalamus, descends through the brainstem to the spinal cord at about the T1 level, then exits the spinal cord to enter the sympathetic chain and synapse in the superior cervical ganglion. From here, the pathway follows first the internal carotid artery and then the ophthalmic division of the trigeminal nerve (cranial nerve V), ultimately terminating in the pupil. Unlike most other pathways, the sympathetic pathway controlling the pupil remains on one side of the nervous system throughout its course. This is often extremely helpful in pinning down the site of a lesion.

Several neurologic deficits with localizing value do not readily lend themselves to a formulation in terms of line segments. For example, coordinated movements involve the interplay of motor cortex, basal ganglia, cerebellum, and brainstem nuclei. The interconnections between these structures result in "double-crossing" and "triple-crossing" pathways that sometimes resemble a tangled ball of yarn. It is often simplest to localize a lesion on the basis of other clinical features, and

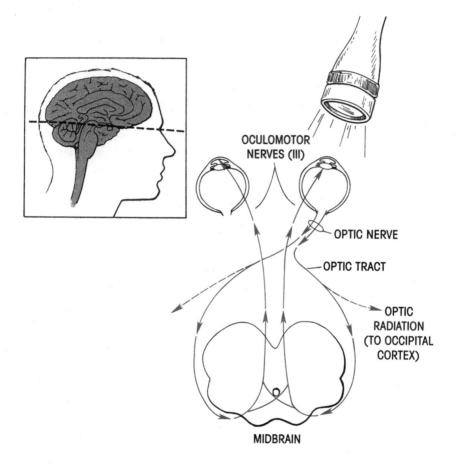

Figure 1-15. *Schematic drawing of the pathway mediating bilateral pupillary constriction in response to light in the right eye.*

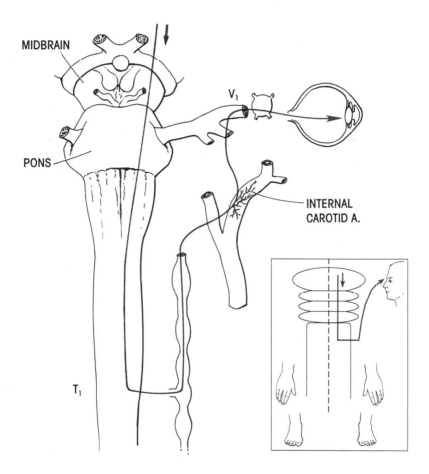

Figure 1-16. *Schematic drawing illustrating the pathway for sympathetic innervation of the left pupil.*

then check to see that the resulting localization is consistent with the patient's movement problem, rather than trying to reason through all the potential sites that could cause that movement abnormality. As another example, selective deficits in distinct cognitive functions result from focal lesions in the cerebral cortex, but the pathways corresponding to these cognitive functions are so complicated that the resulting diagrams would either be incomprehensible or too simplistic to be meaningful.

One exception is language function. Figure 1-17 presents a schematic diagram of the way language function is often conceptualized. Wernicke's area in the posterior temporal cortex is thought to be involved in recognizing the linguistic structures incorporated in a string of sounds. Areas of "higher" association cortex process these linguistic structures to extract meaning. Broca's area in the inferior lateral frontal lobe (just anterior to the region of the motor strip representing the face) is thought to translate linguistic structures into the motor programs necessary for producing speech. Thus, the comprehension of spoken language is represented in Figure 1-17 by pathway 1 from the ear to auditory cortex to Wernicke's area and thence to association areas. The ability to repeat a string of words is represented by pathway 3 from the ear to auditory cortex to Wernicke's area to Broca's area (via the arcuate fasciculus) to the motor strip and thence to the cranial nerves innervating the appropriate muscles of the face, tongue, pharynx, larynx, and diaphragm. This scheme is a gross oversimplification and fails to explain many clinical observations, but it actually proves to have some clinical utility—at least in giving an indication of whether a lesion is likely to be located relatively anteriorly or posteriorly. In fact, an extension of the scheme that includes coding of written symbols in the angular gyrus (just above and behind Wernicke's area at the junction of the occipital, parietal, and temporal lobes) is also useful clinically. In short, this conceptualization is a useful approximation even though it is not an accurate representation of specific linguistic or neurophysiologic mechanisms.

Example 3.   A patient is found to have the following:

1. reduced joint position sense in the left foot

2. reduced pinprick sensation on the palmar surface of the little finger of the right hand

Where's the lesion?

A. LANGUAGE-RELATED STRUCTURES

W = WERNICKE'S AREA
B = BROCA'S AREA

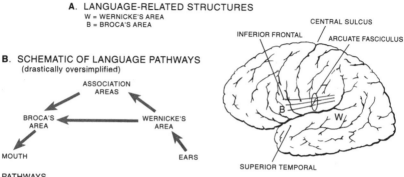

CENTRAL SULCUS
INFERIOR FRONTAL
ARCUATE FASCICULUS

B. SCHEMATIC OF LANGUAGE PATHWAYS
(drastically oversimplified)

ASSOCIATION
AREAS

BROCA'S
AREA

WERNICKE'S
AREA

MOUTH

EARS

SUPERIOR TEMPORAL

PATHWAYS
1. COMPREHENSION: EARS --➤ WERNICKE'S --➤ ASSOCIATION AREAS
2. FLUENCY: ASSOCIATION AREAS --➤ BROCA'S --➤ MOUTH
3. REPETITION: EARS --➤ WERNICKE'S --➤ (VIA ARCUATE FASCICULUS) --➤ BROCA'S --➤ MOUTH

NOTE: Repetition pathway is peri-Sylvian (i.e., involves only structures adjacent to Sylvian fissure). Global hypofusion tends to spare this area, disconnecting it from association areas and producing transcortical aphasias (see Panel C).

C. TRADITIONAL APHASIA CLASSIFICATION SCHEME
(again, oversimplified)

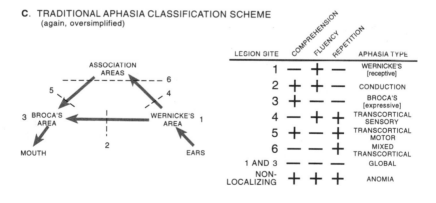

LESION SITE	COMPREHENSION	FLUENCY	REPETITION	APHASIA TYPE
1	−	+	−	WERNICKE'S [receptive]
2	+	+	−	CONDUCTION
3	+	−	−	BROCA'S [expressive]
4	−	+	+	TRANSCORTICAL SENSORY
5	+	−	+	TRANSCORTICAL MOTOR
6	−	−	+	MIXED TRANSCORTICAL
1 AND 3	−	−	−	GLOBAL
NON-LOCALIZING	+	+	+	ANOMIA

ASSOCIATION AREAS

BROCA'S AREA

WERNICKE'S AREA

MOUTH

EARS

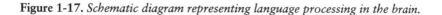

Figure 1-17. *Schematic diagram representing language processing in the brain.*

The line segment corresponding to item 2 has already been discussed (see Figure 1-7). The line segment corresponding to item 1 is shown in Figure 1-11. Both line segments are shown together in Figure 1-18. The two line segments are on opposite sides of the nervous system except for a short segment running from the lower medulla on the left to about the C6/7 level of the spinal cord on the left. This region is the only potential localization site.

Example 4.   A patient is found to have the following:

1.   reduced joint position sense in the left foot

2.   reduced pinprick sensation on the palmar surface of the little finger of the right hand

3.   weakness of left ankle dorsiflexion

4.   hyperreflexia at the left knee

Where's the lesion?

The first two items are the same as in Example 3 and imply a lesion localization somewhere between the low medulla and the C6/7 level of the spinal cord on the left (see Figure 1-18). Within this region, the line segments corresponding to the third and fourth items essentially coincide with the line segment for item 1. Thus, the additional deficits help to confirm the region of potential localization, but they do not help to refine it. One way to narrow the region would be to examine the left biceps reflex. This would be represented by a mirror image of the pathway shown in Figure 1-13. A depressed biceps reflex would imply a lesion in the reflex arc, at the C5 or C6 level of the spinal cord. In contrast, a hyperactive biceps reflex would imply a lesion above the level of C5.

Example 5.   A patient is found to have the following:

1.   reduced joint position sense in the left foot

2.   reduced joint position sense in the right foot

3.   reduced joint position sense in the left hand

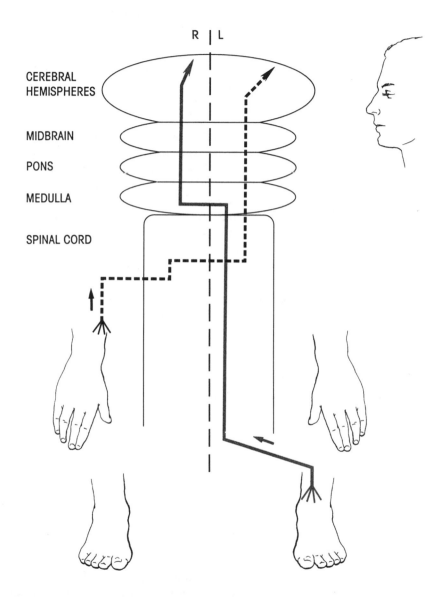

Figure 1-18. *Schematic drawing combining Figures 1-7 and 1-11, corresponding to reduced pinprick sensation in the right upper extremity and reduced joint position sense in the left lower extremity. The only regions common to both pathways lie between the low medulla and the C6/7 level of the spinal cord on the left.*

4.   reduced joint position sense in the right hand

Where's the lesion?

Figure 1-11 shows the line segment corresponding to item 1. Figure 1-19 includes this line segment together with analogous line segments from each of the other three limbs representing items 2, 3, and 4. At first glance, it appears that there is only one level where all these segments intersect: in the medulla, where they all cross. At every other level, two of the segments are on one side of the nervous system and two on the other. On closer scrutiny, however, additional localization sites are evident. Even though the segments lie on both sides of the nervous system, there are two places where they are contiguous across the midline. Thus, while a unilateral lesion could not involve all four line segments, the pattern of deficits could be explained by a bilateral lesion centered on the midline and extending out to each side. The sites where this is possible are in the cervical spinal cord (at the level of C7 and above) and the postcentral gyrus of the cortex. The presence or absence of additional deficits (corresponding to additional line segments) would help to distinguish between these three potential lesion sites (medulla, cervical cord, and cortex).

Example 6.   A patient is found to have the following:

1.   reduced joint position sense in the left foot

2.   reduced pinprick sensation on the palmar surface of the little finger of the right hand

3.   reduced visual acuity in the left eye

Where's the lesion?

The first two items are the same as in Examples 3 and 4 and imply a lesion localization somewhere between the low medulla and the C6/7 level of the spinal cord on the left (see Figure 1-18). This region is not even close to the line segment representing the patient's visual loss (see Figure 1-14). This means that no single lesion site could produce all of this patient's findings. By the rules of the game, the next objective is to explain all of the deficits on the basis of two lesion sites. This can obviously be achieved by assuming that one lesion is in the previously identified region of the medulla or spinal cord and the other lesion is in the left retina or optic nerve. The next step is to decide whether these two

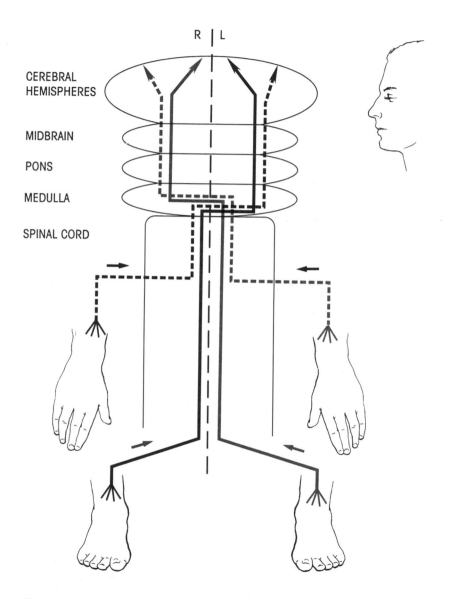

Figure 1-19. *Schematic drawing representing loss of joint position sense in all four limbs. Potential lesion sites lie in the midline and extending bilaterally, at the levels of cortex, low medulla, or high cervical spinal cord.*

lesions are related or coincidental, using the approach to be presented in Chapter 3.

Example 7.   A patient is found to have the following:

1.   reduced joint position and pinprick sensation in the left foot

2.   reduced joint position and pinprick sensation in the right foot

3.   reduced joint position and pinprick sensation in the left hand

4.   reduced joint position and pinprick sensation in the right hand

5.   normal strength and sensation proximally in all four limbs

Where's the lesion?

The deficits in joint position sense in all four limbs were discussed in Example 5. They imply a lesion site lying in the midline and extending bilaterally either in the cortex or in the region extending from the low medulla to the C7 level of the spinal cord. Within this latter region, the line segments representing pinprick sensation lie laterally (see Figure 1-2). Unlike the pathways for joint position sense, they are not contiguous across the midline, and only an extremely large lesion could affect them bilaterally. This is shown in Figure 1-20, which represents a cross section of the spinal cord (the reasoning would be the same for the medulla). Region A is the area corresponding to the loss of position sense in all four limbs and region B is the area corresponding to the loss of pinprick sensation. Because the lateral corticospinal tracts lie between these two regions, a single lesion large enough to encompass both regions A and B would necessarily result in weakness throughout the lower extremities. The preserved proximal strength (item 5) therefore eliminates this potential lesion site.

Similar reasoning eliminates the cortex as a potential localization. The representation of the body surface along the postcentral gyrus is organized in the following order from medial to lateral: distal lower extremity, proximal lower extremity, proximal upper extremity, distal upper extremity, face. The only way a single lesion could produce sen-

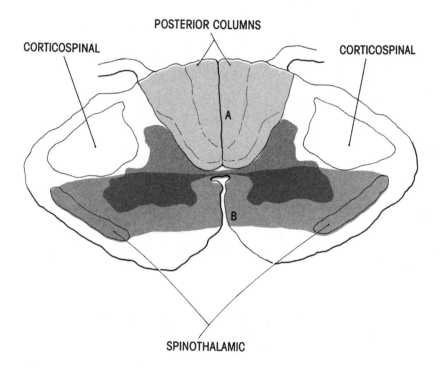

Figure 1-20. *Cross section of the high cervical spinal cord. Region A corresponds to the area that must be affected to produce loss of joint position sense in all four limbs. Region B corresponds to the area that would produce reduced pinprick sensation in all four limbs. Any lesion large enough to affect both region A and region B would also include the lateral corticospinal tracts, resulting in motor symptoms.*

sory deficits in both the distal upper extremity and the distal lower extremity would be to involve the proximal limbs also.

In short, no single lesion site can explain all of the findings in this patient. The findings cannot even be explained by positing two lesions. This patient has a multifocal condition. By the rules of the game, the next goal is to identify some common characteristic unifying all of the lesion sites. In this case, all of the findings are sensory deficits restricted to the distal portions of the limbs. This suggests a process affecting peripheral nerves, specifically involving the longest sensory nerves. **Peripheral poly-neuropathy** is the term for such a condition (see Chapter 6).

VI. Rules for Speed Play

Even in the limited number of examples presented in Part V, several themes emerge repeatedly. Many of these themes can be summarized as general rules that are often sufficient for localizing a lesion without having to perform the kind of systematic analysis presented above. Most neurologists have internalized these rules. When presented with a patient like the one described in Example 4, they immediately think of a spinal cord lesion; in fact, this is even a named syndrome (the **Brown-Sequard syndrome**). The patient described in Example 7 is so typical of a patient with polyneuropathy that no neurologist would require diagrams to reach that conclusion.

The rules given below summarize many of the "shortcuts" used by neurologists in localizing a lesion. They are useful in many clinical situations, but they are simplifications. If they are applied without thinking, they may result in errors or omissions. Even neurologists sometimes fall into this trap. When a case is confusing, it is always best to analyze it systematically as described in Part V. In fact, with more confusing cases, even the analysis of Part V may be inadequate, and the kind of detailed analysis presented in Part IV may be required.

With those caveats, the following rules may be presented. They are derived from the kind of reasoning already presented in analyzing Examples 1–7; a brief explanation follows each rule.

1. **If both strength and pain/temperature sensation are impaired in a single limb, the lesion is either in the periphery (nerve/plexus/root) or in the cortex.**

Explanation: The pathway for pain and temperature sensation crosses soon after entering the spinal cord. The motor pathways cross in the medulla: Below the site of this crossing they are on the opposite side of the nervous system from the sensory pathways; above the site of crossing, they are ipsilateral to the sensory pathways but not aligned with them until the cortex is reached (see Figures 1-3 and 1-8).

2.   If there is reduced pain/temperature sensation in one limb and reduced position/vibration sensation in a contralateral limb, the lesion is somewhere in the spinal cord (on the same side as the position/vibration deficit).

Explanation: The pathway for pain and temperature sensation crosses soon after entering the spinal cord; the pathway for position and vibration sense does not cross until it reaches the low medulla. Between the two sites of crossing (i.e., within the spinal cord), the pathway for pain and temperature in one limb lies on the same side of the nervous system as the pathway for position and vibration sense in the contralateral limbs (see Figure 1-18).

3.   Bilateral sensory and motor deficits throughout the body below a roughly horizontal level on the trunk, with normal function above that level, indicate a spinal cord lesion (at or above that level).

Explanation: A large spinal cord lesion will disrupt all ascending fiber tracts from all parts of the body below the lesion, and it will disrupt all descending fiber tracts traveling to those body parts. A smaller spinal cord lesion may spare portions of those fiber tracts. The tracts are arranged in such a way that the spared portions typically contain the fibers corresponding to the uppermost part of the affected region of the body. Hence, a given sensory/motor level can indicate a large spinal cord lesion at that level, or a smaller lesion higher up in the spinal cord.

4.   Increased reflexes in a symptomatic limb suggest a central lesion; reduced reflexes in a symptomatic limb suggest a peripheral lesion.

Explanation: The nerve root, plexus, peripheral nerve, and muscle are all included in the reflex arc, which is tonically inhibited by descending pathways from above (see Figure 1-13).

5.   Reduced pain/temperature sensation on one side of the face and the opposite side of the body implies a lesion between the pons

and C2 (ipsilateral to the facial numbness). Reduced pain/tempera-ture sensation on one side of the face and the same side of the body implies a lesion in the high brainstem or above.

Explanation: The pathway for pain and temperature sensation from the face enters the pons via the trigeminal nerve, descends on the same side to about the C2 level of the spinal cord, crosses, and ascends on the opposite side. The descending pathway (from the pons to C2) is close to the ascending pathway conveying pain and temperature sensation from the contralateral body. After crossing at the C2 level, the tract conveying facial sensation is on the same side as the tract conveying ipsilateral trunk and limb sensation, but the two tracts are not close to each other until reaching the high brainstem (see Figures 1-5 and 1-10).

6.   Facial weakness ipsilateral to body weakness implies a lesion in the high pons or above.

Explanation: The facial nerve (supplying the muscles of the face) exits from the pons; no lesion below that level can affect facial strength.

7.   Both a third nerve palsy and Horner's syndrome can result in pto-sis and pupillary asymmetry, but with a third nerve palsy, the ptosis is on the side of the large pupil; with Horner's syndrome, the ptosis is on the side of the small pupil.

Explanation: A third nerve palsy often results in dysfunction of para-sympathetic fibers traveling with the third nerve, causing a large pupil because of impaired constriction. Horner's syndrome is due to damage to the sympathetic system, causing inadequate pupillary dilation and therefore a small pupil. With either lesion, the ptosis is always on the same side as the abnormal pupil.

8.   Diplopia is always due to a lesion in the brainstem or periphery (nerve/neuromuscular junction/muscle), but not the cortex. A gaze palsy (impaired movement of both eyes in one direction, but both eyes move congruently and remain aligned in all positions of gaze) is due to a lesion in the cortex or brainstem but not in the periphery.

Explanation: Cortical and brainstem gaze centers control movements of both eyes in parallel; individual eye movements are controlled by brainstem nuclei and mediated by individual cranial nerves. This is discussed further in Chapters 2, 11, and 13.

9. **Visual symptoms restricted to one eye imply a lesion anterior to the chiasm.**

Explanation: At the chiasm and beyond, information from the two eyes is combined in the visual system, so that any lesion will generally affect vision from both eyes. Only prior to the chiasm is this not the case (see Figure 1-14). This point is also discussed in Chapters 2 and 13.

10. **Aphasia or dysphasia (abnormal language processing resulting in difficulty understanding words, recalling words, or organizing words grammatically) implies a lesion in the dominant cerebral hemisphere. Dysarthria (abnormal motor control of speech resulting in disturbances of articulation, rate, rhythm, or voice quality) in the absence of dysphasia suggests a subcortical, brainstem, or cerebellar lesion.**

Explanation: The cognitive processing necessary for language comprehension and production takes place largely in the dominant cerebral hemisphere. The cerebral hemispheres are also involved in the specific motor sequences involved in speech, but there is enough redundancy of function that the unaffected hemisphere can often compensate for a unilateral hemispheric lesion as long as the areas involved in language processing are intact. There is less redundancy at lower levels, so a unilateral subcortical, brainstem, or cerebellar lesion can produce significant dysarthria.

11. **An altered level of consciousness indicates either a brainstem lesion or dysfunction of both cerebral hemispheres.**

Explanation: The physiologic basis of "consciousness" is not well understood. Even if it were, it would surely be too complicated to represent in terms of line segments. Suffice it to say that the reticular activating system in the brainstem is a critical element, but there is no localized region in the cerebral hemispheres essential for maintenance of consciousness. A lesion that completely destroys the function of one cerebral hemisphere will not affect consciousness as long as the other hemisphere is intact.

2

The Neurologic Examination

I. More Localization Problems

Example 1. In the dark, a patient's right pupil is 3 mm larger than the left. In bright light, the right pupil is only 1 mm larger than the left.

Questions:

1. Which pupil is abnormal, the right or the left?

2. Which pathway is abnormal, the sympathetic or the parasympathetic?

3. Is this patient likely to have ptosis? If so, on which side?

Example 2. A patient has weakness of the right face, arm, and leg.

Question:

Which is likely to be weaker, the forehead or the lower face?

Example 3. A patient has weakness of hip flexion, knee flexion, and ankle dorsiflexion in the left lower extremity.

Questions:

1. Is this distribution of weakness consistent with a single root lesion?

2. Is this pattern of weakness suggestive of any other lesion localization?

II. The Neurologic Examination: General Comments

Most of the information necessary to localize a patient's lesion can be obtained by taking a careful history. Even features that are usually considered to be examination findings can be deduced if the right questions are asked. For example, to investigate temperature sensation, patients can be asked whether they have any problems detecting water temperature when washing their hands or stepping into a bathtub. Regarding fine touch discrimination, patients can be asked whether they have problems pulling the correct coin or other objects out of their pockets. Position sense can be explored by asking whether they have problems knowing where their feet are on the accelerator and brake pedals of their cars. Even a history of clonus may sometimes be deduced from patients who experience uncontrollable, rhythmic jerking of the foot when slamming on the brakes. Similarly, precise questions may differentiate between proximal and distal weakness, horizontal and vertical diplopia, monocular and binocular vision loss, aphasia and dysarthria, and so forth.

Even so, some important information can be learned only by examining the patient. Moreover, the information obtained from a history depends on the reliability of the informant. If the informant is a poor observer, has trouble communicating, or for some reason provides misleading information, it is essential to have an independent source of information. The neurologic examination serves this purpose.

The nervous system has many functions, and there are many ways to test each function. The components of a standard neurologic examination are listed in Table 2-1. It would not be practical to perform all pos-

Table 2-1. Organization of the Neurologic Examination

A. Mental status
  1. Level of alertness
  2. Language
    a. Fluency
    b. Comprehension
    c. Repetition
    d. Naming
    e. Reading
    f. Writing
  3. Memory
    a. Immediate
    b. Short-term
    c. Long-term
      i. Recent (including orienta-
         tion to place and time)
      ii. Remote
  4. Calculation
  5. Construction
  6. Abstraction

B. Cranial nerves
  1. Olfaction (CN I)
  2. Vision (CN II)
    a. Visual fields
    b. Visual acuity
    c. Funduscopic examination
  3. Pupillary light reflex (CNs II, III)
  4. Eye movements (CNs III, IV, VII)
  5. Facial sensation (CN V)
  6. Facial strength
    a. Muscles of mastication
       (CN V)
    b. Muscles of facial expres-
       sion (CN VII)
  7. Hearing (CN VIII)

  8. Palatal movement (CNs IX, X)
  9. Dysarthria (CNs IX, X, XII)
  10. Head rotation (CN XI)
  11. Shoulder elevation (CN XI)
  12. Tongue movements (CN XII)

C. Motor
  1. Gait
  2. Coordination
  3. Involuntary movements
  4. Pronator drift
  5. Individual muscles
    a. Strength
    b. Bulk
    c. Tone (resistance to passive
       manipulation)

D. Reflexes
  1. Tendon reflexes
  2. Plantar responses
  3. Superficial reflexes
  4. "Primitive" reflexes

E. Sensory
  1. Light touch
  2. Pain/temperature
  3. Joint position sense
  4. Vibration
  5. Double simultaneous stimu-
     lation
  6. Graphesthesia
  7. Stereognosis

sible tests on each patient. Instead, the examination must be tailored to
the situation. In patients with no neurologic symptoms, a screening
examination is adequate (see Part V of this chapter). In patients who do
have neurologic symptoms, it is best to try to narrow the list of potential
localization sites as much as possible based on the history. It will then be
possible to focus the examination in order to verify the salient features
of the history and to refine the localization even further.

One constraint on the neurologic examination is that it requires
patient cooperation. Some patients are unable or unwilling to cooperate fully with the examination, so findings must be interpreted with
caution and checked for internal consistency. Even when cooperation
is not an issue, variability among normal individuals is often a limiting
factor. It is frequently difficult to determine whether a given finding is
outside the range of normal. For example, one individual may be
much stronger than another, but the weaker individual is not necessarily abnormal. Weakness that has developed recently is a much more
significant indicator of neurologic disease than lifelong weakness. The
same is true of hyperreflexia and many other neurologic findings.
Unfortunately, it is not always clear whether an examination finding is
new or old, because patients usually do not present for examination
until they are already experiencing symptoms. When there is no baseline examination available for comparison, patients can sometimes be
"used as their own controls." If a finding in one region of the body is
different from corresponding findings elsewhere, it is likely to be significant. For this reason, the two sides of the body should be compared
directly at each step of the examination. A finding on the right significantly different from the corresponding finding on the left is strong
evidence of a neurologic lesion. Even when the examination is asymmetric, it can be difficult to determine whether the abnormality is new
or old. It may be completely irrelevant to the patient's current symptoms. Although the examination supplements the history, it cannot
supplant it.

The neurologic examination can be performed in any order. Examiners may even change the sequence of the examination depending on
a patient's symptoms, mobility, and ability to cooperate. Many subtle
abnormalities are most evident by comparing one side of the body to
the other, so it is generally best to follow each test with the same test
on the other side, before moving on to a different test. Sensory testing
and mental status testing are the parts of the examination most likely
to make patients uncomfortable, so it is often wise to perform these
tests last. These are only guidelines, however. Each examiner's style
and preferences will differ.

The sequence in which the neurologic examination is presented is more standardized, primarily to make things easier for a listener or reader. When the findings are presented in a standard sequence, it is easier to focus on the aspects of greatest interest. If a relevant detail is omitted, a listener can interrupt the presentation to ask about it, rather than waiting to see if it will come up eventually. It doesn't really matter what the sequence is, as long as it is consistent. A fairly standard sequence is shown in Table 2-1. It can be thought of as "zooming in" on the patient. The component presented first, mental status, could almost be tested by telephone. Little direct observation of the patient is necessary. Gait is tested by observing the patient, but no physical contact is required. The remainder of the motor examination requires some physical contact, but at a fairly crude level. The component presented last, the sensory examination, requires the closest and most refined physical interactions, such as the small limb movements required for testing joint position sense or the stimuli applied in testing pain sensation. The cranial nerves are inserted as a bridge between mental status and the rest of the examination, and the deep tendon reflexes are positioned between the motor and the sensory exams because the reflex arc includes both sensory and motor components.

The portion of the examination for which presentation in a consistent sequence is most important is the mental status examination. Certain findings on the mental status examination can only be interpreted by knowing a patient's ability to perform other, more fundamental tasks. For example, difficulty with simple calculations may have some localizing significance in a patient who is otherwise cognitively intact, but not in a patient who is unable to answer any questions because of impaired language function or a depressed level of consciousness. This ambiguity is avoided by presenting the level of alertness first, then language function, and then memory. The remainder of the mental status examination can be presented in any order.

III. The Neurologic Examination: How to Do It

Even though the neurologic examination outlined in Table 2-1 is seldom performed in its entirety, one must be able to perform each of the components of the neurologic examination when appropriate. This section presents instructions for doing so. It also provides some basic definitions and standard conventions used to report examination findings, as well as some hints and comments regarding common sources of confusion. Because many of these latter comments reflect my personal observations or opinions, they have been highlighted by setting them in italics and using the first person singular pronoun.

A. Mental Status Examination

1. Level of alertness

No special testing is required. While taking the history and examining the patient, observe whether the patient is alert, attentive, sleepy, or unresponsive.

2. Language

a. Fluency
No special testing is required. Throughout the course of the patient interaction, assess whether the patient's phrases and sentences are of normal length, are spoken effortlessly and at a normal rate, and have normal grammatical structure. Note that fluency is independent of content; speech can be completely fluent and still be incomprehensible.

b. Comprehension
Comprehension is often adequately assessed through the routine history and physical but can also be tested explicitly. Give the patient progressively more complex commands, such as one step (e.g., "Touch your nose."), two steps (e.g., "Touch your nose, then stick out your tongue"), and three steps (e.g., "Touch your nose, then stick out your tongue, and then raise your right foot"). Commands that require a body part to cross the midline (e.g., "Touch your right ear with your left thumb") are more complex than those that don't. Increasingly complex grammatical structures can also be used (e.g., "Touch the coin with the pencil"; "With the comb, touch the coin"). Ask the patient progressively more complex questions, either yes-no (e.g., "Does a stone sink in water?" "Do you put on your shoes before your stockings?") or otherwise. Again, more complex grammatical structures such as passive voice or possessive may be useful (e.g., "Is my aunt's uncle a man or a woman?"; "If a lion was killed by a tiger, which one is still alive?").

c. Repetition
Ask the patient to repeat phrases or sentences of progressively greater length and complexity (e.g., "It is cold outside"; "We all went over there together"; "The lawyer's closing argument convinced the jury"; "The final movement of the symphony was disappointing").

d. Naming

In the course of routine conversation, observe whether the patient frequently pauses and struggles to think of words. In addition, test naming explicitly by asking the patient to name items as you point to them (e.g., shirt, shoe, phone, collar, lapel, shoelace, heel, receiver). Less common objects are generally harder to name, and parts of an object are harder to name than the entire object.

e. Reading

Ask the patient to follow a written command. This can be one of the same commands used to test comprehension of spoken language.

f. Writing

Ask the patient to write an original sentence, and to write a sentence from dictation. Look for omitted or added words, or for word substitutions.

3. Memory

a. Immediate memory

Ask the patient to repeat a string of seven digits immediately after you complete it. Lengthen or shorten the string until you find the longest string the patient can repeat correctly. This is called the **digit span**. Note: Despite its categorization as "immediate memory," this is really more appropriately considered "attention."

b. Short-term memory

Ask the patient to memorize three unrelated words (e.g., baseball, horse, purple), then distract the patient for 5 minutes (usually by performing other parts of the examination). Then ask the patient to recall the list. If the patient misses an item, give clues (e.g., "One was an animal"), and if this isn't enough, offer a multiple choice (e.g., "It was either a cat, a bear, or a horse").

c. Long-term memory

Long-term memory includes both recent and remote memory. Assess **recent** memory by testing the patient's orientation to time (e.g., day, date, month, season, year), place (e.g., state, city, building), and person (e.g., patient's full name) and by asking questions about events of the past few days or weeks, (e.g., "Who are the current candidates for president?" or, assuming an independent source is available for verification, "What did you have for supper last night?"). **Remote** memory can be tested by asking for the names of the presidents in reverse order as far back as the patient can remember, or by asking about important historical events and dates. The patient can also be asked about details of personal life such as birth date, names and ages of children and grandchildren, and work history, assuming independent verification is available.

4. Calculation

Ask some straightforward computation problems (e.g., $5 + 8 = ?$; $6 \times 7 = ?$; $31 - 18 = ?$) and some "word problems" (e.g., "How many nickels are there in \$1.35?" "How many quarters in \$3.75?").

5. Construction

Ask the patient to draw a clock, including all the numbers, and to place the hands at 4:10. Ask the patient to draw a cube; for patients who have trouble doing so, draw a cube and ask them to copy it.

6. Abstraction

Ask the patient to explain similarities (e.g., "What do an apple and an orange have in common?" "... a basketball and a grapefruit?" "... a tent and a cabin?" "... a bicycle and an airplane?" "... a sculpture and a symphony?") and differences (e.g., "What's the difference between a radio and a television?" "... a river and a lake?" "... a baby and a midget?" "... character and reputation?").

Mental Status Examination: Additional Comments

1. Terminology

A number of specialized terms often confuse students. Here is a partial glossary:

abulia: loss of initiative, willpower, or drive.
acalculia: inability to calculate.
agnosia: inability to recognize one or more classes of environmental stimuli, even though the necessary intellectual and perceptual functions are intact.
agraphia: inability to write.
alexia: inability to read for comprehension.
amnesia: inability to retain new information.
anomia: inability to name objects or think of words; in practice, often used as a synonym for *dysnomia.*

anosognosia: inability to recognize one's own impairment.

anterior aphasia: acquired language disorder in which verbal output is *nonfluent* (see "Broca's aphasia," "expressive aphasia," "nonfluent aphasia").

aphasia: literally, a complete loss of language function, but in practice, used as a synonym for *dysphasia*.

aphemia: complete loss of the ability to speak, but retained comprehension and writing ability.

apraxia: inability to perform a previously learned set of coordinated movements even though the necessary component skills (including intellect, language function, strength, coordination, and sensation) remain intact.

Broca's aphasia: acquired language disorder characterized by *nonfluent* verbal output with omission of relational words (prepositions, conjunctions, articles, and minor modifiers) and abnormal *prosody*, impaired repetition, and relatively intact comprehension (see "anterior aphasia," "expressive aphasia," "nonfluent aphasia"; see also Figure 1-17).

conduction aphasia: acquired language disorder characterized by prominent impairment of repetition, relatively intact comprehension, and verbal output that is *fluent* but contains *literal paraphasias* (see Figure 1-17).

delirium: an acute confusional state characterized by clouded, reduced, or shifting attention, often associated with sensory misperception or disturbed thinking.

dementia: acquired impairment of memory and at least one other cognitive function, without clouding of the sensorium or underlying psychiatric disease.

dysnomia: difficulty naming objects or finding the desired words.

dysphasia: acquired disorder of language not due to generalized intellectual impairment or psychiatric disturbance.

expressive aphasia: acquired language disorder in which verbal output is *nonfluent* (see "anterior aphasia," "Broca's aphasia," "nonfluent aphasia").

fluent: an adjective used to describe verbal output that is normal to excessive, easily produced, with normal phrase length (five or more words) and normal *prosody*.

fluent aphasia: acquired language disorder in which verbal output is *fluent* (see "posterior aphasia," "receptive aphasia," "Wernicke's aphasia").

Gerstmann's syndrome: the constellation of (1) *agraphia*, (2) *acalculia*, (3) right-left confusion, and (4) finger *agnosia*; classically associated with lesions in the angular gyrus of the dominant hemisphere (but the subject of endless debate).

jargon: verbal output that contains so many *literal paraphasias* that the words are unrecognizable.

nonfluent: an adjective used to describe verbal output that is sparse, with only one to four words per phrase.

nonfluent aphasia: acquired language disorder in which verbal output is *nonfluent* (see "anterior aphasia," "Broca's aphasia," "expressive aphasia").

paraphasia: a substitution error in which the word produced is similar in sound or meaning to the intended word. A *literal* or *phonemic paraphasia* is a sound substitution error resulting in production of a word that is phonemically related to the intended word (e.g., "greed" or "greeb" instead of "green"). A *semantic* or *verbal paraphasia* is a word substitution error in which the word produced is semantically related to the intended word (e.g., "blue" instead of "green").

posterior aphasia: acquired language disorder in which comprehension is impaired (see "fluent aphasia," "receptive aphasia," "Wernicke's aphasia").

prosody: the rhythm and tempo of speech.

prosopagnosia: inability to recognize faces.

receptive aphasia: acquired language disorder in which comprehension is impaired (see "fluent aphasia," "posterior aphasia," "Wernicke's aphasia").

transcortical aphasia: acquired language disorder in which the ability to repeat is intact (see Figure 1-17).

Wernicke's aphasia: acquired language disorder characterized by markedly impaired comprehension and repetition, with verbal output that is fluent but contaminated by numerous *paraphasias* or, in severe cases, *jargon* (see "fluent aphasia," "posterior aphasia," "receptive aphasia;" see also Figure 1-17).

2. Patient cooperation

Many patients resist formal mental status testing. Some find it threatening. Others are offended by it (e.g., "What do you mean, do I know my name?"). Others just don't see the point, and indeed, I frequently omit formal mental status testing unless there is a specific need for it (see Part V of this chapter). When I do see the need, I usually introduce the mental status examination by saying, "Now I'm going to test your memory. I'm going to ask you to remember three things. Then

I'm going to distract you with a bunch of questions, some of which will be easy and some will be hard. Then I'll test you on the three things." Most patients can understand the need for testing memory, and they are more willing to accept all the other components of the mental status examination if they are presented as "distractions."

Even so, some patients find the mental status examination so annoying that they refuse to cooperate, and some even refuse to proceed with any other portion of the physical examination. For this reason, I usually defer formal mental status testing until I have nearly completed the rest of the examination. By then, I will have observed the patient's ability to respond to some fairly complicated commands (for example, with finger-to-nose testing), and this will help me tailor my examination.

3. Tailoring the examination to the patient

I try to guess the approximate level of performance I expect from a patient and then ask a screening question that I think may be a little too tough. If the patient gets the correct answer, I can skip the easier questions. If the patient doesn't get the correct answer, I can gradually reduce the difficulty of my questions until I have reached the patient's level. This approach saves time. I try to stockpile questions of various levels of complexity, so I don't have to think them up on the spot. For example, it is useful to remember sentences of different word lengths for testing repetition. A reasonably tough math problem that I often use as my initial screening question is "How much change would you get from a dollar if you bought six apples at 12 cents each?"

4. Aphasia terminology

Note the confusing array of synonyms in the list of definitions above. For example, an "expressive aphasia" is one in which expression is impaired, yet a "fluent aphasia" is one in which fluency is preserved. *These terms are often more trouble than they are worth. It is best to describe the pattern of language deficits explicitly, focusing especially on comprehension, fluency, and repetition.*

Dysarthria is an impairment of the motor functions necessary for speech production. Dysarthria is not a language disorder, and it is not a component of the mental status examination.

5. Cultural and educational factors

A patient's background will obviously influence performance on mental status testing, and the examiner must try to take this into account.

There is no reliable way to do this; it is ultimately a matter of gestalt. Some tests are affected more than others by background. For example, the ability to copy a sequence of repetitive hand movements is relatively independent of education. *In contrast, the interpretation of proverbs is so dependent on an individual's cultural and educational background that I consider it useless and instead rely on the interpretation of similarities and differences as an assay of abstract thought.*

6. Reporting findings

It is most informative to report patients' actual responses, rather than interpretations such as "mildly abnormal" or "slightly concrete."

B. *Cranial Nerve Examination*

1. Olfaction

Olfaction need not be tested routinely. It is tested by having the patient occlude one nostril and identify a common scent (e.g., coffee, peppermint, cinnamon) placed under the other nostril.

2. Vision

a. *Visual fields*
Have the patient cover his or her left eye. Stand facing the patient from two arm's-lengths away, close your right eye, and stretch your arms forward and to the sides so that your hands are at the vertical midline of your vision at about "1:30" and "10:30" and just barely visible in your peripheral vision. They should be the same distance from you and the patient. Hold the index finger on each hand extended. Wiggle the finger on either the left, right, or both hands, and ask the patient to identify where the movement occurs while looking directly at your nose. Move your hands down to roughly "4:30" and "7:30" and test again. Then test analogous portions of the visual field of the patient's left eye (using your right eye).

b. *Acuity*
Place a hand-held visual acuity card 14 inches in front of the patient's right eye, while the left eye is covered. The patient should wear his or her usual corrective lenses. Ask the patient to read the lowest line on the chart (20/20). If the patient cannot do so, move up a line, and continue doing so until you reach a line where the

majority of items are read correctly. Note which line this is, and how many errors the patient makes on this line. Repeat the process for the left eye.

c. Funduscopic examination
Funduscopic examination is described in standard physical examination textbooks.

3. Pupillary light reflex

Reduce the room illumination as much as possible. Shine a penlight on the bridge of the patient's nose, so that you can see both pupils without directing light at either of them. Check that they are the same size. Now move the penlight so that it is directly shining on the right pupil, and check to see that both pupils have constricted to the same size. Next, move the penlight back to the bridge of the nose so that both pupils dilate, and then shine the light directly on the left pupil, again checking for equal constriction of the two eyes. Finally, move the penlight rapidly from the left pupil to the right; the pupil size should not change. Swing the light back to the left pupil; again, the pupil size should remain constant. Repeat this "swinging" maneuver several times to be sure there is no consistent tendency for the pupils to be larger when the light is directed at one eye than when it is directed at the other one.

4. Eye movements

Observe the patient's eyelids for **ptosis**. Have the patient fixate on your finger held about two feet away, in the vertical and horizontal midline. Observe for **nystagmus**—a repetitive, quick movement of the eyes in one direction, alternating with a slower movement of the eyes in the opposite direction, several times in a row. Ask the patient to avoid any movement of the head but to continue watching your finger as you slowly move it to the patient's right. Observe the smoothness and range of the patient's eye movements. Keep your finger at the far right of the patient's gaze for several seconds while observing for nystagmus. Move your finger slowly to the patient's left and repeat the observations. Return your finger to the vertical and horizontal midline, then move it slowly up, repeating the observations. Then move your finger slowly down and repeat the observations. Finally, return to the midline position, and move your finger diagonally down and to the left; then return to the midline and move your finger down and to the right.

5. Facial sensation

Lightly touch the patient's right forehead once, and then repeat on the opposite side. Ask the patient if the two stimuli felt the same. Repeat this procedure on the cheek and on the chin. This is usually adequate testing. In some circumstances, the testing should be repeated applying light pressure with a pin. Testing of the **corneal reflex** is not routinely necessary but is useful in uncooperative patients or when the rest of the exam suggests that there may be a problem with facial sensation or strength. It is tested by having the patient look to the far left, then touching the patient's right cornea with a fine wisp of cotton (introduced from the patient's right, outside the field of vision) and observing the reflexive blink that occurs in each eye. The process is then repeated with the left eye.

6. Facial strength

a. Muscles of mastication
Have the patient open the jaw against resistance, then close the jaw against resistance. Have the patient move the chin from side to side.

b. Muscles of facial expression
Have the patient close his or her eyes tightly. Observe whether the lashes are buried equally on the two sides and whether you can open either eye manually. Then have the patient look up and wrinkle the forehead; note whether the two sides are equally wrinkled. Have the patient smile, and observe whether one side of the face is activated more quickly or more completely than the other.

7. Hearing

For a bedside examination, it usually suffices to perform a quick hearing assessment by holding your fingers a few inches away from the patient's ear and rubbing them together softly. Alternatively, you can hold your hand up as a sound screen and ask the patient to repeat a few numbers that you whisper behind your hand while rhythmically tapping the opposite ear to keep it from contributing. Each ear should be tested separately.

8. Palatal movement

Ask the patient to say "aaah" or yawn, and observe whether the two sides of the palate move fully and symmetrically. The palate is most readily visualized if the patient is sitting or standing, rather than supine.

There is generally no need to test the **gag reflex** in a screening neurologic examination. When there is reason to suspect reduced palatal sensation or strength, the reflex can be checked by observing the response when you touch the posterior pharynx on one side with a cotton swab and then comparing to the response elicited by touching the other side.

9. Dysarthria

When the patient speaks, listen for articulation errors, abnormalities of voice quality, and irregularities of rate or rhythm.

10. Head rotation

Have the patient turn the head all the way to the left. Place your hand on the left side of the chin and ask the patient to resist you as you try turning the head back to the right. Palpate the right sternocleidomastoid muscle with your other hand at the same time. Repeat this maneuver in the other direction to test the left sternocleidomastoid.

11. Shoulder elevation

Ask the patient to shrug the shoulders while you resist the movement with your hands.

12. Tongue movement

Have the patient protrude the tongue and move it rapidly from side to side. Ask the patient to push the tongue against the left cheek from inside the mouth while you push against it from outside, then do the same on the right side of the mouth.

Cranial Nerve Examination: Additional Comments

1. Olfaction

I almost never test the sense of smell. It is difficult to know whether patients who cannot identify a particular scent have a disturbance of olfaction or whether they are just not familiar with that scent. When patients give a history of olfactory problems, I take them at their word.

2. Visual fields

There are many alternatives to the technique described here for testing visual fields. You can ask patients to tell you when they first see a test stimulus as you slowly move it in from the periphery at various orientations. You can ask patients to count the number of fingers you hold up at various spots in the field. You can ask patients to tell you when they can detect that a stimulus is red as you move it around the field. You can ask them to tell you when they see a stimulus move. Each of these techniques has advantages and disadvantages, and some neurologists have very strong opinions about which is best. *The reason I prefer the method described here is that the visual stimulus can be presented very briefly, minimizing the opportunity for the patient to shift fixation and maximizing the likelihood that the stimulus is actually in the intended region of the visual field. Regardless of the technique used, each eye must be tested separately. Otherwise, if there is a defect in a portion of the visual field of only one eye, the other eye will be able to compensate and the defect will not be detected. One example of this situation is the bitemporal hemianopia that can occur with a lesion in the optic chiasm (see Chapter 1, Part V): The defective hemifield of each eye corresponds to the intact hemifield of the other eye, so the patient may be completely unaware of the deficit.*

3. Eye movements

Eye movement abnormalities may be masked by convergence if the target is too close to the patient. On the other hand, if you stand too far away, it may be difficult for you to see subtle abnormalities. I often position my head close to the patient and move the target (my finger) back and forth behind me.

4. Corneal and gag reflexes

Because testing of the corneal reflex and the gag reflex is uncomfortable for the patient, I only perform these tests when I am trying to answer a specific question. When I check the gag reflex, I always check it bilaterally. About 20% of normal individuals do not have a gag reflex, so the test is most informative when the responses are asymmetric.

5. Weber and Rinne tests

Most physical diagnosis textbooks advocate the Weber and Rinne tests for distinguishing conductive hearing loss from sensorineural deafness. I do not. I find that patients have difficulty understanding what is being asked, and they give inconsistent responses (especially on the Weber test). Even if these tests gave consistently reliable results, they would still not be as sensitive or as informative as an audiogram.

C. Motor Examination

1. Gait

Observe the patient's **casual** gait, preferably with the patient unaware of being observed. Have the patient walk toward you while walking on the **heels**, then walk away from you walking on **tiptoes**. Finally, have the patient walk in **tandem**, placing one foot directly in front of the other as if walking on a tightrope (i.e., the "drunk driving test"). Note if the patient is unsteady with any of these maneuvers, or if there is any asymmetry of movement. Also look for **festination**, an involuntary tendency for steps to accelerate and become smaller.

2. Coordination

a. Finger tapping
Ask the patient to make a fist with the right hand, and then to extend the thumb and index finger and tap the tip of the index finger on the tip of the thumb as quickly as possible. Repeat with the left hand. Observe for speed, accuracy, and regularity of rhythm.

b. Rapid alternating movements
Have the patient alternately pronate and supinate the right hand against a stable surface (e.g., a table, the patient's own thigh or left hand) as rapidly as possible; repeat for the left hand. Again, observe speed, accuracy, and rhythm.

c. Finger-to-nose testing
Ask the patient to use the tip of his or her right index finger to touch the tip of your index finger, then the tip of his or her nose, then your finger again, and so forth. Hold your finger so that it is near the extreme of the patient's reach, and move it to several different positions during the testing. Repeat the test using the patient's left arm. Observe for accuracy and tremor.

d. Heel-to-shin testing
Have the patient lie supine, place the right heel on the left knee, and then move the heel smoothly down the shin to the ankle. Repeat using the left heel on the right shin. Again, observe for accuracy and tremor.

3. Involuntary movements

Observe the patient throughout the history and physical for **tremor,** **myoclonus** (rapid, shock-like muscle jerks), **chorea** (rapid, jerky twitches, similar to myoclonus but more random in location and more likely to blend into one another), **athetosis** (slow, writhing movements of the limbs), **ballismus** (large amplitude flinging limb movements), tics (abrupt, stereotyped, coordinated movements or vocalizations), **dystonia** (maintenance of an abnormal posture or repetitive twisting movements), or other involuntary motor activity.

4. Pronator drift

Have the patient stretch out the arms so that they are level and fully extended, with the palms facing straight up, and then close the eyes. Watch for five to ten seconds to see if either arm tends to pronate (so that the palm turns inward) and drift downward.

5. Individual muscles

a. Strength

In the upper extremities, test shoulder abduction, elbow extension, elbow flexion, wrist extension, wrist flexion, finger extension, finger flexion, and finger abduction. In the lower extremities, test hip flexion, hip extension, knee flexion, knee extension, ankle dorsiflexion, and ankle plantar flexion.

For each movement, place the limb near the middle of its range, and then ask the patient to resist you as you try to move the limb from that position. For example, in testing shoulder abduction, the patient's arms should be horizontal, forming a letter T with the body, and the patient should try to maintain that position while you press down on both arms at a point between the shoulders and the elbows. When possible, place one hand above the joint being examined to stabilize the joint, and exert pressure with your other hand just below the joint, to isolate the specific movement you are trying to test.

b. Bulk

While testing strength, the muscles active in each movement should be inspected and palpated for evidence of **atrophy. Fasciculations** (random, involuntary muscle twitches) should also be noted.

c. Tone

Ask the patient to relax and let you manipulate the limbs passively. This is harder for most patients than you might imagine, and you may need to try to distract them by engaging them in unrelated conversation, or ask them to let their limbs go limp, "like a wet noodle."

Motor Examination: Additional Comments

1. Grading muscle strength

The most common convention for grading muscle strength is the 0 to 5 Medical Research Council scale:

0 = no contraction
1 = visible muscle twitch but no movement of the joint
2 = weak contraction insufficient to overcome gravity
3 = weak contraction able to overcome gravity but no additional resistance
4 = weak contraction able to overcome some resistance but not full resistance
5 = normal; able to overcome full resistance

The most compelling feature of this scale is its reproducibility. For example, an examiner is unlikely to assign a score of 1 to a muscle that another examiner graded 3 or stronger. A major limitation of the scale is that it is insensitive to subtle differences in strength. In particular, grade 4 covers a wide range, so that in most clinical situations the Medical Research Council scale does not allow precise differentiation of the severity of weakness from one muscle to the next. Similarly, it is not a sensitive tool for documenting moderate changes in strength over time. Many clinicians try to compensate for this by using intermediate grades, such as 3+ or 5−, but this results in less reproducibility, because there is no consensus on how these intermediate grades should be defined.

2. Terminology

a. Patterns of weakness

Monoparesis is weakness of a single limb. **Hemiparesis** is weakness of one side of the body. **Paraparesis** is weakness of both lower extremities. **Quadriparesis** is weakness of all four limbs. **Monoplegia, hemiplegia, paraplegia,** and **quadriplegia** are analogous terms that refer to complete or nearly complete paralysis of the involved limbs. **Diplegia** is a term that is best avoided because it is used differently by different authors.

b. Tone (resistance to passive manipulation)

Several forms of increased resistance to passive manipulation are distinguished. **Spasticity** depends on the limb position and on how quickly the limb is moved, classically resulting in a "clasp-knife phenomenon" when the limb is moved rapidly: The limb moves freely for a short distance, but then there is a "catch" and you must use progressively more force to move the limb until at a certain point there is a sudden release and you can move the limb freely again. Spasticity is generally greatest in the flexors of the upper extremity and the extensors of the lower extremity. This pattern is easy to remember for anyone who has seen patients with long-standing hemiparesis (especially if the patients did not receive physical therapy): They keep the hemi-paretic arm pressed tightly to the chest with flexion at the elbow, wrist, and fingers, and they walk with the hemiparetic leg stiffly extended and the ankle plantar flexed, forcing them to circumduct the leg. **Rigidity,** in contrast to spasticity, is characterized by increased resistance throughout the movement. **Lead-pipe rigidity** applies to resistance that is uniform throughout the movement. **Cogwheel rigidity** is characterized by rhythmic interruption of the resistance, producing a ratchet-like effect. Rigidity is usually accentuated by distracting the patient. **Paratonia** is increased resistance that becomes less prominent when the patient is distracted; without such distraction, the patient seems unable to relax the muscle. This is particularly common in patients who are anxious or demented. Paratonia is also called gegenhalten. When it is prominent, other abnormalities of tone are difficult to assess.

c. Coordination

Coordination testing is often referred to as cerebellar testing, but this is a misnomer. Although the cerebellum is very important in the production of coordinated movements and particular abnormal findings on coordination testing may suggest cerebellar disease, other systems also play critical roles. As an obvious example, severe arm weakness will prevent a patient from performing finger-to-nose testing, even though the cerebellum and its pathways may be intact.

3. Modifications of strength testing

a. Selection of muscles to test

The eight upper-extremity movements and six lower-extremity movements tested in the examination described above are sufficient for a screening examination. If some of these muscles are weak, or if the patient complains of focal weakness, additional testing may be necessary to determine if the weakness is in the distribution of a specific nerve or nerve root.

b. Limb position

The mechanical advantage of the patient relative to the examiner during strength testing is very dependent on the position of the joint. For example, it is much easier to overcome patients when they are trying to extend the elbow from a fully flexed position than it is when they are starting from a position of nearly maximal extension. *In most cases it is reasonable to test the muscle with the joint at about midposition, although positions that increase the patient's mechanical advantage may be preferable for particularly strong examiners or frail patients.*

Some examiners test corresponding muscles on both sides (e.g., the left and right biceps muscles) simultaneously. *I usually do not do this because it prevents me from using one hand to stabilize the joint and palpate the muscle.*

An alternative to the technique presented here for testing strength is to position the patient's limb and then ask the patient to move the limb steadily in a specified direction while the examiner resists the movement. *The main reason I generally prefer to follow the format presented above is that I can give essentially the same instruction (e.g., "Don't let me move your limb") for all movements. This is especially helpful when patients are confused, aphasic, or demented, or when they speak a different language. It may take them a while to understand the instruction initially, but once they understand the task for one or two muscles they usually comprehend it much more readily for subsequent muscles.*

D. Reflex Examination

1. Tendon reflexes

The biceps, triceps, brachioradialis, knee (patellar), and ankle (Achilles) reflexes are the ones commonly tested. The joint under consideration should be at about 90 degrees and fully relaxed. It is often helpful to cradle the joint in your own arm to support it. With your other arm, hold the end of the hammer and let the head of the hammer drop like a pendulum so that it strikes the tendon (specifically, just anterior to the elbow for the biceps reflex, just posterior to the elbow for the triceps reflex, about 10 cm above the wrist on the radial aspect of the forearm for the brachioradialis reflex, just below the patella for the knee reflex, and just behind the ankle for the ankle reflex). You should strive to develop a technique that results in a reproducible level of force from one occasion to the next. When a patient has reflexes that are difficult to elicit, you can amplify them by using reinforcement procedures: Ask the patient to clench his or her teeth or (when testing lower extremity reflexes) to hook together the flexed fingers of both hands and pull. This is also known as the **Jendrassik maneuver.**

Clonus is a rhythmic series of muscle contractions induced by stretching the tendon. It most commonly occurs at the ankle, where it is typically elicited by suddenly dorsiflexing the patient's foot and maintaining light upward pressure on the sole.

2. Plantar response

Using a blunt, narrow surface (e.g., a tongue blade, key, or handle of a reflex hammer), stroke the sole of the patient's foot on the lateral edge, starting near the heel and proceeding along the lateral edge almost to the base of the little toe, then curve the path medially just proximal to the base of the other toes. This should take the form of a smooth J stroke. Always start by applying minimal pressure. This is usually adequate, but if no response occurs, repeat the maneuver with greater pressure.

The normal response is for all the toes to flex (a "flexor plantar response"). When there is damage to the central nervous system motor pathways, an abnormal reflex occurs: the great toe extends (dorsiflexes) and the other toes fan out. This is called an **extensor plantar response**; it is also known as a **Babinski sign.**

3. Superficial reflexes

The abdominal reflexes, cremasteric reflexes, and other superficial reflexes are described in standard physical examination textbooks. They are not usually relevant to standard screening examinations.

4. Primitive reflexes

The grasp, root, snout, and palmomental reflexes are known as primitive reflexes or **frontal release signs.** These tests do not fit easily into any examination category. They are reflex responses, but their pathways are far more complicated than the monosynaptic arcs of the deep tendon reflexes. *I do not test these reflexes. They have very little localizing value, and, in particular, there is no convincing evidence that they reflect frontal lobe pathology. They are not even reliable indicators of abnormal function, and except for the grasp, all of these reflexes are seen in a substantial proportion of normal individuals.*

Reflex Examination: Additional Comments

1. Grading reflexes

The most common convention for grading deep tendon reflexes is simple but imprecise:

0 = absent
1 = reduced (hypoactive)
2 = normal
3 = increased (hyperactive)
4 = clonus

Some examiners use a grade of 5 to designate sustained clonus, reserving 4 for unsustained clonus that eventually fades after 2–10 beats. Also, some examiners include a reflex grade of 1/2 to indicate a reflex that can only be obtained using reinforcement.

The obvious limitation of this scheme is that it provides no guidelines for determining when reflexes are reduced, normal, or increased. This is left up to individual judgment, based on the examiner's sense of the range of reflexes present in the normal population.

2. Detection of subtle asymmetry

Comparison between reflexes in one part of the body and another is much more important than the absolute reflex grade. The most important comparison is between corresponding reflexes on the right and left, where even subtle asymmetry may be significant. For example, patients with an S1 radiculopathy may have an ankle jerk that would be considered normal, yet it is clearly less brisk than the ankle jerk on the other side. This is another limitation of the reflex grading scale: It does not express subtle distinctions that may be clinically important. For this reason, many examiners augment the scale by using + or – to designate intermediate grades. These grades have very little reproducibility from one examiner to another (or even for a single examiner from one examination to the next). They are only useful for indicating that asymmetry exists, not for quantifying it in any meaningful way.

When reflexes are brisk, it is difficult to detect slight asymmetry. For the most sensitive comparison, it is best to reduce the stimulus until it is just barely above threshold for eliciting the reflex. I typically set aside my reflex hammer and use my fingertips for this purpose. I look for two manifestations of asymmetry. First, is the threshold stimulus the same on each side, or do I consistently need to hit harder on one side than the other? Second, if the threshold stimulus is the same on each side, does it elicit the same magnitude of response on each side? Such subtle distinctions are most readily made by testing the reflex on one side immediately after testing the corresponding reflex on the other side, rather than testing all reflexes in one limb before testing the contralateral limb.

Another technique I use to heighten sensitivity to subtle reflex asymmetry is to place my finger on the patient's tendon and strike my finger rather than striking the tendon directly. This helps me aim more accurately and allows me to feel the tendon contraction. Moreover, it demonstrates to patients that I am willing to "share the pain," thereby gaining their sympathy and cooperation.

3. Relaxing the patient

Relaxation is critical in the reflex examination. Tendon reflexes are difficult to elicit when patients tense the muscles being tested. It is helpful to distract patients by engaging them in conversation while testing their reflexes. I take this opportunity to ask questions that have come to me during the rest of the examination. When I have forgotten a significant aspect of the social history, this is a convenient time to ask about it. If I have decided that formal mental status testing is necessary, I often do it while testing reflexes.

4. Significance of a Babinski sign

The Babinski sign is not graded. It is an abnormal finding that is either present or not. It is one of the few neurologic examination findings that can be interpreted without comparison to the contralateral response or consideration of patient compliance.

E. Sensory Examination

1. Light touch sensation

To test for light touch sensation, have the patient close his or her eyes and tell you whether you are touching the left hand, right hand, or both simultaneously. Repeat this several times, using as a stimulus a single light touch applied sometimes to the medial aspect of the hand and sometimes to the lateral aspect. Note whether the patient consistently fails to detect stimulation in one location. Also note whether the patient consistently "extinguishes" the stimulus on one side of the body when both sides are **stimulated simultaneously.** Next, touch the patient once lightly on the medial aspect of each hand simultaneously, and ask if they feel the same. Ask the same question for the lateral aspect of each hand. If any abnormalities are detected, extend your region of testing proximally in the limb to map out the precise area of abnormality. Perform analogous testing on the feet.

2. Pain/temperature sensation

When preparing to test pain and temperature sensation explain to the patient that you will be touching each finger with either the sharp or the dull end of a safety pin, and demonstrate each. Be sure the safety pin is previously unuscd. Then, with the patient's eyes closed, lightly touch the palmar aspect of the thumb with the sharp point of the pin, and ask the patient to say "sharp" or "dull." Repeat this for each finger of each hand, usually using the sharp point but including one dull stimulus on each hand to be sure the patient is paying attention. Next, touch the patient with the pin once lightly on the medial aspect of each hand, and ask if they feel equally sharp. Ask the same question for the lateral aspect of each hand. If any abnormalities are detected, extend your region of testing proximally in the limb to map out the precise area of abnormality. Perform analogous testing on the feet.

It is not usually necessary to test both pain and temperature, as either will suffice. You can test temperature in a fashion analogous to pain; a reasonable stimulus is the flat portion of a tuning fork after it has been immersed in cold water and dried.

3. Joint position sense

With the finger and thumb of one hand, stabilize the distal interphalangeal joint of the patient's left hand by holding it on the medial and lateral aspects. With the finger and thumb of your other hand, hold the medial and lateral aspects of the tip of the thumb and move it slightly up or down. Have the patient close his or her eyes and identify the direction of movement. Repeat several times. Most normal patients can identify movements of a few degrees or less. Perform analogous testing of the patient's right thumb and both great toes. If abnormalities are detected, proceed to more proximal joints in the same limb until a joint is found where position sense is intact.

The **Romberg test** also helps to assess position sense. Have the patient stand with both feet together, and then note whether the patient can maintain balance after closing his or her eyes.

4. Vibration sense

Vibration sense can be tested by tapping a 128-Hz tuning fork lightly against a solid surface to produce a slight (silent) vibration. With the patient's eyes closed, hold the nonvibrating end of the tuning fork firmly on the distal interphalangeal joint of the patient's left thumb and ask the patient if the vibration is detectable. Let the vibration fade until the patient no longer detects it, then apply the tuning fork to your own thumb to see if you can still feel any vibration. Repeat this testing on the patient's right thumb and both great toes. For one of the limbs, stop the vibration before applying the tuning fork to the limb to be sure that the patient is paying attention. If not, clarify to the patient that you are only interested in actual vibration, not just pressure. If any abnormalities are detected, apply the tuning fork to progressively more proximal joints until one is found where the vibration is detected normally.

5. Double simultaneous stimulation

The test for double simultaneous stimulation is performed while testing light touch sensation (see above).

6. Graphesthesia

To test for graphesthesia, ask the patient to close the eyes and identify a number from 0 to 9 that you draw on his or her index finger using a ballpoint pen (with the stylette in). Repeat with several other numbers and compare to the other hand. There is rarely any need to test graphesthesia in the feet.

7. Stereognosis

To test for stereognosis, ask the patient to close the eyes and identify a small object (e.g., nickel, dime, quarter, penny, key, paper clip) you place in his or her right hand. Test the left hand in the same way.

Sensory Examination: Additional Comments

The sensory examination is often the most frustrating part of the neurologic examination. The instructions often must be repeated several times or more before patients understand what they are being asked to do. Even then, some patients overinterpret insignificant distinctions while significant abnormalities go undetected in other patients who have difficulty attending to the task. This part of the examination is also tiresome and somewhat uncomfortable for patients. *For these reasons, the sensory examination is usually one of the last things I test. That way, I have a fairly good sense of whether the patient is likely to overinterpret small differences, and I can adjust accordingly. Furthermore, if a patient gets exasperated and refuses to proceed with the examination (which sometimes happens), I already have most of the other information I need.*

IV. The Neurologic Examination: How to Interpret It

The general principles governing lesion localization were discussed in Chapter 1. This section presents some additional principles that are often helpful in deducing lesion localization based on specific examination findings.

A. Mental Status Examination

Cognition is poorly understood. All of the categories used to describe mental status (e.g., calculation, abstraction) are convenient simplifications, but they do not necessarily reflect the way in which the brain actually functions. For example, it is very unlikely that any region or circuit in the brain is devoted specifically to calculation.

This complicates the interpretation of the mental status examination. For example, when patients are asked to subtract serial sevens (i.e., "Count backwards from 100 by 7"), they must (1) be alert, (2) comprehend language well enough to understand a fairly abstract command, (3) retain the command in memory long enough to process it, (4) possess the necessary calculation skills, (5) be able to verbalize the response, and (6) maintain attention on the task so that the current result can be taken as the basis for generating the next one. Students often ask whether this task is a test of calculation or of attention. The answer is both, and neither. It is not possible to assign a one-to-one correlation between a task on the mental status examination and a single cognitive function in the same way that abduction of an eye correlates to the function of a single lateral rectus muscle. When a patient is unable to perform a specific task, there are always several possible explanations. The examiner must observe the response to a variety of tasks, determine which ones are difficult for the patient, and try to determine the kinds of cognitive processing common to those tasks. Inferences about lesion localization are then possible.

Decreased level of alertness occurs only with dysfunction of both cerebral hemispheres or of the reticular activating system in the brainstem (see Speed Rule 11 in Chapter 1). The usual cause is a generalized metabolic abnormality, such as hypoxia or hyperglycemia. Less commonly, appropriately placed structural lesions (especially expanding ones) may produce the same result. The implications and management options are very different for structural causes and metabolic causes, and the examination is primarily aimed at distinguishing between these two possibilities (see Chapter 11).

Mental status changes in alert patients can result from either focal or generalized processes. Generalized processes usually affect all cognitive functions about equally, although early on the main manifestations may just be inattention or word-finding difficulty. Focal lesions typically affect some cognitive functions more than others, and the pattern of cognitive deficits can have some localizing significance.

The most common examples of selective mental status abnormality involve language function. As discussed in Chapter 1, language fluency, comprehension, and repetition each have rough anatomical correlates within the dominant cerebral hemisphere. Language disorders can be separated into broad categories depending on the degree to which each of these three functions is involved. For example, a classic Wernicke's aphasia (lesion site #1 in Figure 1-17) is characterized by fluent speech but impaired comprehension and repetition. Any aphasia in which repetition is spared is called transcortical (transcortical sensory when comprehension is impaired, transcortical motor when speech is nonfluent, and mixed transcortical when both comprehension and fluency are abnormal) (lesion sites #4, #5, and #6 in Figure 1-17).

Other cognitive abnormalities that may be seen in relative isolation include acalculia, agraphia, alexia, and apraxia. Each of these deficits is associated with focal lesions in the dominant hemisphere. The left hemisphere is dominant for language in almost all right-handed individuals. The left hemisphere is also language-dominant in most left-handed subjects, but the relationship is less predictable.

Neglect of one side of the environment can be seen with a focal lesion in either hemisphere, but it is much more common and tends to be more severe when the lesion is in the nondominant hemisphere. Nondominant parietal lesions may also produce anosognosia, which is the inability to recognize the existence or severity of one's own impairment.

Unilateral disease of prefrontal cortex often has surprisingly few clinical consequences, but bilateral prefrontal disease is typically associated with difficulty maintaining and shifting attention. Such patients will demonstrate both **impersistence** (an inability to stick with a task or topic of conversation) and **perseveration** (a tendency to continue returning to tasks and topics of conversation even when they are no longer appropriate).

None of these focal findings has any localizing significance unless it occurs out of proportion to other cognitive deficits. Each of them can occur as part of a general dementing illness such as Alzheimer's disease. In fact, it is often impossible to assess language function or other "focal" functions when significant dementia is present, or when there is reduction in the level of alertness. Patients with generalized cognitive impairment perform poorly on all aspects of the mental status examination, and it is usually futile to try to determine if one function is more severely affected than another.

B. Cranial Nerve Examination

1. Visual field defects

Because of the precise spatial organization of the visual pathways throughout their course, visual field defects can be exquisitely localizing at times. The most basic principles of visual field defects and their localizing value were discussed in Chapter 1 (see Figure 1-14).

2. Pupillary abnormalities

a. Asymmetric pupils (anisocoria)

The sympathetic and the parasympathetic pathways that determine pupillary size were discussed in Chapter 1 (see Figures 1-15 and 1-16). The question remains: when one pupil is larger than the other ("anisocoria"), which pupil is abnormal? For example, assume the left pupil is larger than the right. This could be caused either by a lesion in the sympathetic pathway on the right or by a lesion in the parasympathetic pathway on the left. To decide, the pupils should be examined both in bright light and in the dark. If the pupillary asymmetry is greatest in the dark, then the lesion is in the sympathetic system, because this is the system responsible for dilating the pupils, and darkness induces maximal dilation. In the present example, this indicates a lesion in the sympathetic pathway on the right (Figure 2-1A). Conversely, pupillary asymmetry that is greatest in the light indicates a lesion in the parasympathetic pathway on the left (Figure 2-1B). When

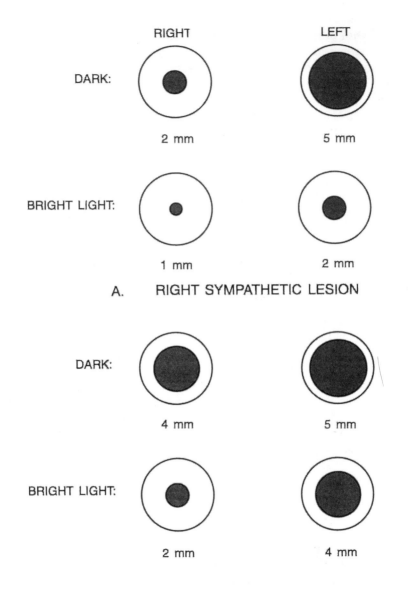

Figure 2-1. *Diagram illustrating the distinction between sympathetic and parasympathetic lesions producing anisocoria. When the left pupil is larger than the right, it could mean a right sympathetic lesion (**A**) or a left parasympathetic lesion (**B**). With sympathetic lesions, the pupillary asymmetry is greatest in the dark, whereas with parasympathetic lesions, the asymmetry is greatest in bright light.*

the pupillary asymmetry is of equal magnitude in dark and in light, it is generally **physiologic** (i.e., a normal variant).

Another clue to the lesion site in a patient with anisocoria may be provided by ptosis. Because the parasympathetic fibers travel with the third cranial nerve for much of their course, a parasympathetic lesion often produces other signs of third nerve dysfunction, including eye movement abnormalities or pronounced ptosis (because the levator palpebrae muscle is innervated by the third nerve). Sympathetic lesions also produce ptosis, because they innervate Müller's muscle in the eyelid, but this is a much smaller muscle than the levator palpebrae, so the ptosis is much less dramatic. Thus, ptosis on the side of the larger pupil indicates a parasympathetic lesion on that side. Mild ptosis on the side of the smaller pupil indicates a sympathetic lesion on that side (Horner's syndrome). This is a restatement of Speed Rule 7 (see Chapter 1).

b. Afferent pupillary defect

Anisocoria indicates a lesion in the efferent fibers supplying the pupillary sphincter muscles. A lesion in the afferent limb of the pupillary reflex (i.e., in the retina or optic nerve) does not produce anisocoria. Such a lesion is best appreciated on the "swinging flashlight test." To understand this test, one must recognize two facts. First, pupillary size is determined by an average of the illumination detected by each eye. For a simple demonstration of this, observe a normal subject's right pupil while covering the left eye: the pupil enlarges, because the average illumination has been effectively halved. Second, the efferent limb of the pupillary reflex is bilateral, so that both pupils receive the same command and they are always the same size. They are only unequal when the efferent pathways are not working properly.

Now consider what happens when a patient has an optic nerve lesion. For purposes of illustration, assume the lesion is in the left optic nerve and that it reduces the perceived illumination in that eye by 50%. A bright light directed at the left eye will still increase the perceived illumination in that eye compared to the ambient room light. The average of the perceived illumination in the two eyes will thus increase also, and both pupils will constrict. Assume that this produces a change in pupil size from 5 mm to 3 mm (Figure 2-2A,B). A bright light directed at the right eye will produce a similar response: In this case, the change in perceived illumination from ambient room light will be even greater, resulting in even stronger pupillary constriction, producing a change in pupil size from 5 mm to 2.5 mm, for example (Figure 2-2C). It is difficult for an examiner to appreciate this subtle a distinction in the magnitude of the pupillary response. But now consider what happens when the bright light

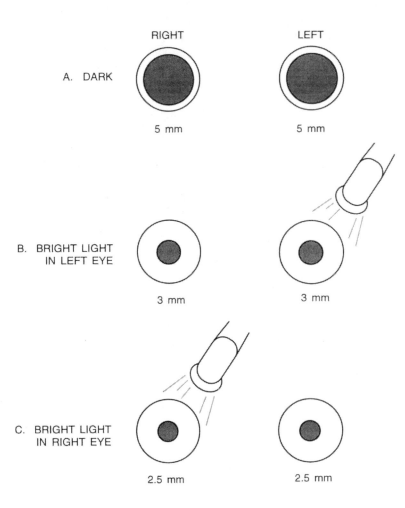

Figure 2-2. *Diagram illustrating a left afferent pupillary defect. The left pupil is the same size as the right under all conditions of illumination, because the efferent pathways are intact, but both pupils are smaller when light is directed at the right eye than when it is directed at the left eye, because light is detected better by the right eye. Alternate swinging of the light between the two eyes therefore produces dilation each time the light is directed to the left eye.*

is swung back and forth between the two eyes. When it is directed at the left eye, both pupils are 3 mm. When swung to the right eye, both pupils constrict to 2.5 mm. When swung back to the left eye, both pupils dilate back to 3 mm, and so forth. Because the examiner usually can observe the pupil under the bright light more readily than the other pupil, the examiner notes the left pupil dilating each time the light is directed at it. This result might seem paradoxical, as if the pupil were dilating in response to bright light, but not when one recognizes that the dilation only occurs when the light is swung from the right eye to the left one. In effect, by swinging the bright light back and forth, the examiner is simply varying the intensity of the light perceived by the brain, and the pupils are constricting and dilating appropriately in response. This finding is termed a left **afferent pupillary defect,** or a left Marcus-Gunn pupil.

3. Eye movement abnormalities

a. Gaze palsy

An eye movement abnormality in which the two eyes move conjugately but they have limited movement in one direction is called a gaze palsy. It is due to malfunction of one of the "gaze centers" (cortical and brainstem regions responsible for conjugate gaze) or to interruption of the pathways leading from them. When the lesion is in a brainstem gaze center, the neurons there cannot be activated either voluntarily or by reflex (such as the oculocephalic reflex or "doll's eyes response"). This is called a **nuclear gaze palsy.** When the lesion is in a cortical gaze center, only voluntary gaze is impaired; reflexes can still activate the brainstem neurons responsible for gaze. This is called a **supranuclear gaze palsy.**

b. Internuclear ophthalmoplegia

Lesions distal to the brainstem gaze centers (for example, in the nucleus of cranial nerve VI, or in the inferior oblique muscle on one side) produce disconjugate abnormalities of eye movements. Specific patterns of eye movement abnormalities and their localizing significance are discussed in Chapter 13. One particular eye movement abnormality merits special recognition. Isolated impairment of adduction in one eye could conceivably result from a focal neuromuscular junction problem or damage to a single medial rectus muscle, but it is much more commonly due to a lesion in the ipsilateral **median longitudinal fasciculus** (MLF). This pathway runs from the sixth nerve nucleus on one side up to the third nerve nucleus on the other. This allows one eye's lateral rectus muscle and the other eye's medial rectus muscle to be activated synchronously, producing conjugate horizontal gaze (whether activated voluntarily or by reflex). A lesion in the MLF unlinks these two nuclei, so that the brainstem gaze center is able to get its message to the sixth nerve nucleus but not to the contralateral third nerve nucleus. The third nerve and medial rectus muscle continue to function normally in situations that do not require conjugate eye movements (e.g., convergence on a near object), but they cannot be activated by the horizontal gaze center. A lesion of the MLF is termed an **internuclear ophthalmoplegia**. The adduction difficulty is accompanied by nystagmus in the other eye as it abducts; in fact, in subtle cases, this may be the most prominent finding.

4. Facial weakness

Just as hyperactive deep tendon reflexes or a supranuclear gaze palsy indicate a central lesion whereas hypoactive reflexes or disconjugate eye movement abnormalities imply a peripheral lesion, the pattern of facial weakness can help differentiate between central and peripheral lesions. When one entire side of the face is weak, the lesion is usually peripheral. With a central lesion (such as a stroke in one cerebral hemisphere), the forehead muscles are often spared. This is because the portion of the facial nerve nucleus representing the forehead typically gets input from the motor strips of both cerebral hemispheres, so it can still be activated by the cortex contralateral to the lesion. The portion of the facial nerve nucleus representing the lower face does not have the same bilateral input; its input is predominantly from the contralateral cortex.

5. Hearing loss and vertigo

As explained in Chapter 1, a central lesion affects hearing in both ears almost equally. The only way to produce hearing loss restricted to one ear is with a peripheral lesion. Examination findings that help to distinguish between central and peripheral vertigo are discussed in Chapter 14.

6. Dysarthria and dysphagia

Unilateral weakness of muscles of the palate, pharynx, or larynx indicates a peripheral lesion (i.e., at the level of lower motor neuron, neuromuscular junction, or muscle). These muscles are innervated by fibers that originate in the nucleus ambiguus in the medulla and that travel in the glossopharyngeal and vagus nerves (CNs IX and X, respectively). The nucleus ambiguus receives descending input from both cerebral hemispheres. A unilateral central lesion does not produce focal palatal, pharyngeal, or laryngeal weakness, because input to the nucleus ambiguus from the other hemisphere remains intact.

Dysarthria and dysphagia are prominent symptoms of lower motor neuron lesions of CNs IX and X. These symptoms tend to be less prominent after unilateral central lesions because of the bilateral cortical input to the nucleus ambiguus. Bilateral central lesions often produce dramatic speech and swallowing problems, however. This is known as pseudobulbar palsy because the interruption of descending input to the brainstem simulates a lesion in the brainstem itself (a "bulbar" lesion). On close examination, the character of the dysarthria is different in patients with upper motor neuron lesions and patients with lower motor neuron lesions. There is classically a strained, strangled character to the speech of the former, for example, while the latter typically sound breathy, hoarse, and hypernasal. In fact, dysarthria can result from any conditions that damage motor control of the structures necessary for speech production, including cerebellar or basal ganglia disorders, and the specific characteristics of the dysarthria may be useful in localization and differential diagnosis.

7. Neck weakness

The accessory nerve (CN XI) is a prime candidate for the most confusing cranial nerve. The motor nerves innervating the sternocleidomastoid (SCM) and trapezius muscles originate in the cervical spinal cord (at the C1-2 level for the SCM and the C3-4 level for the trapezius). They then ascend alongside the spinal cord and enter the skull through the foramen magnum, only to exit the skull again through the jugular foramen. The descending cortical input to the nuclei controlling the trapezius muscle originates almost exclusively in the contralateral cerebral hemisphere. The cortical input to the nucleus for the SCM muscle comes from both hemispheres, but predominantly the ipsilateral one. An additional confounding feature is that the left SCM rotates the head to the right (and vice versa).

As a result, peripheral lesions produce weakness of the ipsilateral SCM and trapezius muscles, resulting in weakness of shoulder elevation on that side but impaired head rotation to the opposite side. Central lesions produce weakness of the ipsilateral SCM but the contralateral trapezius. When a central lesion is large enough to cause more extensive weakness (i.e., hemiparesis) there is weakness of shoulder elevation on the side of the hemiparesis and weakness of head rotation toward the side of the hemiparesis.

8. Tongue weakness

The hypoglossal nerve (CN XII) receives descending cortical input from both hemispheres about equally, except that the fibers destined for the genioglossus muscle receive their cortical input only from the contralateral hemisphere. There appears to be variability in this pattern, so unilateral central lesions sometimes produce ipsilateral tongue weakness, more often produce contralateral tongue weakness, and most often produce no significant tongue weakness at all. Unilateral peripheral lesions produce weakness of the ipsilateral tongue muscles, resulting in difficulty protruding the tongue to the opposite side. Atrophy and fasciculations are often prominent with peripheral lesions, as with lower motor neuron lesions throughout the body (see the following section on motor examination).

C. Motor Examination

1. Upper motor neuron vs. lower motor neuron lesions

Several examination findings help to distinguish central from peripheral lesions in the motor system. Deep tendon reflexes provide one clue, as discussed in Chapter 1 (Speed Rule 4): reflexes are typically hyperactive with a central lesion and hypoactive with a peripheral one. The Babinski sign is a reliable indicator of a central lesion. Atrophy and fasciculations are common with lower motor neuron disease and unusual with upper motor neuron disease. The pattern of muscle involvement is also helpful. A central lesion usually results in weakness that is more pronounced in the flexors of the lower extremities than in the extensors, but in the upper extremities the extensors are weaker than the flexors. This is often called pyramidal weakness, but it does not occur with pure lesions of the pyramidal tracts. Instead, it is the net result of disrupting all the descending motor tracts and is probably most appropriately called an **upper motor neuron** (UMN) pattern of weakness. The UMN pattern of weakness also causes supination of the upper extremity to be weaker than pronation; this accounts for the finding of a pronator drift, in which the arm pronates and drifts downward when the patient is asked to hold it extended with palms up (supinated). This is a fairly sensitive indicator of subtle UMN weakness. It is also useful as a test for internal consistency, because patients with nonorganic weakness will often allow their arm to drift downward but fail to pronate it.

Another feature distinguishing a central lesion from a peripheral one is the resistance of the limbs to passive manipulation (muscle tone). A central lesion is characterized by spasticity, whereas tone is normal or reduced with a peripheral lesion.

To summarize, an UMN lesion is characterized by the pattern of weakness (most prominent in the extensors of the upper extremity and the flexors of the lower extremity), spasticity (most pronounced in the opposite muscles), hyperreflexia, and the Babinski sign. A lower motor neuron lesion is characterized by weakness, hypotonia, hyporeflexia, atrophy, and fasciculations.

2. Patterns of lower motor neuron weakness

For patients with weakness due to diffuse disease of the peripheral nervous system, the specific pattern of muscle involvement often provides useful localizing information (see Chapter 6). For example, predominantly distal weakness usually suggests a disease of peripheral nerves, but predominantly proximal weakness typically occurs in muscle disorders and neuromuscular junction diseases.

For patients with weakness due to focal lesions in the peripheral nervous system, the most reliable approach to localization is to consult a reference book, but in most cases adequate localization can be achieved by remembering a few simple patterns. In each extremity, consider three principal joints: the hip, knee, and ankle in the lower extremities, and the elbow, wrist, and knuckle in the upper extremities (it really doesn't matter which knuckle; the pattern applies equally well to interphalangeal joints and metacarpophalangeal joints). At each joint, consider flexion and extension separately. This gives six principal movements in each limb. Most localization problems can be solved by remembering the innervation patterns for these six principal movements (plus shoulder abduction and finger abduction in the upper extremities).

Figure 2-3 shows which nerve roots provide innervation for each of these principal movements. In the upper extremities, the pattern can be remembered by ordering the movements in a kind of spiral that proceeds down the arm: shoulder abduction (A), elbow flexion (B), elbow extension (C), wrist extension (D), wrist flexion (E), finger flexion (F), finger extension (G), and finger abduction (H). The corresponding roots then proceed in order: C5 (A), C5-6 (B), C6-7 (C), C6-7 (D), C7-8 (E), C8 (F), C8 (G), and T1 (H).

In the lower extremities, the pattern is even simpler (Figure 2-4). The movements can be ordered in sequence down the front first and

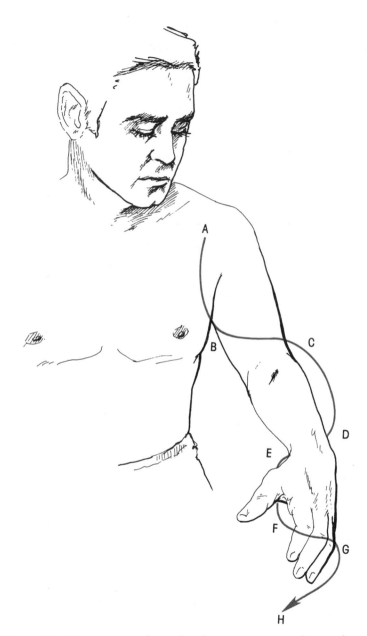

Figure 2-3. *Nerve roots and peripheral nerves corresponding to the principal movements of the upper extremity. The letters labeling the movements form a spiral down the extremity. The nerve roots and peripheral nerves corresponding to each movement are listed in the accompanying table.*

then the back: hip flexion (A), knee extension (B), ankle dorsiflexion (C), hip extension (D), knee flexion (E), and ankle plantar flexion (F). The corresponding roots are: L2-3 (A), L3-4 (B), L4-5 (C), L4-5 (D), L5-S1 (E), and S1-2 (F).

The peripheral nerves providing innervation for these same principal movements are listed in Figures 2-3 and 2-4. There is no simple pattern, but fortunately, there aren't many nerves to remember. In the upper extremities, all the extension movements in the figure (C, D, and G) are innervated by the radial nerve. The two distal flexion movements (E and F) are supplied by the median nerve, and the proximal one (elbow flexion, B) by the musculocutaneous nerve. The axillary nerve supplies the deltoid muscle, which is the main shoulder abductor (A), and the interosseous muscles (H) are innervated by the ulnar nerve.

In the lower extremities, the sciatic nerve innervates the muscles responsible for knee flexion (E); its peroneal branch supplies ankle dorsiflexion (C), while its tibial branch supplies ankle plantar flexion (F). Knee extensor muscles are innervated by the femoral nerve. The innervation of the iliopsoas muscle, which flexes the hip, arises very proximally from the L2 and L3 nerve roots; some consider this to be part of the femoral nerve, and others simply call it the "nerve to iliopsoas." The gluteus muscles, responsible for hip extension (D), are innervated by the gluteal nerves.

The nerve root corresponding to each commonly tested deep tendon reflex can also be derived from Figures 2-3 and 2-4. In particular, the biceps and brachioradialis reflexes are mediated by the C5-6 roots, the triceps reflex by the C6-7 roots (mainly C7), the knee jerk by the L3-4 roots (mainly L4), and the ankle jerk by the S1 root. The internal hamstring reflex is less often tested, but it is mediated by the L5 nerve root.

Table for Figure 2-3

	Movement	Roots	Peripheral Nerve
A.	Shoulder abduction	5	Axillary
B.	Elbow flexion	5/6	Musculocutaneous
C.	Elbow extension	6/7	Radial
D.	Wrist extension	6/7	Radial
E.	Wrist flexion	7/8	Median
F.	Finger flexion	8	Median
G.	Finger extension	8	Radial
H.	Finger abduction	T1	Ulnar

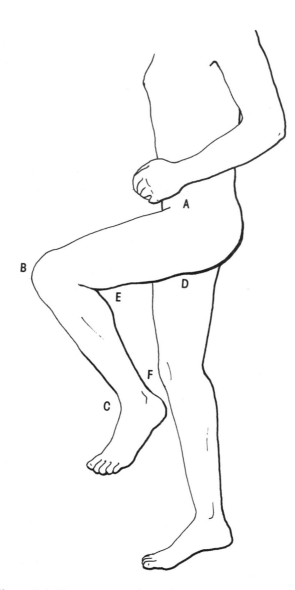

Figure 2-4. *Nerve roots and peripheral nerves corresponding to the principal movements of the lower extremity. The letters labeling the movements proceed in order from proximal to distal down the front of the limb, and then repeat from proximal to distal down the back of the limb. The nerve roots and peripheral nerves corresponding to each movement are listed in the accompanying table.*

D. Reflex Examination

The localizing significance of the tendon reflexes is discussed above and in Chapter 1.

E. Sensory Examination

As explained in Chapter 1, the pathways for different sensory modalities cross at different levels in the nervous system, making them very useful for localizing lesions. Unlike the distinction between UMN and lower motor neuron lesions in the motor pathways, there are not really any examination findings that help to confine a lesion to a specific portion of a sensory pathway.

For most localization problems, precise knowledge of the sensory fields of specific peripheral nerves and nerve roots is unnecessary. It is usually sufficient to remember the following facts (refer to Figures 2-5 and 2-6).

1.   Sensation travels from the thumb and index finger via the C6 nerve root, from the middle finger via the C7 root, and from the fourth and fifth fingers via the C8 root.

2.   For the remainder of the upper extremity, the root innervation "fans out" from the hand (see Figure 2-5).

3.   These innervation patterns cover both the anterior and posterior aspects of the upper extremity.

4.   The _L_5 dermatome includes the _l_arge toe and the _l_ateral _l_ower _l_eg; the _S_1 dermatome includes the _s_mall toe and _s_ole. Roots L4, L3,

Table for Figure 2-4

	Movement	Roots	Peripheral Nerve
A.	Hip flexion	2/3	Femoral ("nerve to iliopsoas")
B.	Knee extension	3/4	Femoral
C.	Ankle dorsiflexion	4/5	Peroneal
D.	Hip extension	4/5	Gluteal
E.	Knee flexion	5/1	Sciatic
F.	Ankle plantar flexion	1/2	Tibial

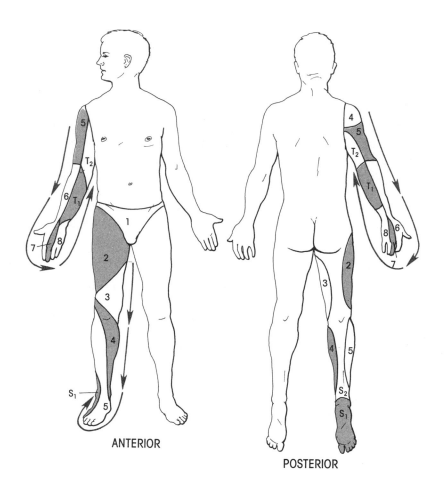

Figure 2-5. *Diagram illustrating the nerve roots corresponding to the principal dermatomes in the upper and lower extremities.*

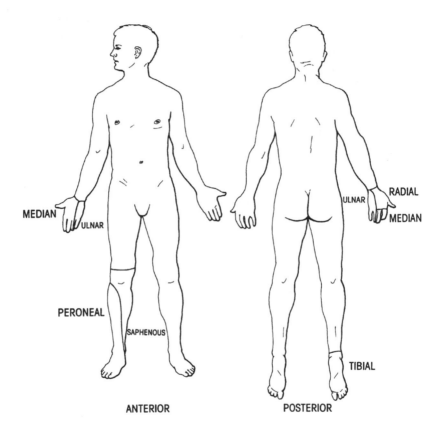

MEDIAN

ULNAR

RADIAL

MEDIAN

ULNAR

PERONEAL

SAPHENOUS

TIBIAL

ANTERIOR

POSTERIOR

Figure 2-6. *Diagram illustrating the territories of sensory innervation for the principal peripheral nerves of the distal upper and lower extremities.*

and L2 cover the region fanning out medially and proximally from the L5 dermatome. The S2 dermatome extends from the S1 dermatome up the back of the leg (see Figure 2-5).

   5.   The median nerve carries sensation from all fingers except the fifth finger and half of the fourth, which are served by the ulnar nerve. These nerve territories extend proximally up to the wrist on the palmar aspect of the hand. On the dorsal aspect, the ulnar nerve territory still extends to the wrist, but the median nerve territory fades into radial nerve territory at the metacarpal phalangeal joints (see Figure 2-6).

   6.   The common peroneal nerve innervates the lateral leg and the dorsum of the foot; the tibial nerve innervates the sole.

For the peripheral nerve innervations of more proximal limb regions, it is best to consult diagrams in reference books.

V. The Neurologic Examination: How to Modify It

A. Screening Neurologic Examination

Medical students should always try to perform complete physical examinations (including complete neurologic examinations) on all patients they evaluate, so they can gain a sense of the range of normal variation and ask questions about the findings they observe. House officers and practicing physicians usually do not have the time to perform complete examinations on all patients, however. They must be able to perform a rapid examination that screens for most common abnormalities. They can then use the results of this screening examination together with the history to decide whether certain components of the examination must be conducted in more detail. For such screening purposes, the following neurologic examination is generally adequate and can be completed in 5 minutes or less. This examination is offered as a suggestion for students to use in future practice; it is not adequate for students examining patients on a neurology service.

Mental status

Test patients for orientation to person, place, and time. Make sure they can follow at least one complicated command, taking care not to give them any nonverbal cues. If their responses are appropriate and they are able to relate a detailed and coherent medical history, no further mental status testing is necessary (unless they have cognitive complaints).

Cranial nerves

Test visual fields in one eye, both pupillary responses to light, eye movements in all directions, facial strength, and hearing to finger rub.

Motor system

Test strength in the following muscles bilaterally: deltoids, triceps, wrist extensors, hand interossei, iliopsoas, hamstrings, ankle dorsiflexors. Test for a pronator drift. Test finger tapping, finger-to-nose, and heel-knee-shin performance. Test tandem gait and walking on the heels.

Reflexes

Test plantar responses and biceps, triceps, patellar, and ankle reflexes bilaterally.

Sensation

Test light touch sensation in all four distal limbs, including double simultaneous stimulation. Test vibration sense at the great toes.

Remember, this examination must be expanded when an asymmetry or other abnormality is found. For example, if the triceps muscle is weak in one arm, other muscles innervated by the radial nerve must be tested, as well as other muscles in the distribution of the C7 nerve root. The examination must also be expanded to focus on patients' specific complaints. For example, patients complaining of memory loss need thorough mental status testing even if their performance on the screening examination is perfectly normal.

B. Examination of Stuporous or Comatose Patients

People in coma cannot answer questions or follow commands, making it necessary to modify or eliminate many parts of the neurologic examination. Fortunately, there is no great mystery regarding the region of nervous system disorder in these patients; it is in the brainstem or above. The neurologic examination is directed mainly at determining whether this pathology is due to a structural lesion or due to metabolic dysfunction (including drug effects). The basis for this determination is discussed in Chapter 11; the most pertinent examination findings are abnormal reflexes that indicate dysfunction in specific regions of the brainstem or a consistent asymmetry between right- and left-sided responses.

Mental status

The mental status examination in a comatose patient is simply an assessment of the patient's responses to visual, auditory, and noxious stimuli. In addition to local reflex responses (summarized below in the discussion of motor and sensory systems), a comatose patient may demonstrate motor responses that reflect more generalized reflex activity. Two specific patterns of motor activity are classically described. **Decorticate posturing** consists of upper-extremity adduction and flexion at the elbows, wrists, and fingers, together with lower-extremity extension. **Decerebrate posturing** consists of upper-extremity extension, adduction, and pronation together with lower-extremity extension. This terminology reflects the analogy that has been drawn between these postures and the postures maintained by experimental animals after specific lesions, but in fact, these postures do not have reliable localizing value in human patients. In general, patients with decorticate posturing in response to pain have a better prognosis than those with decerebrate posturing.

Cranial nerves

Visual acuity cannot be tested and formal testing of visual fields is impossible. A rough assessment of visual field defects may be obtained by assessing response to visual threat, such as a finger or small object introduced suddenly into the visual field. Pupillary reflexes can be tested in the same manner as in an awake person.

Eye movements can be assessed by activating them through reflexes. The **oculocephalic reflex**, or "doll's eyes reflex," is tested by turning the patient's head from side to side. If there is any chance that there has been a traumatic injury to the cervical spine, plain films of the cervical spine must be obtained before testing this reflex. When the oculocephalic reflex is present (positive doll's eyes), the eyes do not turn with the head; it is as if the patient is maintaining fixation on a single point in space. The eyes thus appear to be moving relative to the head in the direction opposite to the head movement. This reflex is usually suppressed (and therefore not usually tested) in conscious patients, but it is a normal finding in comatose patients. Absence of this reflex in a comatose patient indicates dysfunction somewhere in the reflex pathway: in the afferent limb (from the labyrinth and vestibular nerve, and also from neck proprioceptors), the efferent limb (CNs III and VI and the muscles they innervate), or the pathways connecting them in the pons and medulla.

Another reflex that activates eye movements even more strongly is the vestibulo-ocular reflex (cold calorics). The patient is supine, with the head or upper body tilted forward so that the neck forms an angle of 30 degrees with the horizontal. A syringe is filled with 50–100 ml of ice-cold water with a small catheter attached. The water is injected against the tympanic membrane (checking with an otoscope first to be sure the membrane is intact). In this position, this stimulus has the same effect on the horizontal semicircular canal as sustained turning of the head in the opposite direction; this results in sustained deviation of both eyes toward the ear being stimulated. Absence of this reflex indicates dysfunction of the pons, medulla, or (less commonly) CNs III, VI, or VIII. Unlike the oculocephalic reflex, this reflex is also present in conscious people, producing not only deviation of the eyes toward the stimulated ear but also nystagmus, with the fast component away from the stimulated ear. There is usually no reason to test this reflex in conscious patients, however, because caloric stimulation can cause severe vertigo and nausea, and the same elements of the nervous system can be tested in much less noxious ways.

CNs V and VII can be assessed in comatose patients by testing corneal reflexes and by observing facial grimacing in response to noxious stimulation (supraorbital pressure or nasal tickle, for example). CNs IX and X can be assessed by testing the gag reflex, but remember that the gag reflex may be absent in 20% of normal subjects.

Motor and sensory systems

Formal strength testing is impossible in comatose patients, but deep tendon reflexes and resistance to passive manipulation can still be tested in the usual manner. The strength with which the patient moves each limb in response to pain should be assessed, and also the degree to which the movement is purposeful. Noxious stimulation of the lower extremity (produced by squeezing a nailbed or pinching the skin) may produce **triple flexion** (dorsiflexion of the ankle, with flexion of the knee and hip) purely as a local withdrawal reflex. To look for purposeful withdrawal, the stimulus should be applied in a location where triple flexion would be an inappropriate response, such as the anterior thigh: Hip flexion would indicate purely reflex withdrawal, whereas hip extension would indicate a purposeful movement. In contrast, hip flexion in response to a noxious stimulus applied to the posterior thigh could be either a reflex or a purposeful response. In both upper and lower extremities, reflex withdrawal produces limb adduction, so to differentiate reflex withdrawal from purposeful movement, the noxious stimulus should be applied to the medial aspect of the limb.

Pain sensation in comatose patients can be assessed by observing the response to noxious stimulation (and noting whether the response varies depending on which limb is stimulated). Other sensory modalities cannot be tested.

VI. Discussion of Localization Problems

Example 1.   The magnitude of this patient's pupillary asymmetry is greatest in the dark, so the sympathetic system is not functioning normally. The smaller pupil is therefore the abnormal one (see Figure 2-1A). Thus, this patient has a sympathetic lesion on the left, and left-sided ptosis would be expected.

Example 2.   For a patient to have face, arm, and leg weakness all on the same side of the body, there must be an upper motor neuron lesion (see Chapter 1, Speed Rule 6). An upper motor neuron lesion typically spares forehead muscles, because there is bilateral cortical input to the portion of the facial nerve nucleus controlling those muscles.

Example 3.   The L2-3 roots correspond to hip flexion, the L5-S1 roots to knee flexion, and the L4-5 roots to ankle dorsiflexion (see Figure 2-4). Thus, no single root lesion could produce this pattern of weakness. This pattern is typical of an upper motor neuron lesion, which usually produces more weakness in the flexors of the lower extremity than in the extensors.

3

What's the Lesion?

James W. Albers and Douglas J. Gelb

I. Case Histories

For each of the following cases, answer the following questions:

1. Where's the lesion?
2. Is the lesion focal, multifocal, or diffuse?
3. Is this a mass lesion or a nonmass lesion?
4. What is the temporal profile?
5. What diagnostic category is most likely?

Case 1. A 55-year-old woman has been brought to the emergency room by her husband because she seems confused and is having progressively more difficulty expressing her thoughts. For at least the last 10 weeks she has had some increasing clumsiness and weakness in her right arm and leg, and she is bumping into objects in her home. On examination, she has a right visual field defect (homonymous hemianopia), aphasia, a mild right hemiparesis (face, arm, leg), and increased reflexes on the right side with an extensor plantar response (Babinski sign) on the right.

Case 2. A 72-year-old right-handed man noted the abrupt feeling of heaviness in his left arm while watching television. His left leg gave out when he tried to stand, and he fell to the floor. He called for help, and when his wife came into the room, she noted that the left corner of his face was sagging. He could still speak. He had no symptoms other than the weakness of his entire left side. Over the next several hours he improved slightly.

Case 3. A 22-year-old man was well until 2 days ago, when he developed fever, severe headache, nausea, and vomiting. He became progressively more obtunded over the next day. He had two generalized seizures in the morning and was brought to the emergency room, where he was found to have a fever and stiff neck. He was stuporous, and had generalized hyperreflexia and bilateral Babinski signs.

Case 4. A 47-year-old man developed ringing in his right ear several years ago, and it has grown worse over time. His hearing in that ear also has gradually deteriorated. Over the same time period, he experienced weakness and loss of feeling in the right side of his face, and he now notes stiffness, weakness, and numbness of his left arm and leg.

Case 5. A 28-year-old accountant and part-time boxer has been brought to the urgent care clinic by his wife because he has become irritable and abusive. She reports that he has had intermittent headaches for 3 months that have become more severe and constant in the past month. He has been unable to work for about a week because of excessive drowsiness, and he sleeps for up to 24 hours if not awakened. The patient is poorly cooperative and says only that he has a headache.

On neurologic examination, he is drowsy and irritable but able to follow commands. He has mild to moderate weakness in his left arm and leg and a left pronator drift. Tendon reflexes are hyperactive on the left. There is a left Babinski response. The lower part of his face droops slightly on the left side.

Case 6. A 21-year-old right-handed woman experienced a sensation of numbness and tingling over her abdomen and in her legs. The next day, her legs began to feel stiff and tight, and she experienced incomplete voiding and difficulty in initiating her urinary stream. As the day progressed, the numbness and tingling became more pronounced in her mid-abdomen and below, and she noted difficulty in walking. She went to bed early that evening, and when she awoke the next morning, she was unable to stand.

Case 7. A 69-year-old right-handed retired executive is seeing her internist for a routine checkup. Her husband mentions that she has undergone a marked personality change over the past several months. He also notes that she has been forgetful for about a year and keeps asking the same things over and over. She no longer seems interested in her personal appearance. The mental status examination confirms these observations. Her speech is fluent, but she frequently pauses because she can't think of a word. She has difficulty following complicated commands. She can only remember one of three items after a 5-minute delay, and she recalls no current events. She is unable to subtract two-digit numbers in her head. The remainder of her examination is normal.

Case 8. A 44-year-old left-handed woman suddenly developed a severe bitemporal-occipital headache. She also complained of a stiff neck. When she tried to lie down, she experienced severe nausea and vomited twice. She was taken immediately to the hospital, where she was noted to be somnolent. She responded appropriately when stimulated, however, and moved all four limbs equally. Her level of consciousness deteriorated over the next 4 hours, to the point where she could not be aroused even with vigorous stimulation.

Case 9. A 57-year-old woman has come to the emergency room because in the middle of a business meeting earlier today she suddenly became dizzy and experienced nausea and vomiting. On examination, she has dysarthria, dysphagia (with weakness of the left palate), loss of pinprick sensation over the left side of her face and the right side of her body, and ataxia of her left arm and leg. Four hours have passed, and there has been no progression or improvement.

Case 10. A 30-year-old man with Hodgkin's disease began to experience severe pain beginning in his back and encircling the left side of his chest in a band 3 cm wide just below his breast. The pain was very intense at first but subsided somewhat, coincident with a rash that appeared in precisely the same distribution. He is still having pain in that area 2 weeks later and notes diminished touch sensation in the region of pain.

Case 11. A patient describes a pain that is similar to the one noted in Case 10. The pain involves the left side of her chest. No rash is present, and for many months, the pain has been getting worse. It remains localized to a narrow and circumscribed area of her chest, making her think that it might be "heart trouble." In addition, she complains of difficulty walking and says that her left leg seems to be weak and stiff.

II. Beyond Localization

Although lesion localization is fundamental to the process of generating a differential diagnosis, it is only the first step. It might seem as if the next step, once the lesion site has been identified, would simply be to obtain an imaging study of that region. This is not always the most appropriate diagnostic strategy, however. Even when it is, a prior determination of the diagnoses that are plausible on clinical grounds will be important for guiding decisions regarding which imaging modality to order, how urgently to do it, and how to interpret ambiguous results. Anyone who has ever read a radiologist's report knows that "clinical correlation is required." In most cases, a reasonable hypothesis about etiology can be generated by addressing the following three issues:

> A. **Localization:** Where's the lesion?
> B. **Temporal profile:** How did the symptoms begin, and how have they changed over time?
> C. **Epidemiology:** Does the patient have risk factors for specific conditions?

Before explaining how this information is used to draw conclusions about etiology, a few terms must be defined.

A. Localization

The principles of localization were presented in Chapters 1 and 2. When considering potential etiologies, the most important question is whether the lesion is focal, multifocal, or diffuse.

A **focal lesion** is confined to a single circumscribed area. Focal lesions are usually unilateral, but not always; a lesion that extends from one side to the other across the midline is also focal.

A **multifocal lesion** is made up of two or more focal lesions distributed randomly. These lesions may all be at the same level of the nervous system (for example, many different cortical lesions, or many lesions of individual peripheral nerves), or they may be at different levels (for example, one in the spinal cord and one in the cerebral cortex).

A **diffuse lesion** is made up of two or more focal lesions distributed nonrandomly. For example, two lesions situated symmetrically on the right and left sides of the nervous system without extending across the midline would constitute a diffuse lesion. Diseases causing generalized dysfunction of neurons, or just of peripheral nerves, or just of sensory nerves, or just of long nerves, would all be examples of diffuse lesions.

B. Temporal Profile

The first consideration in describing the temporal profile is determining whether symptoms are transient or persistent. **Transient** symptoms resolve completely; **persistent** symptoms do not. There are three types of persistent time course:

Static (stationary) symptoms reach a maximum level of severity and then do not change.

Improving symptoms reach a maximum level of severity and then begin to resolve.

Progressive symptoms continue to worsen.

These categories are mutually exclusive at any instant, but over time a patient's category may change. For example, consider a patient who develops symptoms that continue to get worse for a week, remain unchanged for a month, and then start to improve so that by 6 months the patient is completely back to normal. If evaluated at 3 days, the symptoms would be progressive, but at 3 weeks they would be static, and at 3 months they would be improving. For diagnostic purposes, the most important information about the temporal profile is the rapidity with which changes occur:

Acute symptoms evolve over minutes to days.

Subacute symptoms evolve over days to weeks.

Chronic symptoms evolve over months to years.

C. Epidemiology

Lesion localization and temporal profile are the most important factors in generating a list of potential etiologies. Epidemiologic considerations are used mainly to arrange the list in order of likelihood. For example, thyroid disease and brucellosis can both cause subacute diffuse processes, but a physician treating an affluent adult patient in an urban area would be much more concerned about thyroid disease because it is much more common in that setting. As another example, an adult patient with a stroke is more likely to have atherosclerotic disease than an arterial dissection, but dissection becomes a serious consideration if the same patient has recently sustained trauma to the neck. The relevant epidemiologic factors vary from one disease to the next, so they will not be discussed in detail in this chapter.

III. Etiology

There are seven general categories of persistent neurologic disease that can be distinguished, each with a characteristic spatial-temporal profile.

A. Degenerative Diseases

In degenerative disorders, one or more components of the nervous system begin to malfunction after functioning normally for many years. Once the deterioration begins, it doesn't stop. The two most common examples are Alzheimer's disease and Parkinson's disease. Degenerative diseases are **diffuse, chronic,** and **progressive.**

B. Neoplastic Diseases

In practice, the term *neoplasm* is applied mainly to collections of cells that are multiplying uncontrollably because of some genetic transformation (i.e., cancer). The rules presented here apply to the more general, literal meaning of neoplasm, "new growth." This means that any new structural lesion that is growing (including a slowly enlarging hematoma or a herniating intervertebral disk) will be classified as a neoplasm. This makes sense clinically, because when these processes are in the differential diagnosis, cancer is usually a possibility also, and it is appropriate to direct the diagnostic evaluation at the most serious potential diagnosis. Neoplastic diseases are characterized as **focal**, **chronic** (or, less often, subacute), and **progressive**.

C. Vascular Diseases

Disruption of the cerebrovascular system can produce either ischemia (resulting from obstructed blood vessels) or hemorrhage (resulting from ruptured blood vessels). Either way, the symptoms are almost always **acute**. Ischemic lesions are always **focal**. Hemorrhagic lesions may be either **focal** or **diffuse**, depending on whether the blood escapes into a freely interconnecting space (e.g., subarachnoid hemorrhage) or a confined space (e.g., subdural hematoma, parenchymal hemorrhage). Ischemic events are typically **static** or **improving**, while hemorrhagic events are typically **progressive**.

D. Inflammatory Diseases

Inflammation in the nervous system is most often a response to an infection or some other insult. As with hemorrhage, infection in a confined space (i.e., abscess) results in a **focal** lesion, whereas in an unrestricted space the result is a **diffuse** lesion (e.g., meningitis or encephalitis). Either way, the time course is usually **subacute** and **progressive**. In some cases, the immune system appears to become activated even without external provocation (e.g., autoimmune diseases); **multifocal** deficits typically result, with a **chronic** or **subacute** time course. The most common examples are multiple sclerosis and vasculitis.

E. Toxic and Metabolic Diseases

In one sense, all diseases are metabolic, because the only way to damage any organ is to interfere with cellular metabolism. For example, occlusive vascular disease deprives cells of oxygen and energy sources, ultimately resulting in complete termination of all cellular processes. This would not generally be considered a metabolic disease, however, because there is an underlying structural lesion: an obstructed blood vessel. The term *metabolic disease* is reserved for processes that disrupt cellular metabolism at a molecular level without any underlying structural lesion evident macroscopically. Diseases caused by toxic substances, both endogenous (e.g., uremia) and exogenous (e.g., drug overdose), are included in this category. Diabetes mellitus, thyroid disease, vitamin B_{12} deficiency, abnormal liver function, electrolyte abnormalities, and hypoxemia are some other metabolic disorders that commonly produce neurologic symptoms. Since structural lesions are excluded by definition, metabolic diseases are **diffuse**. Their time course can be **acute**, **subacute**, or **chronic**.

F. Traumatic Diseases

The main feature distinguishing traumatic disease from vascular disease is an epidemiologic consideration: the onset in the setting of head trauma. Traumatic disorders are always **acute** in onset. Nonhemorrhagic traumatic lesions are generally **static** or **improving**; they may be **diffuse** (concussion) or **focal** (contusion, encephalomalacia). Traumatic hemorrhage has the same spatial-temporal profile as nontraumatic hemorrhage: it is **progressive** and may be **diffuse** or **focal**.

G. Congenital and Developmental Diseases

Congenital and developmental disorders are conceptually very similar to degenerative diseases, except that the deterioration begins early in life. In some cases, the affected element of the nervous system never develops at all. Like degenerative disease, developmental disorders are characteristically **chronic** and **diffuse**. They may be **progressive** or (unlike degenerative disease) they may be **static**.

Table 3-1 summarizes the way in which these diagnostic categories can be distinguished on the basis of focality and time course.

It is often helpful to distinguish between mass lesions and nonmass lesions. **Mass lesions** alter cellular function not only at the site of the lesion but also in the surrounding area, by compression or destruction of neighboring cells. **Nonmass lesions** alter cellular function at the site of the lesion but spare adjacent cells. Mass lesions cause **focal, progressive** symptoms. **Diffuse** processes, regardless of time course, are nonmass lesions; so are lesions that are focal but not **progressive**. It is clear from Table 3-1 that circumscribed hemorrhages, abscesses, and neoplasms are all mass lesions; all the other processes listed in the chart are nonmass lesions.

The categories listed in Table 3-1 easily generalize to multifocal conditions. Thus, an acute multifocal process that is static or improving is still most likely vascular (and probably embolic, in particular).

Table 3-1. Characteristic Spatial-Temporal Profiles of Major
Diagnostic Categories

	Acute: Static or Improving	Acute: Progressive	Subacute	Chronic
Focal	1. Vascular (ischemic)	1. Vascular (intra-parenchymal hemorrhage)	Inflammatory (abscess)	Neoplasm
	2. Traumatic (contusion, encephalomalacia)	2. Traumatic (intraparenchymal, subdural, or epidural hemorrhage)		
Diffuse	1. Toxic-metabolic (including anoxic)	1. Vascular (subarachnoid hemorrhage)	1. Inflammatory (meningitis, encephalitis)	1. Degenerative
	2. Traumatic (concussion)	2. Toxic-metabolic	2. Toxic-metabolic	2. Congenital-developmental
		3. Traumatic (subarachnoid hemorrhage)		3. Toxic-metabolic

Trauma can also produce multifocal lesions with this temporal profile, just as it can produce focal lesions. Acute, progressive multifocal lesions are rare, but the analogy with focal lesions still applies: This combination of focality and temporal course suggests multifocal hemorrhage, which in turn suggests a bleeding diathesis. Just as subacute focal processes are generally inflammatory, so are subacute multifocal processes. Multiple sclerosis is the most common specific diagnosis when the lesions are all in the central nervous system. Other diagnoses in this category include vasculitis and endocarditis. Finally, when symptoms are chronic, and multifocal rather than focal, neoplastic disease remains the prime diagnostic consideration. Specifically, a metastatic tumor is the most likely diagnosis in this setting.

This approach is less useful for transient symptoms, where the distinction between acute, subacute, and chronic symptoms becomes less meaningful. Moreover, the symptoms often resolve so quickly that it is impossible to distinguish between multifocal and diffuse lesions.

Even so, it is often possible to distinguish focal transient symptoms from diffuse transient symptoms, especially in patients with paroxysmal disorders, who have episodic recurrence of transient symptoms and over time may learn to identify and describe their symptoms in detail. The three most common causes of focal transient symptoms are seizures, transient ischemic attacks, and migraines. Diffuse transient symptoms are most often caused by transient hypoperfusion (e.g., a cardiac arrhythmia), but seizures and certain metabolic processes must also be considered (e.g., hepatic encephalopathy, hypoglycemia, and intoxication).

IV. Discussion of Case Histories

Case 1. The aphasia, right hemianopia, and right hemiparesis localize the lesion to the left cerebral cortex (if this is not clear, review Chapter 1). The lesion is therefore **focal**. It is also **progressive**, so it is a mass lesion. The time course is **chronic**, making a **neoplasm** most likely.

Comment: An appropriate summary note might read: "55-year-old woman with a 10-week history of progressive symptoms and neurologic findings suggestive of a left cortical mass lesion, likely neoplasm." In this case, magnetic resonance imaging and surgical biopsy confirmed the diagnosis of glioma. The patient was treated with radiation therapy and chemotherapy.

Case 2. Facial weakness ipsilateral to body weakness suggests a **focal** lesion in the high pons or above (see Speed Rule 6 in Chapter 1). There has been no progression, so this is not a mass lesion. The symptoms developed **acutely**. A focal lesion that developed acutely and is improving is usually an **ischemic vascular** lesion (unless there is a history of trauma).

Comment: A computed tomography (CT) scan demonstrated a small infarct in the right internal capsule. The patient had his antihypertensive medications adjusted and was started on aspirin.

Case 3. The altered level of consciousness indicates either a brainstem lesion or involvement of both cerebral hemispheres (see Speed Rule 11 in Chapter 1). The generalized seizures also are indicative of bihemispheric disease. All of the abnormal neurologic findings (e.g., hyperre-flexia and Babinski signs) are symmetric. Thus, the condition is **diffuse**. It follows that it is not a mass lesion. The symptoms developed over 2 days, making them **subacute**. A diffuse, subacute process could either be **toxic-metabolic** or **inflammatory** (meningitis or encephalitis). In this case, the fever and stiff neck make meningitis or encephalitis most likely.

Comment: The patient was started empirically on ceftriaxone and a lumbar puncture was performed immediately. Cerebrospinal fluid examination demonstrated greater than 200 white blood cells, pre-dominantly lymphocytic. Acyclovir was added, and when cerebrospi-nal fluid cultures remained negative at 48 hours, the ceftriaxone was stopped. The patient gradually recovered, and polymerase chain reac-tion testing of the spinal fluid eventually confirmed the diagnosis of herpes simplex encephalitis.

Case 4. The right facial numbness and left body numbness indicate a lesion on the right between the pons and the C2 level of the spinal cord (see Speed Rule 5 in Chapter 1). The left arm and leg weakness and stiffness further restrict the possible localization to the region between the pons and the low medulla (if this is not evident, draw the pathways). Finally, the tinnitus and hearing loss in the right ear local-ize the lesion further, to the right pons or pontomedullary junction. Such a precise unilateral localization implies a **focal** lesion. It is pro-gressive, so it is a mass lesion. The progression has taken place over several years, making it **chronic**. A focal, chronic lesion is a **neoplasm**.

Comment: In this case, the neoplasm was a schwannoma—a benign tumor. It was resected, and the patient continues to do well 15 years later.

Case 5. As with Case 2, the weakness of left face, arm, and leg imply a right-sided **focal** lesion at the level of the high pons or above. It is a mass lesion, because it is **progressive**. The time course is **chronic** (3 months). Again, a focal, chronic lesion signifies a **neoplasm**.

Comment: In this case, a CT scan demonstrated a right subdural hematoma (SDH). This shows how the rules are only approximations. Still, SDH represents a "new growth" that slowly expands, so for practical purposes it behaves like a benign tumor. The patient had the SDH evacuated, and he recovered fully.

Case 6. Even though no information about the physical examination is available, the likely lesion localization can be inferred from this patient's history alone. The abnormal sensory and motor function below a level in the mid-abdomen indicates a **focal** lesion in the spinal cord, at the thoracic level or above (see Speed Rule 3 in Chapter 1). Since the symptoms are **progressive**, this is a mass lesion. The time course is subacute. A focal, **subacute** lesion is typically **inflammatory**—specifically, an abscess.

Comment: An MRI scan of the cervical and thoracic spine failed to demonstrate an abscess, but a lumbar puncture revealed a pleocytosis in the spinal fluid. All cultures were negative. This patient was thought to have transverse myelitis, an inflammatory (possibly autoimmune) disorder that behaves like a mass lesion in the spinal cord. Her symptoms gradually resolved without treatment. This is another example of how the rules can fail. In this case, they pointed to the correct diagnostic category but the wrong specific diagnosis. As it happens, it is often impossible to distinguish between transverse myelitis and a spinal cord abscess on clinical grounds, so it is appropriate to direct the evaluation at the possibility of an abscess, which would require urgent treatment.

Case 7. This patient has personality changes and deficits in several different cognitive functions, including language comprehension, short-term and long-term memory, and calculations. This implies a **diffuse** cortical localization. Since it is diffuse, this is not a mass lesion. The deficits have progressed over several months, making this a **chronic** problem. A diffuse, chronic disorder can be a **degenerative** disease, a **congenital/developmental** problem, or a **toxic-metabolic** disorder. The patient is too old for a congenital or developmental disease, and there is nothing to suggest any specific metabolic abnormality, so a degenerative disease is most likely.

Comment: Even though a degenerative disease is the most likely diagnosis, potential toxic-metabolic causes should be investigated. In fact, neoplasms can sometimes break the rules and produce a diffuse picture rather than focal. This patient had a head CT scan and a number of blood and urine tests to investigate these possibilities. All of the tests were normal, and her subsequent course was consistent with Alzheimer's disease.

Case 8. This case is similar to Case 3, except that the time course is acute rather than subacute. The lesion is **diffuse** (and therefore not a mass lesion), and it is **progressive**: This means it is either **vascular** (specifically, subarachnoid hemorrhage), **toxic-metabolic**, or **traumatic**. There is no history of trauma and no reason to suspect a toxic-metabolic disorder, so subarachnoid hemorrhage is the most likely diagnosis.

Comment: A head CT scan was normal, but a lumbar puncture revealed subarachnoid hemorrhage. A cerebral angiogram demonstrated a large aneurysm of the anterior communicating artery. The aneurysm was successfully clipped, and the patient has returned to her baseline level of function.

Case 9. The reduced pinprick sensation over the left face and right body imply a **focal** lesion on the left, between the pons and the C2 level of the spinal cord (see Speed Rule 5 in Chapter 1). The weakness of the left palate confines the lesion to the medulla, because only lower motor neuron lesions produce unilateral palatal weakness (see Chapter 2). Ataxia of the left arm and leg is also consistent with a lesion in this location, because a lesion in the medulla can disrupt cerebellar connections. The symptoms began **acutely**, but they have not progressed, so this is not a mass lesion. A focal, acute lesion with a static time course implies either a **vascular (ischemic)** or a **traumatic** etiology, and there is no history of trauma in this case.

Comment: This patient had a normal head CT scan, but MRI revealed a small infarction in the left lateral medulla. In the emergency room, she was found to have atrial fibrillation, which had never been noted before. The stroke was presumed to be embolic, so anticoagulant therapy was begun. Further evaluation revealed hyperthyroidism. She was converted to normal sinus rhythm, her hyperthyroidism was treated, and after 6 months the anticoagulation was stopped. By that time, her symptoms had completely resolved except for minimal ataxia of the left arm.

Case 10. This patient has symptoms confined to the distribution of a single nerve root. This makes a lesion in the nerve root itself most likely, but theoretically the lesion could be anywhere from the level of the nerve root on up the sensory pathway to the cortex. Additional symptoms would be expected with any of these higher localizations, however. In any case, the lesion is **focal**. It is not progressive, so it is not a mass lesion. The time course is **subacute**, so the process is probably **inflammatory**, and specifically, an abscess.

Comment: This is another situation in which the rules indicate the correct diagnostic category (inflammatory) but the wrong specific diagnosis. In this case, epidemiologic factors are important. A rash in a dermatomal distribution is very suggestive of Herpes zoster reactivation, which can produce sensory symptoms (especially pain) in the same distribution. This occurs particularly often in immunocompromised individuals, including those receiving chemotherapy for cancer. The patient received famciclovir and pain treatment, and the symptoms gradually resolved.

Case 11. In addition to chest wall symptoms like those described by the patient in Case 10, this patient has left leg weakness, which could not be explained by a lesion in a thoracic nerve root. Instead, the most plausible localization is within the thoracic spinal cord on the left, in the one or two segments where the spinothalamic pathway has not yet crossed to the right side of the cord. This is a **focal** lesion, and since it is progressive, it is a mass lesion. The time course is **chronic**. A chronic focal lesion is a **neoplasm**.

Comment: An MRI scan revealed a meningioma compressing the left T4 nerve root and the spinal cord at that level. This benign tumor was resected, and the patient's only residual symptom was mild stiffness of the left leg.

II

Common Diseases

4

Stroke

Douglas J. Gelb and Marc I. Chimowitz

I. Case Histories

Case 1. A 65-year-old man drove himself to the emergency room at 9 AM after experiencing a 4-minute episode of word-finding difficulty and right hand weakness. He had experienced four similar episodes in the last 3 weeks. He had undergone coronary bypass surgery for unstable angina a year ago, and he had a long history of hypertension and diabetes. He was taking aspirin, propranolol, and glyburide daily. He was afebrile, his blood pressure was 140/80, his pulse was 85 per minute and regular, and a left carotid bruit could be heard in systole and diastole. There were no murmurs and his neurologic examination was normal.

Case 2. A 59-year-old woman came to the emergency room at her family's insistence at 9 PM after she mentioned that she had been having trouble seeing out of the left eye since awakening that morning. She had been in good health except for long-standing hypertension and occasional "rapid heart beats." She denied previous visual symptoms or other episodic neurologic symptoms. She was taking nifedipine. The patient was alert, her blood pressure was 170/95, her pulse was 130 per minute and irregular, and there were no murmurs or bruits. The only abnormality on neurologic exam was a left homonymous hemianopia.

Case 3. A 73-year-old man was brought to the emergency room by paramedics after he fell down on the way back from the bathroom and discovered that he could not move his left side. His symptoms had not progressed in the 90 minutes that had elapsed since the initial event. He had been hypertensive for 20 years and was taking hydrochlorothiazide, and he had been taking lovastatin for a year because of hyperlipidemia. He denied previous episodes of focal neurologic symptoms. He was alert, with a blood pressure of 180/100 and a pulse that was 80 per minute and regular. There were no bruits or murmurs. Neurologic exam showed awareness of his neurologic deficit; slurred speech; left hemiparesis involving face, arm, and leg; left-sided hyperreflexia; a left extensor plantar response (Babinski sign); and normal sensation.

Questions:

1. What are the causes of these patients' symptoms?

2. How would you manage these patients in the emergency room?

3. Would you admit these patients to the hospital?

4. What tests would you order?

5. What treatment would you initiate?

II. Background Information

A. *Definitions*

stroke: A focal neurologic deficit of sudden onset caused by central nervous system ischemia (80%) or hemorrhage (20%).

transient ischemic attack (TIA):   A focal neurologic deficit of sudden onset caused by transient ischemia and resolving within 24 hours. The vast majority of TIAs last less than 15 minutes.

B. *Pathophysiology*

Ischemic stroke occurs when the brain is deprived of glucose and oxygen because of inadequate cerebral blood flow. The severity of injury is a function of how much the blood flow has been reduced and for how long. In the center of a region of focal ischemia, blood flow is typically less than 20–30% of normal. If this degree of ischemia persists for more than an hour, complete necrosis of all tissue elements occurs. This maximally affected zone is surrounded by a region known as the ischemic penumbra where the blood flow reduction is less profound and the tissue damage is reversible for a longer time. A variety of factors mediate the damage that occurs during this interval, including increased tissue lactate, hydrogen ions, and inorganic phosphate concentrations because of reversion to anaerobic glycolysis; release of excitatory amino acids into the extracellular space; increased calcium influx into cells; increased extracellular potassium; release of arachidonic acid and its metabolites due to increased lipolysis; free radical production; and possibly specific derangements of genomic expression ("programmed cell death"). Many of these same biochemical processes mediate cellular injury in hemorrhagic stroke.

C. Classification of Strokes by Etiology

Cerebral ischemia may be global, as in the case of cardiac arrest, or focal, as a result of cerebrovascular occlusive disease. Cerebrovascular occlusive disease is a heterogeneous disorder. Many vascular pathologies, each with a distinct natural history, may cause focal ischemic stroke. Common examples of these include thromboembolism from atherosclerotic lesions in large extracranial or intracranial arteries, embolism from a variety of cardiac sources, and atherosclerosis or lipohyalinosis of small arteries that penetrate the brain substance. Lipohyalinosis is a vasculopathy that occurs in patients with hypertension. Occlusion of a single penetrating artery to the brain results in a small (less than 1.5 cm) subcortical infarct, often called a lacune.

Less common causes of ischemic stroke include carotid or vertebral artery dissection, arteritis, fibromuscular dysplasia, migraine, antiphospholipid antibody syndrome, procoagulant states, and sickle cell disease.

Hemorrhage into the subarachnoid space usually occurs after rupture of a berry aneurysm (a congenital aneurysm that is typically located on a major artery in the circle of Willis), whereas hemorrhage into the parenchyma of the brain usually results from the bursting of small aneurysmal dilatations of penetrating arteries in the brain, which are often caused by hypertension. An arteriovenous malformation can hemorrhage into the subarachnoid space or into the brain parenchyma.

III. Approach to Stroke

Three questions are fundamental in managing a patient who has had a stroke (listed in order of decreasing urgency):

1. What can be done to reverse the damage?

2. What can be done to limit the damage?

3. What can be done to prevent the patient from having another stroke in the future?

Question 3 has two components. They apply not only to patients who have had a stroke, but to all individuals at risk for stroke.

3a. **Secondary prevention:** How can strokes be prevented in patients with established cerebrovascular disease?

3b. **Primary prevention:** How can vascular disease itself be prevented or at least minimized?

Questions 1 and 2 are addressed in Part IV. Question 3a is discussed in Part V and Question 3b in Part VI.

IV. Management of Acute Stroke

A. Reversal of Deficits

Patients who receive recombinant tissue plasminogen activator (rt-PA) intravenously within 3 hours of the onset of ischemic stroke symptoms are 30–50% more likely than untreated patients to have minimal or no neurologic deficit 3 months later. Although rt-PA treatment also increases the likelihood of intracerebral hemorrhage in the first 36 hours, the beneficial effect of the treatment outweighs the risk.

Unfortunately, it is often difficult to evaluate and treat patients within 3 hours of symptom onset. Unlike patients with myocardial ischemia, whose pain often convinces them of the urgency of their condition, patients with cerebral ischemia may misinterpret or minimize their symptoms. In some cases, the time of symptom onset is unknown. For example, patients whose symptoms are first noticed on awakening could have suffered their stroke at any time during their sleep. They are only eligible to receive rt-PA if they were awake and asymptomatic at some point in the preceding 3 hours. Even when patients receive medical attention quickly, their evaluation (including a CT scan to be sure there is no intracerebral hemorrhage or prominent edema) must be rapid and efficient if they are to receive treatment within the required time frame.

It may eventually be possible to extend the time window during which reperfusion therapy is beneficial, either by modifying the treatment protocol or by using other agents. For example, preliminary results indicate that intra-arterial administration of prourokinase directly into an intracranial thrombus may be beneficial if treatment is begun within 6 hours of symptom onset. Even so, there are limits to the results that can be expected with reperfusion therapy. Many of the biochemical processes that mediate cell injury in the ischemic penumbra continue even after adequate blood flow is restored, so therapy directed at counteracting free radical formation, excitatory amino acid release, transmembrane ion shifts, or programmed cell death may be critical for the preservation of brain function. This is currently the subject of intense study, but every agent tried so far has been disappointing.

Aspirin provides a small but statistically significant benefit in the treatment of acute stroke. Promising results have also been reported with a novel antiplatelet agent (abciximab), a defibrinogenating agent (ancrod), and low-molecular-weight (heparin), but all of these agents require further study.

B. *Limitation of Deficits*

Even though the neuronal injury that results from a stroke cannot yet be treated successfully, factors that exacerbate the damage can be addressed. Both neurologic and systemic complications must be considered.

1. Neurologic complications

The most important neurologic complication of acute stroke is increased intracranial pressure. Strokes produce significant edema, which may result in mass effect on the brainstem, affecting level of consciousness and autonomic functions. There is debate about whether the typical measures used to treat increased intracranial pressure (see Chapter 11) are effective in the setting of ischemic stroke, but they may be lifesaving in the setting of hemorrhagic stroke. In addition, some clinicians advocate evacuation of the blood clot in patients with hemorrhagic stroke, at least in certain circumstances. This approach is most widely accepted in the setting of a large parenchymal hemorrhage in the cerebellum, because swelling in this location can rapidly compress the brainstem and impair life-sustaining autonomic functions. There is much less acceptance of this approach for hemorrhage in other locations, but no carefully controlled clinical trials have addressed this issue. Hemicraniectomy has been used as a last resort to relieve severely increased intracranial pressure in patients with large ischemic strokes in the nondominant hemisphere. A study of this treatment is in progress.

Infarcted or hemorrhagic brain regions may serve as seizure foci. Seizures may even be the presenting symptom of infarction or hemorrhage on rare occasions. Seizures produce a transient rise in intracranial pressure, and this can be particularly dangerous in stroke patients who already have increased intracranial pressure due to edema. Status epilepticus is even more ominous in that regard and requires urgent treatment (see Chapter 5).

Any patient with an intracranial lesion is at risk for syndrome of inappropriate secretion of antidiuretic hormone. Hyponatremia may in turn produce further neuronal injury, either directly or by provoking seizure activity. Serum sodium should be measured regularly, and appropriate testing and treatment undertaken if hyponatremia develops.

Patients who have suffered strokes (especially left hemisphere strokes) develop depression at a rate higher than would be predicted simply on the basis of a situational response to their deficits. It appears that depression may be a direct manifestation of injury to particular regions of the brain. When severe, the depression may significantly impede clinical recovery from a stroke. Some studies indicate that these patients respond to antidepressant medications, while others fail to observe a reliable response to any of the usual treatments for depression.

2. Systemic factors

Hypoxia, hypotension, hyperthermia, and hyperglycemia may all exacerbate the neuronal injury that results from stroke. Patients should be monitored closely for the development of any of these conditions and treated appropriately if they occur. Stroke patients often have impairment of their airway protection mechanisms and may need elective intubation to limit aspiration.

Patients who are rendered nonambulatory by a stroke should be treated prophylactically to prevent deep venous thrombosis. They should also receive vigorous skin care to prevent skin breakdown and decubitus ulcers.

C. Rehabilitation

Patients should be trained to maximize their function based on their current abilities. Speech pathologists can teach patients strategies to improve communication skills. They can also evaluate the ability of patients to swallow and suggest interventions to reduce the risk of aspiration. Physical therapists can teach patients exercises designed to increase range of motion and prevent contractures in weak muscles, as well as exercises to strengthen both the affected muscles and the unaffected muscles that may be required to compensate for the weak muscles. Occupational therapists can determine whether patients might benefit from facilitative or prosthetic devices.

V. Secondary Prevention

Patients who have had TIAs or strokes are at risk for additional strokes, with potentially devastating consequences. A major focus in managing patients with established cerebrovascular disease is the identification of the site (or sites) of pathology so that appropriate preventive therapy can be provided.

A. Diagnosis

It is not always possible to find the source of a patient's stroke. In some cases, no cerebrovascular abnormalities or risk factors are found; in other cases, there are several possible sources, all equally plausible. Even so, the likely source can often be identified based on clinical features and the results of diagnostic tests.

1. Nature of neurologic deficit

Some neurologic signs or syndromes may exclude certain causes of stroke from the differential diagnosis. For example, a cerebellar stroke could not be caused by carotid stenosis, since the cerebellum is supplied by the posterior circulation. As another example, penetrating artery disease rarely produces hemianopia, aphasia, or apraxia. Other signs increase the likelihood of a specific cause of stroke. Wernicke's aphasia, for example, most often results from an embolus from the heart or a proximal large artery; the same is true of alexia without agraphia and "top of the basilar" syndrome. In contrast, pure sensory stroke is usually caused by penetrating artery disease. While there are exceptions to many of these rules, they serve as useful guidelines.

2. Transient ischemic attacks

If untreated, a large proportion of patients with TIAs subsequently have strokes. If the cause of the TIAs can be determined and effective secondary prevention instituted, the patient may be protected from experiencing any permanent neurologic deficit. Thus, a TIA should be evaluated aggressively. It provides the patient and physician with an urgent warning, and a brief opportunity to act on it. Most of the major etiologic subtypes of cerebrovascular occlusive disease may cause TIAs, but the characteristics of the TIAs differ depending on the etiology.

Approximately 50–75% of patients who have stroke because of carotid occlusive disease have preceding TIAs. These usually consist of recurrent, brief (typically less than 10 minutes) episodes of ipsilateral transient monocular blindness, contralateral hand and face weakness, or disturbed speech. The TIAs frequently recur over a period of weeks to months.

In patients with cardioembolic stroke, TIAs preceding the infarction are rare, and they usually last longer than 1 hour. Approximately 20–30% of patients who have stroke because of penetrating artery disease have preceding TIAs, often occurring in a flurry within a week of the stroke.

3. Temporal profile of neurologic deficit

The hallmark of an embolic mechanism (cardiac or artery-to-artery) is maximal neurologic deficit at onset. Approximately 80% of patients with cardioembolic stroke have a maximal deficit at onset, whereas 38–45% of patients with large-artery disease or penetrating artery disease have a maximal deficit at onset. Other temporal profiles are more common with large- or small-artery occlusive disease and rarely are associated with embolism. These include a stuttering or stepwise course, a smoothly progressive course, or a fluctuating course.

4. Specific risk factors

Although hypertension, diabetes, smoking, and hyperlipidemia are established risk factors for large-artery atherosclerotic cerebrovascular disease, they are also direct risk factors for penetrating artery disease and indirect risk factors for cardioembolic stroke. For example, patients with one or more of these conditions are at increased risk for myocardial infarction, which in turn is a relatively common cause of cardioembolic stroke. It is certainly important to evaluate patients for these risk factors and to treat any risk factors found (see Part VI), but they are not very useful in identifying the specific cause of a patient's stroke.

Patients with mitral stenosis, a prosthetic heart valve, or atrial fibrillation are predisposed to cardioembolic stroke. Thorough evaluation is necessary, however, because these patients sometimes have other potential sources of stroke as well. For example, the frequency of greater than 50% carotid stenosis is significantly higher in patients with nonvalvular atrial fibrillation than in patients without nonvalvular atrial fibrillation who are matched for age and other vascular risk factors.

In patients with few risk factors for atherosclerosis, penetrating artery disease, or cardioembolic disease, less common alternative causes of stroke should be considered. This is particularly relevant in young patients who have had strokes. Such patients should be carefully evaluated for coagulopathy, hematologic disorders, arterial dissection, connective tissue diseases, and particular infections (especially syphilis).

5. Associated features (bruits and headaches)

A carotid bruit provides useful evidence that a patient may have carotid occlusive disease. This may or may not be related to the patient's symptoms. For example, carotid stenosis should be considered asymptomatic if the patient's deficits have all been most consistent with ischemia in a different vascular territory or penetrating artery disease. Just as presence of a bruit does not prove that a patient's symptoms are due to carotid disease, absence of a bruit does not exclude this possibility. A carotid bruit may be absent because of low flow through a tight stenosis (or because the artery has become completely occluded).

Headache is a relatively common accompaniment of stroke caused by atherosclerotic large artery occlusive disease, nonatherosclerotic large-artery disease (e.g., dissection), cardioembolism, and hemorrhage, but headache is uncommon in patients with stroke caused by penetrating artery disease.

6. Computed tomography or magnetic resonance imaging features

Ischemic strokes are usually not evident on standard CT or MRI scans until 24 to 48 hours after the event and sometimes only appear after 1 week or more. Diffusion-weighted MRI permits detection of ischemic stroke within minutes of the event, but it is generally not necessary to make decisions regarding secondary prevention quite so urgently. In the acute setting, the most important question is not what kind of stroke the patient had, but whether the patient had a stroke at all. This question can usually be answered clinically, and the main role of imaging studies is to eliminate mass lesions (primarily hemorrhage, but occasionally tumor or abscess) that can mimic stroke. A standard CT scan is generally adequate for this. More advanced imaging techniques may eventually be helpful in determining which patients are most likely to respond to reperfusion therapy or other acute interventions, but such applications are purely investigational at this point.

With regard to determination of the source of a stroke, imaging studies may supplement clinical inferences. For example, if the stroke is visualized by CT or MRI in an area supplied by the posterior circulation, carotid occlusive disease is clearly not the cause. As another example, penetrating artery disease does not produce a lesion larger than 2 cm in diameter, whereas a subcortical lesion less than 1.5 cm is highly predictive of penetrating artery disease (though there is debate about this latter point). Infarcts caused by penetrating artery disease tend to be round or oval shaped, whereas infarcts caused by large-artery disease or cardioembolism tend to have more irregular shapes and margins.

Comma-shaped lesions, 2–5 cm in size, involving the internal capsule and caudate, putamen or globus pallidus are called striatocapsular infarcts. These lesions are usually caused by occlusive disease of, or an embolism to, the middle cerebral artery proximal to or at the origins of the lateral lenticulostriate arteries.

Wedge-shaped cortical infarcts, particularly in the distribution of the middle cerebral artery, are usually caused by an embolic mechanism (either cardioembolism or artery-to-artery embolism), whereas irregular, patchy infarcts in the border zones between the territories of the middle cerebral artery and the anterior cerebral artery or posterior cerebral artery are typically caused by low flow from carotid occlusive disease or global hypoperfusion.

Multiple cortical infarcts in different vascular territories are most suggestive of cardio-embolism. Rarer causes of multiple infarcts are diffuse atherosclerosis, coagulopathy, or vasculitis.

Cardioembolism is associated with hemorrhagic infarction on CT in up to 40% of cases, which is substantially higher than the rates of hemorrhagic infarction associated with other causes of ischemic stroke. The probable explanation for the high rate of hemorrhagic infarction associated with cardioembolism is that reperfusion after spontaneous lysis of the embolus leads to bleeding from vessels injured by the preceding ischemia.

7. Cardiac and vascular imaging

Although the clinical and imaging features described above may provide compelling evidence for a specific cause of stroke, the carotid arteries and heart must still be imaged directly. Echocardiography enables identification of cardiac lesions predisposing to embolism. These include mitral stenosis, left ventricular aneurysm or dyskinesia, atrial or ventricular clot, valvular vegetations, and interatrial shunts.

Transesophageal echocardiography is a more sensitive and specific test for many of these lesions than conventional transthoracic echocardiography, and it has been shown to be more cost-effective.

Intra-arterial angiography is still the gold standard for imaging extracranial and intracranial arteries, although the resolution of magnetic resonance angiography is steadily improving. Duplex carotid ultrasound is a useful screening test for detecting carotid occlusive disease (sensitivity = 85%, specificity = 90%). Normal carotid ultrasound results are usually reliable and may eliminate the need for more invasive vascular studies in some patients. Patients with abnormal carotid ultrasound results usually need cerebral angiography, however, because ultrasound estimates of the magnitude of stenosis are sometimes inaccurate, and more detailed definition of the cerebral vascular anatomy may be needed if endarterectomy is a consideration.

The development of transcranial Doppler ultrasound has enabled measurement of blood flow velocities in all the major cerebral arteries. This technique has a variety of clinical applications including detection of intracranial arterial stenoses, arteriovenous malformations, and vasospasm after subarachnoid hemorrhage.

Positron emission tomography, single photon emission computed tomography, and functional MRI techniques (diffusion-weighted imaging, perfusion imaging, magnetic resonance spectroscopy, and activation studies) enable measurement of cerebral blood flow and metabolism, but the clinical utility of these techniques for evaluating patients with stroke remains to be determined.

B. Treatment

1. Antiplatelet medications: general comments

In addition to therapy directed at the specific cause of stroke, patients with cerebrovascular disease are generally treated with medications intended to reduce the risk of subsequent thromboembolism. Unless there is a compelling reason for the patient to take warfarin, antiplatelet agents are typically used for this purpose. Aspirin, ticlopidine, clopidogrel, and dipyridamole are the antiplatelet medications currently available.

Aspirin is the antiplatelet agent that has been used most extensively. Studies have shown that aspirin reduces the risk of stroke and cardiovascular disease in patients presenting with TIAs or minor stroke. Unfortunately, these studies failed to characterize the patients' underlying vascular pathology with precision, so the specific situations in which aspirin might provide particular benefit are unknown. The ideal dose also remains unknown. Laboratory research has suggested that doses on the order of 30 mg per day should be adequate to block the thromboxane pathway, as desired, whereas higher doses also block the prostacyclin pathway, which may partially negate the beneficial effect. The dose of aspirin used in many of the large clinical stroke trials, however, was 1,300 mg per day. This dose of aspirin reduces the risk of stroke by about 22% compared with placebo. A few studies have shown that aspirin is also effective for preventing stroke at doses of 50 mg per day or less. Although meta-analyses suggest that high and low doses of aspirin are equally effective in preventing stroke, there has never been a definitive study comparing the two regimens. Many clinicians opt for a convenient compromise dose of 325 mg per day, which has the advantage of being relatively well-tolerated by patients. Enteric-coated preparations should be used to lower the risk of gastrointestinal side effects.

Ticlopidine, which inhibits platelet aggregation by blocking the binding of adenosine diphosphate to its receptor on platelets, was shown to be slightly more effective than aspirin in reducing stroke risk in patients with TIA or minor stroke, but ticlopidine is expensive and can be associated with severe neutropenia. Clopidogrel is a chemically related drug that also blocks adenosine diphosphate–induced platelet aggregation. In one study comparing clopidogrel to aspirin, patients who were treated with clopidogrel had a lower combined risk of ischemic stroke, heart attack, or vascular death than did patients treated with aspirin. The difference was statistically significant, but small, and the largest benefit occurred in patients whose primary problem was peripheral vascular disease. For cerebrovascular disease per se, it is still not known whether clopidogrel is more or less effective than aspirin. Clopidogrel is nearly as expensive as ticlopidine but has not been associated with neutropenia.

Possible mechanisms by which dipyridamole inhibits platelet function include inhibition of phosphodiesterase in platelets or inhibition of red blood cell uptake of adenosine (which suppresses platelet reactivity). Early studies of dipyridamole in cerebrovascular disease revealed no benefit relative to placebo, and the combination of dipyridamole with aspirin was no more effective than aspirin alone. In a study that included many more patients than previous studies and that used a higher daily dose in a slow-release preparation, the opposite results were found: the use of either aspirin or dipyridamole alone produced a statistically significant reduction in the risk of stroke or death, and the combination of aspirin and dipyridamole was more effective than either drug alone.

In short, there are several antiplatelet agents that can be used for secondary prevention of stroke, and the optimal regimen has not been established. Many clinicians use aspirin as the initial agent because of its overall safety and well-established efficacy for vascular disease in general. For patients who continue to have symptoms despite aspirin therapy, one of the other agents is often prescribed. Although there have been no studies directly comparing the efficacy of clopidogrel and ticlopidine, the similar chemical structure of the two drugs and favorable side-effect profile of clopidogrel favor its use. Combination therapy (e.g., with aspirin and clopidogrel) is another option, either as initial treatment or as a treatment for patients who remain symptomatic despite treatment with individual drugs, but further studies are necessary to clarify the safety and efficacy of this approach.

2. Carotid stenosis

Patients who have had a TIA or stroke in the distribution of a carotid artery with a **high-grade stenosis** (70–99%) have a very high risk of recurrence: 26% of such patients will have another stroke on the same side within 2 years, even if they receive appropriate medical therapy. Carotid endarterectomy, in which the plaque is removed surgically, reduces this risk to 9% over 2 years.

In patients with only **moderate stenosis** (50–69%), endarterectomy also reduces the risk of subsequent stroke, but the magnitude of the benefit is much smaller: 22% of patients treated medically will have another stroke on the same side within 5 years, compared to 16% of patients treated with endarterectomy. This is an absolute risk reduction of 6% over 5 years, or 1.2% per year, which is low enough that individual circumstances must be considered carefully in deciding whether to recommend the surgery. For example, these statistics come from a study that was done at centers selected for their high level of expertise, where the risk of disabling stroke or death from the endarterectomy was 2%. In centers with less experience, a higher complication rate could easily negate the small benefit of surgery. Similarly, patients with multiple medical problems may have a greater than average risk of surgical complications that would outweigh the benefit of the procedure. Such considerations are much less important for patients with high-grade stenosis, because endarterectomy results in an absolute risk reduction for ipsilateral stroke that is much more robust (17% over 2 years or 8.5% per year). For patients with less than 50% stenosis, endarterectomy does not provide a significant benefit.

There is some debate about the appropriate time for performing endarterectomy after a stroke. The blood vessels in an area of ischemic brain are fragile and have an increased propensity to hemorrhage. A sudden surge of blood at high pressure after an endarterectomy might exacerbate this risk. For this reason, some physicians delay endarterectomy until at least 6 weeks after a stroke (yet this is a period when the risk of recurrence is high). In general, it appears that except for especially large strokes, the benefit of early endarterectomy exceeds the risk of hemorrhagic conversion of an ischemic stroke.

The statistics for patients with **asymptomatic high-grade** carotid stenosis (i.e., patients who have never experienced symptoms in the distribution of the stenotic artery) closely resemble the results for patients with moderate symptomatic stenosis: endarterectomy provides a statistically significant benefit, but the magnitude of benefit is small. With medical management, 11% of patients with greater than 60% carotid stenosis will experience an ipsilateral stroke or die within 5 years, compared to 5% of patients who receive an endarterectomy. This is an absolute risk reduction of 6% over 5 years, or 1.2% per year, a benefit that could easily be negated in circumstances in which the surgical morbidity is less than ideal.

There is no consensus regarding the correct management of patients with symptomatic, high-grade stenosis in whom endarterectomy is not an option (such as patients who are poor surgical risks because of severe chronic obstructive pulmonary disease or heart disease). Promising results have been reported with endovascular techniques, namely carotid angioplasty with or without stent placement, but until large, controlled trials establish a benefit, these procedures remain experimental.

Regardless of whether an endarterectomy is performed, all patients with symptomatic or asymptomatic carotid disease should receive antiplatelet therapy. Aspirin is typically used. For patients who have had an endarterectomy, one study found aspirin doses of 325 mg per day or less to be more effective than doses of 650 mg per day or more.

3. Cardioembolic disease

Chronic anticoagulation with warfarin is generally accepted as the most effective treatment for prevention of stroke in a patient with a cardiac source of emboli. This finding has been most convincingly demonstrated in the setting of chronic atrial fibrillation, where randomized, controlled, prospective studies have been conducted. There is also evidence supporting the use of warfarin in patients with artificial heart valves and in patients who have recently experienced myocardial infarctions. There is less information available about anticoagulation for other kinds of cardioembolic disease, but it is still commonly used, primarily on the basis of analogy and anecdotal evidence. Bacterial endocarditis (in a patient without an artificial heart valve) is the one cardioembolic condition for which anticoagulation is generally considered to be contraindicated, because of a high risk of cerebral hemorrhage (see Chapter 10).

Anticoagulation should be maintained as long as the cardioembolic source remains; for many patients this means life-long anticoagulation. These patients need to be monitored regularly to maintain the correct degree of anticoagulation. An INR in the range of 2.0–3.0 is the usual goal, although a target range of 2.5–4.0 is standard for patients with mechanical heart valves.

In patients who have just had a stroke, some clinicians advocate a delay of hours, days, or even weeks before initiating anticoagulation with heparin because the propensity for hemorrhagic transformation is particularly high after cardioembolic strokes. The increased risk from acute anticoagulation appears to be low, however, except when patients are overanticoagulated, which most often occurs when patients receive a bolus of heparin to initiate therapy. Given the lack of consensus on the proper time to begin therapy and the possibility that an initial bolus may increase the risk of hemorrhage, immediate heparinization should be initiated only in patients with a clear embolic source; no bolus should be given and the dose should be titrated upward gradually.

Patients with cardioembolic disease who cannot take warfarin (e.g., patients who fall frequently because of disequilibrium) are usually treated with aspirin, which has been shown to reduce the risk of stroke relative to placebo in patients with atrial fibrillation. It is less effective than warfarin but produces fewer bleeding complications. The role of other antiplatelet agents in this setting is unknown.

It is difficult to interpret the finding of a patent foramen ovale (PFO) in a patient with a TIA or stroke. On the one hand, a PFO can be demonstrated on surface echocardiography in 10–18% of normal adults, suggesting that most patients with PFO are asymptomatic. On the other hand, the incidence of PFO is higher in patients with stroke than in the general population, especially in patients with stroke and no other identifiable cause. It remains to be determined whether such patients should be treated with chronic anticoagulation, antiplatelet agents, cardiac surgery, or percutaneous transcatheter closure of the PFO.

4. Occlusive disease of large intracranial arteries

The large intracranial arteries (such as the carotid siphon, middle cerebral artery, and basilar artery) are not accessible for endarterectomy. Endovascular procedures, especially angioplasty with or without stenting, are a promising alternative, but they remain investigational, as discussed earlier. At one time, extracranial-intracranial bypass surgery was popular for intracranial disease in the anterior circulation, but a large, prospective, randomized study showed no difference between patients treated with bypass surgery plus aspirin and patients treated with aspirin alone. Bypass surgery has also been performed on the extracranial vertebral arteries, but the efficacy of this procedure has never been studied in a controlled way. As a result, bypass surgery is rarely considered in patients with occlusive disease of the large intracranial arteries, and secondary preventive therapy is usually limited to pharmacologic measures. Unfortunately, there are no prospective data on the effectiveness of any of the available agents (warfarin or the antiplatelet medications—aspirin, ticlopidine, clopidogrel, or dipyridamole) in patients with angiographically proven intracranial disease. There is retrospective evidence that warfarin may be beneficial for patients with more than 50% stenosis of a major intracranial artery; a prospective study comparing warfarin to aspirin in this setting is in progress. Some physicians currently use warfarin to treat these patients, whereas others use aspirin first, changing to clopidogrel if patients continue to have TIAs or strokes despite aspirin, and changing to warfarin if symptoms persist despite clopidogrel.

5. Penetrating artery disease

As with disease of the large intracranial vessels, there is no surgical option in patients with occlusive disease of the penetrating arteries. Endovascular techniques are not feasible either. The same pharmacologic options exist, and again, their efficacy remains unproved. There is no reason to presume that the optimal treatment for intracranial large vessel disease (e.g., atherosclerosis of the middle cerebral artery) will be the same as the optimal treatment for penetrating artery disease, but the issue has not been adequately studied. Because there is no compelling reason to choose one medication over another in the setting of penetrating artery disease, most clinicians treat these patients with aspirin, primarily because of its safety. Patients who have recurrent symptoms despite aspirin are often switched to one of the other agents.

6. Uncommon causes of ischemic stroke

For other causes of stroke, such as coagulopathies, hematologic disorders, vasculitis, or neurosyphilis, treatment is aimed at the underlying disorder. For example, patients with polycythemia vera are typically treated with phlebotomy and hemodilution; patients with lupus are treated with steroids or cytotoxic agents. With modern imaging techniques, arterial dissection is being recognized with increasing frequency. This is most common in the setting of neck trauma or chiropractic manipulation, but the trauma may be surprisingly mild (such as an abrupt neck movement), and there is often no history of trauma at all. The optimal management approach has not been established, but these patients are often anticoagulated for 3–6 months to allow time for thrombotic material to organize and be recanalized.

Atherosclerotic disease of the aortic arch is also increasingly recognized as a cause of stroke. Although optimal treatment is unknown, anticoagulation is commonly used rather than antiplatelet agents in patients with large plaques in the aorta, particularly if they are mobile.

Patients with significantly elevated titers of antiphospholipid antibodies are commonly treated with warfarin, but the only evidence to support this practice is retrospective. Warfarin is also typically used to treat patients with other hypercoagulable states, including protein C deficiency, protein S deficiency, and antithrombin 3 deficiency.

7. Cerebral hemorrhage

The diagnostic and therapeutic approach to patients with subarachnoid hemorrhage is discussed in Chapter 12. The principal means of avoiding recurrent subarachnoid hemorrhage from an aneurysm is to clip the aneurysm, although coils are sometimes used to promote thrombosis. Techniques aimed at reducing the risk of recurrent hemorrhage from an arteriovenous malformation include resection, embolization, and radiation. In patients with hypertension-related intraparenchymal hemorrhage, blood pressure control is the key to reducing the risk of recurrent hemorrhagic events.

VI. Primary Prevention

Primary prevention is directed toward the early recognition and treatment of risk factors that predispose to the development of vascular disease and cardiac disease. These risk factors include hypertension, diabetes, smoking, and hyperlipidemia. There is convincing evidence that control of mild as well as severe hypertension substantially reduces the risk of stroke. The use of HMGcoA reductase inhibitors to reduce cholesterol also results in a decreased incidence of stroke. In fact, in patients who have had a prior heart attack, this beneficial effect occurs even if the total cholesterol and low-density lipoprotein cholesterol levels are in the normal range. There is also strong evidence that cessation of smoking lowers the risk of ischemic stroke. Although there is no convincing evidence that stroke risk can be reduced by rigorous control of blood glucose in diabetics, intensive therapy has been shown to delay the onset and slow the progression of other complications of the disease. An elevated homocysteine level is a risk factor for premature atherosclerosis. Folic acid supplementation can lower homocysteine levels, and studies are in progress to evaluate whether this treatment helps to prevent stroke and other vascular events.

VII. Discussion of Case Histories

Case 1. A 65-year-old man drove himself to the emergency room at 9 AM after experiencing a 4-minute episode of word-finding difficulty and right-hand weakness. He had experienced four similar episodes in the last 3 weeks. He had undergone coronary bypass surgery for unstable angina a year ago, and he had a long history of hypertension and diabetes. He was taking aspirin, propranolol, and glyburide daily.

Comment: Episodic focal neurologic symptoms can be vascular, epileptic, psychogenic, metabolic, or migrainous in origin. In a 65-year-old "vasculopath," however, these spells most likely represent TIAs. Furthermore, the characteristics of the spells (occurring over 3 weeks, brief episodes, stereotypical nature with involvement of language and right hand) suggest large-artery occlusive disease as the cause.

He was afebrile, his blood pressure was 140/80, his pulse was 85 per minute and regular, and a left carotid bruit could be heard in systole and diastole. There were no murmurs and his neurologic examination was normal.

Comment: The bruit is on the side appropriate to his symptoms and the diastolic component suggests a high-grade stenosis. The normal neurologic examination signifies that the patient has not had a stroke. All the data point to carotid disease as the cause of the patient's TIAs.

An intravenous (IV) line was inserted and normal saline was infused at 75 ml per hour. A CT scan of the head and carotid ultrasound were performed that day. The CT scan was normal and the carotid ultrasound suggested greater than 80% stenosis of the left internal carotid artery. The patient was admitted to the neurology service and a cerebral angiogram was scheduled for the next day.

Comment: Patients with cerebral ischemia should be well hydrated to avoid hypotension. The IV fluid should not contain dextrose (even in nondiabetics) because hyperglycemia is associated with increased infarct size in patients who suffer stroke. This patient has a high risk of stroke in the near future, and admission to the hospital will facilitate rapid evaluation and definitive treatment to prevent stroke. Hospital admission will also make it easier to evaluate the patient for treatment with rt-PA within the appropriate time window if his symptoms recur and persist while his evaluation is in progress (there is no indication for rt-PA at this point, because his symptoms have resolved). Some neurologists use heparin in patients with TIAs and high-grade arterial stenosis, hoping to prevent thrombosis at the stenotic site, but this has not been adequately studied. Furthermore, if he were to develop a stroke while on heparin, an elevated partial thromboplastin time would make him ineligible to receive rt-PA, for which there is more compelling evidence of benefit.

Angiography showed 90% stenosis of the left internal carotid artery, mild plaque without stenosis of the right internal carotid artery, and normal intracranial vessels bilaterally. Surgery was planned for the following day. The surgery was successful and the patient was discharged 5 days later. In addition to the medications he was taking on admission, he was discharged on pravastatin given his history of heart disease and a borderline elevation of his total and low-density lipoprotein cholesterol. He reported no new symptoms at a follow-up visit 6 weeks later.

Case 2. A 59-year-old woman came to the emergency room at her family's insistence at 9 PM after she mentioned that she had been having trouble seeing out of the left eye since awakening that morning. She had been in good health except for longstanding hypertension and occasional "rapid heart beats." She denied previous visual symptoms or other episodic neurologic symptoms. She was taking nifedipine. The patient was alert, her blood pressure was 170/95, her pulse was 130 per minute and irregular, and there were no murmurs or bruits. The only abnormality on neurologic exam was a left homonymous hemianopia.

Comment: Patients with homonymous hemianopia frequently think their visual loss is monocular. Covering one eye at a time will often reveal the binocular visual loss to the patient. This patient had an acute, focal lesion with no history of trauma. This suggests a vascular etiology. The absence of prior TIAs, the irregular heartbeat (possibly atrial fibrillation), and the location of the lesion (probably right occipital lobe) suggest a cardioembolic mechanism.

An IV line was inserted and normal saline was infused at 75 ml per hour. An electrocardiogram confirmed atrial fibrillation, and a CT scan of the head was normal. Heparin was begun at 800 units per hour and the patient was admitted to the neurology service. Her blood pressure remained slightly elevated at 170–180/90–100.

Comment: Even if this patient had come to the emergency room as soon as she noticed her problem, rt-PA would not have been an option because her stroke could have occurred at any time after she fell asleep. Heparin was begun because the probable cause of stroke was cardioembolism related to atrial fibrillation. If the CT scan had shown intracranial hemorrhage, heparin would have been contraindicated. The mildly elevated blood pressure was left untreated to avoid relative hypotension and diminished cerebral perfusion.

The following day, transesophageal echocardiography showed spontaneous contrast in the left atrium but no clot. Heparin was continued, and the patient's partial thromboplastin time was maintained at 1.2–1.5 × control. Warfarin (5 mg orally) was started the same day.

Comment: Transesophageal echocardiography was performed to rule out valvular disease, vegetations, or thrombus. It showed spontaneous contrast (also termed smoke), which is thought to represent a precursor of thrombus in patients with sluggish left atrial flow. Warfarin was begun for long-term stroke prophylaxis.

The patient's hemianopia persisted, and a repeat CT scan 3 days after admission showed a right occipital infarct without hemorrhagic transformation. Heparin was discontinued when the patient's INR was therapeutic (2.0–3.0). The patient was discharged on nifedipine for blood pressure control, digoxin to control the heart rate associated with atrial fibrillation, and warfarin for stroke prophylaxis. The patient was given specific instructions to obtain a repeat INR in 1 week.

Comment: Patients with acute ischemic stroke usually have a normal CT scan on the day of the stroke, but by 2 or 3 days later, most large infarcts are visualized on CT. A diffusion-weighted MRI is a much more sensitive test for acute ischemic stroke, but it is not as widely available, especially in the acute setting. If the repeat CT scan had shown a hemorrhage, warfarin would have been discontinued.

Warfarin is a potentially dangerous drug. All patients discharged on warfarin should know who is going to monitor their warfarin therapy as an outpatient. They should be given clear instructions on what dose to take daily, and they should be told when to get blood drawn for the next INR measurement.

Case 3. A 73-year-old man was brought to the emergency room by paramedics after he fell down on the way back from the bathroom and discovered that he could not move his left side. His symptoms had not progressed in the 90 minutes that had elapsed since the initial event. He had been hypertensive for 20 years and was taking hydrochlorothiazide, and he had been taking lovastatin for a year because of hyperlipidemia. He denied previous episodes of focal neurologic symptoms. He was alert, with a blood pressure of 180/100 and a pulse that was 80 per minute and regular. There were no bruits or murmurs. Neurologic exam showed awareness of his neurologic deficit; slurred speech; left hemiparesis involving face, arm, and leg; left-sided hyperreflexia; a left extensor plantar response (Babinski sign); and normal sensation.

Comment: **The neurologic examination suggests a right-sided lesion at the level of the pons or above. An acute, focal, non-progressive lesion is generally ischemic. The absence of cortical signs (such as neglect) suggests a small lesion, and this makes penetrating artery disease a prime consideration. This is supported by the absence of TIAs, bruits, and arrhythmia.**

The patient was a candidate to receive rt-PA, so blood was sent for electrolytes, glucose, platelet count, and coagulation studies. He was taken immediately for a CT scan, which showed an old, small (1 cm) basal ganglia infarct on the left. The blood test results were normal, and IV rt-PA was administered. He was admitted to the neurology service, and his blood pressure was monitored in an intensive care unit for the next 24 hours, following an institutional protocol. By the time the patient was transferred out of the intensive care unit, he had recovered "approximately 75%" of the function on his left side but he still had significant weakness.

Carotid ultrasound performed the next day was normal. An MRI scan of the brain 2 days after admission showed a small (1 cm) infarct in the right internal capsule and the previously noted left basal ganglia infarct. The patient was transferred to the rehabilitation service, and a calcium channel blocker was prescribed in addition to the diuretic for better long-term blood pressure control.

Comment: **This patient might very well have improved even without rt-PA, but his chances of improvement were better with treatment. The second brain imaging study requested was an MRI scan because MRI is more sensitive than CT for detecting small subcortical infarcts. The use of rt-PA is recommended in acute stroke regardless of the underlying cause. Carotid ultrasound confirmed the absence of carotid** disease, and there was nothing to suggest a cardioembolic source. Long-term stroke prophylaxis in this patient consisted of aspirin and better control of blood pressure.

5

Seizures

Ivo J. Drury and Douglas J. Gelb

I. Case Histories

Case 1. A 7-year-old boy was noted by his teacher to be intermittently inattentive in the classroom. He would stare with a blank expression on his face for several seconds at a time. He would not respond to his name being called and sometimes had rapid fluttering movements of his eyelids. Once the staring ceased, he would immediately become his usual self. His pediatrician was able to provoke one of the spells by having the child hyperventilate in the office.

Questions:

1. What is the most likely diagnosis in this patient?

2. What other diagnoses need to be considered?

3. What is the drug of choice in this syndrome?

Case 2. A 27-year-old woman in the second trimester of her first pregnancy was referred to the epilepsy clinic from the high-risk obstetrics clinic. As a college student at age 19 years she had her first generalized tonic-clonic seizure. She had three more seizures during her early twenties, each beginning with an unpleasant sensation in her abdomen, followed on one occasion by staring and picking at her blouse buttons before progressing into a generalized tonic-clonic seizure. She was the product of a normal pregnancy and delivery with normal developmental milestones. At age 15 months she had experienced two prolonged seizures with high fever, both lasting approximately 15 minutes and associated with transient paralysis of her right arm. She had continued to develop normally and had been successful both athletically and scholastically. Since age 24 years she had taken phenytoin, 200 mg twice a day.

Questions:

1. What type of seizures does this patient have?

2. What diagnostic tests does this patient need?

3. What are the drugs of choice for this patient?

4. How should this patient be managed

   a. through the rest of her pregnancy? and

   b. thereafter?

Case 3. A 55-year-old woman had a generalized tonic-clonic seizure while grocery shopping one afternoon. She had been experiencing moderately severe headaches early every morning for approximately 1 week but had been well previously. When the emergency medical service arrived, the patient was having a second generalized tonic-clonic seizure. A witness reported generalized stiffening of all four extremities followed by clonic movements associated with cyanosis, frothing at the mouth, and urinary incontinence. The patient had two more seizures without recovering consciousness before reaching a local emergency room. The emergency room physicians diagnosed convulsive status epilepticus.

Questions:

1. Do you agree with the emergency room doctors' diagnosis?

2. How should this patient be managed in the emergency room?

3. How should this patient be investigated after her seizures are controlled?

II. Background Information

A. Definitions

seizure: the clinical phenomena experienced by a patient or witnessed by an observer during an abnormal electric discharge from neurons in the brain.
seizure disorder (epilepsy): a condition of recurrent seizures.
status epilepticus: a state of continued or frequent seizures with failure to return to a baseline of alertness between the seizures.

B. Clinical Characteristics of Seizures

The manifestations of a seizure are a function of where the abnormal neuronal hyperactivity starts and the pathway by which it spreads. For some seizures, the pathway of spread can be readily deduced from the clinical manifestations. The best known example is *Jacksonian spread*, in which a patient exhibits abnormal motor activity (usually shaking) in a portion of one limb, with progression of the movement to other areas on the same side of the body in an order consistent with the organization of the body's representation in the cortical motor strip. Seizures originating in a region of sensory cortex may present as sensory symptoms that spread in an analogous fashion. Visual hallucinations of various types may occur with seizure activity in the occipital cortex, and olfactory hallucinations are commonly experienced in seizures involving medial temporal cortex. More complex experiences, such as a rising sensation in the epigastric area, feelings of depersonalization, or an overwhelming sense of déjà vu (the impression that the current situation is an exact repetition of a situation in which the patient has participated previously), typically indicate involvement of limbic cortex. Seizures involving the prefrontal cortex may produce complex sequences of coordinated movements. The common characteristic of all these seizures is that they originate in a focal region of a single hemisphere. Such seizures are classified as **partial seizures.**

In some cases, the abnormal neuronal activity of a partial seizure ultimately spreads to involve both hemispheres. Such a seizure is called a **partial seizure with secondary generalization.** Once a seizure has generalized, it produces an alteration of consciousness because of the bilateral hemispheric involvement. Even without generalizing, some partial seizures result in altered consciousness, typically because of limbic system involvement. These are called **complex partial seizures.** These seizures are brief (usually no longer than 2–3 minutes), stereotyped episodes that may consist only of altered consciousness and motionless staring (which can be clinically indistinguishable from an absence seizure; see below) or may be accompanied by involuntary motor behaviors called automatisms. Partial seizures that are not associated with altered consciousness are called **simple partial seizures.**

With some seizures, the clinical manifestations indicate involvement of both cerebral hemispheres from the outset; these are called **generalized seizures.** The diffuse synchronization is presumed to be mediated by deep, midline structures that either modulate overall excitability of the cortex or serve as a focus of abnormal activity that propagates out to both hemispheres simultaneously. The following are examples of generalized seizures:

1. **Tonic seizures** are characterized by sudden muscular rigidity that may be either in extension or flexion. The rigidity can be generalized and result in a fall.

2. **Generalized tonic-clonic seizures** begin suddenly without warning. Tonic activity (rigid position of limbs, usually in extension) involves all axial and appendicular muscles. An epileptic cry may occur due to tonic spasm in truncal muscles. Shortly afterward the clonic (jerking) activity develops as the tonic rigidity is interrupted by brief periods of muscle relaxation. Apnea during the tonic and clonic phases may lead to cyanosis. The ictal activity itself usually lasts no longer than 1–2 minutes. Incontinence may occur at the beginning of the postictal phase, which is characterized by flaccidity and gradual return to normal consciousness. In the early postictal phase the patient will be disoriented and may complain of a headache, sore mouth from oral trauma, and muscular aching.

3. **Clonic seizures** involve generalized rhythmic jerking of muscles without an initial tonic phase.

4. **Atonic seizures** are characterized by a brief loss of muscle tone. This can be generalized and result in a fall, or it can be localized and produce focal loss of postural control, such as a head-drop.

5. **Absence seizures**, formerly called petit mal seizures, consist of a few seconds of staring with a blank look, unresponsiveness, cessation of any ongoing activity, and sometimes fluttering of the eyelids. They may be readily provoked by hyperventilation in the untreated child.

6. **Myoclonic seizures** consist of localized or widespread, nonrhythmic, rapid, jerking movements of muscles. Myoclonus may also be nonepileptic; the most common example is the isolated limb jerk that commonly occurs in normal individuals as they fall asleep. More diffuse and disabling nonepileptic myoclonus sometimes occurs in patients who have suffered anoxic brain injury.

C. Electroencephalogram Characteristics of Seizures

An electroencephalogram (EEG) is a recording of the brain's electric activity monitored by electrodes placed at standard locations along the scalp. The activity recorded by each electrode represents the summated activities of many individual neurons. Consistent patterns can be identified in normal individuals, and brain damage can distort these patterns. Seizures, in particular, may produce very distinctive patterns, because they represent coordinated activity throughout much larger areas of the brain than would occur in normal individuals. For example, absence seizures characteristically are associated with a pattern described as regular spike-and-wave activity at a frequency of 3 Hz.

For this reason, the EEG is most useful when it is recorded while the patient is experiencing a clinical spell. Most patients cannot predict when their spells will occur, however. Because their events occur much less frequently than a 30-minute EEG recording is likely to capture by chance, the majority of recordings are obtained between spells (*interictally*). Interictal EEGs often show characteristic "epileptiform" abnormalities in patients with seizure disorders. A single interictal EEG will show epileptiform activity in 50–70% of patients with a seizure disorder. The yield of interictal EEG can be increased by repeated studies or use of activation procedures such as hyperventilation (especially useful for provoking absence seizures) or sleep deprivation. A small number of patients with clinically unequivocal seizure disorders have consistently normal interictal EEGs. Moreover, epileptiform activity is not 100% specific: Some subjects with interictal abnormalities on EEG never have any symptoms consistent with a seizure. Thus, while EEG can supply useful information, the diagnosis of seizures still rests on clinical judgment.

In some circumstances it is desirable to characterize seizures as carefully as possible. This involves continuous EEG monitoring and concurrent videotaping of the patient, in the hopes of recording the patient's actual spells (rather than just interictal activity). This approach is only feasible if the patient is known to have spells fairly frequently.

D. Classification of Seizures and Seizure Disorders

The main principles of the classification of seizures can now be summarized. Seizures are partial when there is behavioral or EEG evidence to indicate that they begin in a part of the brain limited to one hemisphere and generalized when they begin bilaterally. Partial seizures are considered complex when there is alteration in awareness and simple when there is not. Simple partial seizures can progress to become complex partial seizures. Either can evolve to a secondarily generalized seizure.

The current recommended classification scheme for seizure disorders is based on three features: whether the seizures are partial or generalized, whether the disorder is primary (idiopathic) or secondary (a known or suspected underlying disturbance), and the age at onset of seizures.

III. Approach to Seizures

Four questions must be addressed in a patient being evaluated for seizures:

1. Is the patient in status epilepticus?

Status epilepticus is an *emergency*! It is discussed in Part V of this chapter. Except for status epilepticus, seizures do not represent an emergency situation (even though they may be very anxiety-provoking for all concerned), so the remaining questions can be addressed thoroughly and deliberately.

2.   Has the patient really had a seizure?

3.   Does the patient need to be evaluated for underlying causes of seizures?

4.   What treatment, if any, is indicated?

Although unnecessary delay should be avoided, some of these questions may be unanswerable until additional spells have occurred. This can obviously be disconcerting to patients and family members, but the physician must avoid treating each individual seizure as a catastrophic event requiring revision of the diagnosis or abandonment of the management plan. The goal is to treat the seizure disorder, not the individual seizures. Ultimately, of course, the aim in treating the seizure disorder is to block individual seizures completely, but this cannot always be accomplished immediately, and in some patients complete seizure control may not be achieved.

IV. Seizure Management

A. Determining If the Patient Has Had a Seizure

A variety of conditions produce recurrent spells that can be confused with seizures. It is important to keep these conditions in mind and to be aware of the features that help to distinguish seizures from nonepileptic spells.

1. Spells involving loss of consciousness

The most common cause of temporary loss of consciousness is syncope, which occurs when a transient reduction in cardiac output produces generalized cerebral ischemia. Many different conditions can produce syncope, including cardiac arrhythmia, obstructed cardiac outflow (such as occurs with aortic stenosis), sudden cardiac failure from a large myocardial infarction, or impaired autonomic reflexes (e.g., orthostatic hypotension). Excessive parasympathetic tone, often called *vasovagal syncope* or *vasodepressor syncope*, is the most common cause. It occurs when there is excessive parasympathetic response to a sudden increase in sympathetic activity, most often in the setting of stress or excitement. Excessive parasympathetic responses may also be responsible for *micturition syncope* and *defecation syncope*.

Most episodes of syncope are preceded by a premonitory state known as *presyncope*, consisting of light-headedness and sometimes nausea, diaphoresis, tinnitus, and change in skin color. These premonitory symptoms may be helpful in distinguishing a syncopal spell from a seizure; unfortunately, the presyncopal symptoms themselves may sometimes be confused with partial complex seizures. Another useful distinguishing feature may be the setting in which the spells occur. For example, people who lose consciousness when having their blood drawn probably have vasovagal syncope; orthostatic syncope commonly occurs during religious services, when there is venous pooling in the legs due to prolonged sitting or standing. Patients are usually only briefly confused, if at all, after syncope, whereas more prolonged confusion or focal signs would suggest a seizure. Incontinence is also more common with seizures, though it can occur with syncope. Spells that include rhythmic motor activity are usually seizures, but myoclonic jerks may occur with restitution of blood flow after a syncopal episode, making distinction from a seizure difficult in some cases.

2. Spells without loss of consciousness

Both transient ischemic attacks (TIAs) and migraines may produce transient neurologic symptoms that spread in a manner similar to a partial seizure (see Chapters 4 and 12). Accompanying headache helps to distinguish migraine from seizure, but some patients with otherwise typical migraine never experience headache (so-called migraine equivalents), and some patients who have seizures have severe headaches afterward. The motor or sensory symptoms that occur with migraine tend to evolve more slowly than the symptoms of a seizure, which, in turn, tend to evolve more slowly than the symptoms of a TIA. The sensory and motor manifestations of TIAs and migraines tend to be "negative" phenomena, such as numbness or weakness, whereas seizures are more likely to produce "positive" symptoms, such as paresthesias or jerking movements.

3. Spells of psychogenic origin

Psychological conditions or malingering can result in spells that resemble seizures. This diagnosis should be suspected when there is a high degree of variability in the clinical manifestations of a patient's spells. Spells that involve one limb on one day and a different limb the next, or visual symptoms on some occasions and auditory symptoms on other occasions, or spells lasting 2 minutes sometimes and 2 days at other times are all atypical of a seizure disorder in which the symptoms are generally very stereotyped for any individual patient. Another clue that the condition might be psychogenic is when the spells occur only when the patient is in a psychologically stressful situation. There are exceptions to all of these generalizations, however. Caution should be exercised before concluding that spells have a psychogenic origin simply because they are unusual or seem inconsistent. All fields of medicine abound with examples of organic conditions that were initially thought to be psychogenic. In many cases, clinical features are inadequate to determine if a patient's spells are seizures or not. This is one of the situations in which continuous EEG monitoring with concurrent videotaping may be helpful. If a patient has spells during the monitoring and there is no EEG abnormality before, during, or after the spells, they are not seizures (with rare exceptions). Of course, the patient could have other spells that are seizures—some patients with epilepsy also have nonepileptic spells of psychogenic origin.

Because seizures are transient and patients have usually returned to baseline by the time of evaluation, accurate diagnosis depends on obtaining as detailed a history as possible. Patients often have little or no recollection of the spell, so witnesses' accounts are especially important. It is best to have patients and witnesses describe in an open-ended fashion everything they observed before, during, and after the spell in question (as well as any other episodes of unusual behavior they may have witnessed). It is helpful to know the exact sequence of events and how long each stage lasted, with special emphasis on determining whether the symptoms suggest a partial or generalized onset. If adequate detail cannot be obtained by asking several open-ended questions (e.g., "How did you feel when you regained consciousness?" "Were you immediately able to resume what you had been doing before the spell?"), directed questions may be necessary. In particular, some of the most characteristic symptoms of complex partial seizures can seem embarrassing to patients, or they may have considered them so strange that they passed them off as "something I ate." Unless patients volunteer the information, they should be explicitly asked whether they have ever experienced unusual visceral sensations, smells, visual or auditory hallucinations, feelings of depersonalization, or déjà vu phenomena. Similarly, it may be necessary to inquire explicitly about incontinence, because patients may be too embarrassed to mention it. Directed questions may also be necessary to determine if the patient had any persistent focal deficits after the spell ended. Such deficits usually indicate a partial seizure, although they can occasionally occur when a generalized seizure unmasks an otherwise asymptomatic area of previous injury.

In addition to the information derived from the history, EEGs can provide evidence useful for determining whether a seizure disorder is likely, and if so, the type of seizures involved. The EEG cannot substitute for historic information, however (see Part II, Section C of this chapter).

B. Determining the Cause of Seizures

Seizures occur when large groups of neurons engage in repetitive, entrained activity. Inhibitory processes prevent such activity in normal individuals, but these protective mechanisms can be defective as a result of genetic abnormalities or because a region of brain tissue has sustained structural or metabolic injury. This injury may have been early in life, at a time when normal developmental processes allowed intact regions of brain to compensate for the injured tissue, with no clinical consequences except for the potential to serve as a source of seizures months, years, or even decades later. Less often, seizures are a manifestation of ongoing pathologic processes that might require specific treatment. Stroke is the most commonly identified structural cause of seizures in older individuals. Mass lesions are also more likely to be the cause of seizures in middle-aged and elderly patients than in patients who present at a younger age. Clinical and radiologic evidence of the lesion may not be detectable until months or years after seizure onset. One clue that a patient's symptoms may be due to an active structural lesion is the presence of concurrent neurologic symptoms, such as headaches.

The most common metabolic causes of seizures are hypoxia, hyponatremia, hyperglycemia, hypoglycemia, hypocalcemia, and hypomagnesemia. Seizures may also occur with severe uremia or hepatic failure. Prescription drugs and recreational drugs are common causes of seizures, especially antidepressants and antipsychotic medications (particularly when doses are increased too rapidly), aminophylline and other methylxanthines, lidocaine, penicillins, narcotic analgesics, cocaine, heroin, and phencyclidine. Withdrawal from alcohol may produce seizures, which almost always occur after 6–48 hours of abstinence. Withdrawal seizures may also occur in patients who have been abusing barbiturates or benzodiazepines.

Some historic features provide evidence that a patient's seizures are caused by a remote injury. All patients with seizures should be asked if there was anything unusual about their mother's pregnancy or method of delivery and if they required prolonged neonatal hospitalization. Patients' developmental milestones should be reviewed. Delayed milestones relative to siblings may be a clue to a neurologic insult early in life. On similar grounds, febrile seizures should be documented; complicated febrile seizures (such as seizures of long duration or those followed by focal weakness) increase the likelihood of seizures later in life. Patients with significant closed-head injury have an increased incidence of seizures. Scholastic and athletic achievements in comparison with other children, especially siblings, can be valuable information in identifying subtle deficits.

Historic information is often sufficient to determine the cause of seizures, but additional diagnostic testing may be required. A complete neurologic examination may identify subtle deficits that could indicate previous or ongoing brain injury. At least one brain imaging study should be performed in most epileptic patients, especially those with partial seizures, to exclude an underlying structural lesion such as a brain tumor. An MRI scan performed with and without gadolinium is the imaging procedure of choice. Serum electrolytes (including calcium and magnesium, which are not routinely included in some screening blood panels), glucose, blood urea nitrogen, creatinine, liver enzymes, and blood counts should be measured to determine if the seizures are a manifestation of a systemic disturbance. Patients who present acutely with seizures should be evaluated for infection (including a lumbar puncture), and a urine toxin screen should be obtained.

Before these investigations, patients should be advised that the evaluation often fails to identify a specific underlying reason for seizures, so they should not be distressed if the search is unrevealing. There is usually no need to repeat the evaluation, even if the patient continues to have seizures. The most important reasons to repeat part or all of the evaluation are recent onset of focal seizures (in which case the imaging study should be repeated at some point, because it is possible that the initial study failed to detect an early mass lesion), a significant change in seizure characteristics, or consistent failure to respond to treatment.

C. Determining If Seizures Require Treatment

When a clear underlying cause of seizures can be identified, there may be no need for specific treatment of the seizures if the underlying problem can be corrected. For example, seizures occurring in the setting of severe hyperglycemia or uremia are best addressed by treating the underlying metabolic abnormality, and seizures related to drug toxicity or alcohol withdrawal require management of the underlying substance abuse problem. The main exception is status epilepticus due to an underlying toxic/metabolic disorder, for which antiepileptic drugs (AEDs) may be required acutely until the underlying abnormality can be corrected.

When no underlying cause of seizures can be identified, or when the identified cause is untreatable, AEDs provide the main management option. Seizure frequency is the principal determinant of whether these drugs should be used. A few patients have seizures very infrequently, perhaps once every few years, and they would rather live with these rare seizures than take medication on a regular basis. Because there is no proof that such rare seizures produce any long-term adverse consequences, this choice can be reasonable for some patients. This situation is quite rare, however. Most patients with epilepsy have more than one seizure a year. Even patients whose seizures are infrequent often find the experience so disturbing that they will go to great lengths to avoid even a single seizure. Thus, patients with seizure disorders usually receive AEDs. The principles governing their use are discussed below (see Section D).

A more difficult question arises when a patient has had a single seizure for which no underlying cause can be found. By definition, such patients do not have a seizure disorder. Although approximately 30% will go on to have further seizures (i.e., they will prove to have a seizure disorder), the rest will not. There is debate about the relative risk of prolonged medication use when it is not necessary versus the risk of delay in treating a seizure disorder. If the history suggests a focal onset, if there are abnormal findings on neurologic examination or imaging studies, if there is epileptiform activity on EEG, or if the patient had a history of seizures in the remote past, it may be justifiable to initiate treatment after a single episode. Under other circumstances, however, continued observation without institution of AEDs may be preferable.

D. Antiepileptic Drugs

Table 5-1 lists the most commonly used AEDs, the seizure types for which they are indicated, typical dosage regimens, and side effects. Choice of the optimum AED for a patient's particular seizure disorder depends on an accurate classification of the underlying syndrome. When a patient has a disorder that includes several types of seizures, he or she should be prescribed a single medication that is effective against all the varieties of seizures the patient experiences.

As indicated in Table 5-1, there is considerable overlap in the drugs that are effective for some types of seizures. There have been very few studies directly comparing one drug to another in specific clinical settings, so the selection of a specific drug from among several effective alternatives is based primarily on issues such as side effect profiles, ease of administration, and cost. Taking such factors into consideration, the following general guidelines can be proposed:

Table 5-1. Antiepileptic Drugs

Drug	Seizure Types	Administration Routes	Typical Daily Doses	Oral Half-Life [Dose Schedule]	Side Effects
Ethosuximide	Absence	PO	750 mg	30 hrs [daily or b.i.d.]	Nausea, sedation, bone marrow suppression, skin rash
Phenobarbital	Tonic-clonic, partial	PO, IV	60–120 mg	96 hrs [daily]	Sedation, behavioral disturbances (children), rash
Primidone	Tonic-clonic, partial	PO	500–1,000 mg	Primidone 5–18 hrs; phenobarbital 96 hrs [daily or b.i.d.]	Sedation and impotence
Phenytoin	Tonic-clonic, partial	PO, IV	300–400 mg	22 hrs [daily]	Nystagmus, ataxia, sedation, rash, gingival hyperplasia, hepatitis, lymphadenopathy
Fosphenytoin	Tonic-clonic, partial	IV, IM	Given primarily as initial load; maintenance is usually with phenytoin	NA	Same as oral phenytoin (fewer than IV phenytoin)
Carbamazepine	Tonic-clonic, partial	PO	800–1,600 mg	15 hrs [t.i.d.] (modified release: [daily or b.i.d.])	Ataxia, nystagmus, diplopia, hyponatremia, leukopenia, movement disorders
Valproic acid	Tonic-clonic, absence, myoclonic, partial	PO, IV	1,000–2,500 mg	8 hrs [t.i.d. or q.i.d.]	Tremor, weight gain, nausea, sedation, idiosyncratic hepatitis, asymptomatic change in liver function test results, thrombocytopenia, or platelet dysfunction

Continued

Table 5-1. *Continued*

Drug	Seizure Types	Administration Routes	Typical Daily Doses	Oral Half-Life [Dose Schedule]	Side Effects
Gabapentin	Partial (adjunctive therapy)	PO	900–2,700 mg	6 hrs [t.i.d. or q.i.d.]	Somnolence, ataxia, dizziness, fatigue, nausea, nystagmus
Lamotrigine	Partial, tonic-clonic, absence, myoclonic	PO	300–500 mg	30 hrs [b.i.d.]	Rash (sometimes severe), dizziness, sedation, diplopia
Topiramate	Partial (adjunctive)	PO	400 mg	22 hrs [b.i.d.]	Somnolence, mental slowing, dizziness, ataxia
Tiagabine	Partial (adjunctive)	PO	32–56 mg	4–8 hrs [t.i.d. or q.i.d.]	Dizziness, sedation, tremor, nausea, irritability
Oxcarbazepine	Partial	PO	1,200–2,400 mg	9 hrs [b.i.d.]	Dizziness, somnolence, diplopia, nausea, ataxia, hyponatremia
Levetiracetam	Partial (adjunctive)	PO	1,000–4,000 mg	7–8 hrs [t.i.d.]	Mild dizziness, mild somnolence

NA = not applicable.

1. **Partial seizures (simple or complex, with or without generalization).** Initial treatment is usually with carbamazepine or phenytoin. If the seizures cannot be controlled with either of these agents, any of the other medications except ethosuximide can be tried.

2. **Absence seizures.** Ethosuximide is the agent of choice. Valproic acid is the best alternative. If the patient has other types of seizures in addition to absence, valproic acid is preferable to ethosuximide because valproic acid is more likely to be effective against a broad range of seizure types.

3. **Myoclonic seizures.** Valproic acid is the agent of choice; clonazepam (not listed in Table 5-1 because it is rarely used) is the best alternative.

4. **Tonic-clonic seizures.** This is probably the category about which there is the least consensus. Phenytoin is a reasonable choice as initial treatment. Alternatives would include valproic acid or carbamazepine.

The following general principles apply to the institution of any antiepileptic drug:

• Unless a patient is having frequent and uncontrolled seizures, the drug should be introduced slowly to allow the patient time to adjust to the sometimes troubling initial symptoms such as sleepiness and a slight reduction in mental sharpness. The dose should be increased gradually until seizure control is achieved or the patient can't tolerate any further increase because of toxic symptoms. Serum drug levels should not be the principal basis for making dose adjustments. The published "therapeutic range" for any drug is based on a population average. There is a great deal of variability in individual patients' responses to these drugs. Some patients achieve complete seizure control with levels considerably below the therapeutic range, while others require levels higher than the upper limit of the range. Some patients experience unacceptable toxic effects at the lowest possible doses of a medication, while others have no problems at levels above the therapeutic range. Drug levels thus provide only approximate guidelines for therapy. They are useful for monitoring drug compliance, however, and they may also be helpful in determining why a patient who was previously well controlled has resumed having seizures. If there is a record of the drug level during the period of good control, it can be compared to the current drug level. Superimposed medical illnesses or drug-drug interactions may cause changes in AED levels despite a stable dosing regimen.

• One drug should be used at a time. If a patient's seizures remain uncontrolled at the highest dose a patient can tolerate, the medication should be gradually tapered while a different AED is introduced at gradually increasing doses. This maneuver should be repeated until a medication is found that controls the patient's seizures without producing unacceptable side effects. If no such agent is found, it is sometimes appropriate to use two AEDs simultaneously, especially if they have different modes of action. There are very few circumstances that require the use of more than two AEDs at one time.

• Four of the most recently introduced medications for epilepsy—gabapentin, topiramate, tiagabine, and levetiracetam—have only been approved as adjunctive agents for use in combination with other AEDs. This is because new agents cannot be tested as single-drug therapy for ethical reasons. There is now at least some evidence that each of these three agents may also be effective in isolation, so one or more of them may eventually be approved for use as monotherapy. Lamotrigine is an example of a drug that was initially approved only as an adjunctive agent but is now approved for single-drug use also.

Patients must be educated about strict compliance and possible side effects. For certain drugs, periodic laboratory testing is necessary to monitor for potential toxicity (such as bone marrow suppression or liver damage). These laboratory tests should also be checked before starting the patient on the medication so that a baseline is available for comparison.

When seizure control is achieved, patients should be informed that they must remain on the AED until instructed otherwise by their physician. It is often reasonable to attempt to withdraw AEDs after complete seizure control has been achieved for periods varying from two to four years, but this should always be performed under the close supervision of a physician. The medication taper should be gradual (over approximately 3–6 months). Seizures are most likely to recur within the first year after drug withdrawal. Factors that favor successful withdrawal from AEDs include a normal neurologic examination, idiopathic seizure type, a low overall number of seizures, and probably a normal EEG or an EEG that is improved over the baseline tracing.

E. Surgical Options in Epilepsy Management

The majority of patients with epilepsy can achieve seizure control with AEDs. Surgical approaches are reserved for patients in whom medical control is inadequate. In some cases, the goal of surgery is to render patients seizure-free; in other cases, the aim is merely to reduce the frequency or severity of seizures.

Surgical resection of the seizure focus is the procedure most likely to eliminate seizures in properly selected patients. The chances of success are greatest for patients who have medically refractory partial seizures with onset in the temporal lobe. Evaluation of such patients is directed at identifying as precisely as possible the site of onset of seizure activity, typically through long-term video/EEG recording of ictal activity. This study may include invasive recording of EEG activity through depth or subdural electrodes. Other investigations are aimed at determining whether this portion of brain may be safely removed without causing serious neurologic deficits (such as severe memory loss, language disturbance, or major motor deficits). In carefully selected groups of patients, resective surgery may produce complete seizure resolution in up to 80% of patients in whom medical therapy has failed.

Other surgical approaches include hemispherectomies in young children with widely distributed epileptic disturbances over one hemisphere, especially when there is a contralateral hemiparesis. Section of the corpus callosum can be of benefit in a small number of patients with refractory seizures characterized by frequent falls and sometimes other seizure types. Such patients may achieve elimination of one seizure type but generally do not become seizure free.

Vagus nerve stimulation is another surgical approach that can be tried in patients who are refractory to medical therapy. Two helical electrode coils are wrapped around the left vagus nerve in the carotid sheath and connected to an infraclavicular pulse generator. The generator is then programmed to deliver pulses of a specified duration, frequency, and amplitude. Patients treated in this way have on average a 25–30% reduction in seizure frequency, and 25–30% of patients have at least a 50% reduction in seizure frequency, which is comparable to the results obtained with most adjunctive medications. Patients also have the option of using an external magnet to activate the device when they start to experience a seizure; for some patients, this can abort the seizure or reduce its severity. The mechanism of action is unknown.

F. Patient Education

Education of patients and family members is a critically important part of the management program. Historically, the diagnosis of epilepsy has had a negative connotation, and epileptics have been shunned by society. Patients should be informed that this stigma is based on a misunderstanding. Many epileptic patients conduct normal and productive lives, and prominent people in the worlds of art, literature, music, and sport have had epilepsy. As discussed earlier (see Section B), the need to pursue a thorough investigation of the underlying basis for the seizures should be explained to the patient, making it clear at the outset that in the majority of patients with seizures, no underlying cause is found. Explaining the indications for, side effects of, and planned duration of treatment with AEDs will help in achieving compliance. A major cause of poor patient compliance is poor patient education.

Certain restrictions apply to a patient once seizures have been diagnosed. In 43 states, any person who has experienced an unprovoked episode of altered consciousness is forbidden to drive for a set period of time. The required seizure-free interval is 1 year in 22 states and varies from 3–18 months in the other 21 states. There is no specified time requirement in the remaining seven states; instead, patients must submit statements from physicians or advisory boards indicating that they should be allowed to drive. In most states, the physician is required to inform the patient of the law regarding driving and to document in writing in the medical record that the patient has been informed. In six states, physicians are required to notify the Department of Motor Vehicles directly. Other commonsense restrictions also apply. No epileptic patient should swim alone. Epileptic patients should shower and not bathe, as it is possible to drown in just a few inches of water. They should avoid situations that might put them at risk if they were to have a seizure, such as working at heights or using power equipment.

V. Special Clinical Problems

A. Convulsive Status Epilepticus

Status epilepticus is a medical emergency with significant mortality (10%) and major morbidity. The prognosis is closely related to the cause. The most common cause of status epilepticus is poor medication compliance in patients previously diagnosed with epilepsy; in this situation, status epilepticus is readily responsive to reinstitution of AEDs and the outlook for the patient is favorable. Patients with no prior history of epilepsy who present in status epilepticus are most likely to have meningitis, encephalitis, hypoxic-ischemic encephalopathy, or a large stroke. The prognosis for these patients is worse. The longer a patient is in status, the worse the outcome. This is partly because the duration is more likely to be prolonged in patients with more severe underlying disease, but there is also a great deal of experimental evidence that status epilepticus itself damages the brain and that the degree of damage is a function of duration.

The medications that are most commonly used to treat status epilepticus are benzodiazepines, barbiturates, propofol, and phenytoin or its prodrug, fosphenytoin. In the absence of any clear demonstration that one of these agents is more effective than another, the most important factor in treating status epilepticus appears to be how quickly treatment is initiated, not which drug is used. Almost any order of drug administration could be defended. The physician should simply choose one protocol and commit it to memory so that the treatment of status epilepticus becomes practically a matter of reflex response. This will prevent wasting valuable moments while trying to decide which agent to use or where to find it. Treatment should be initiated whenever seizure activity persists significantly longer than usual for the patient. If the patient's baseline is not known, treatment should be initiated whenever seizure activity persists beyond 5 minutes. One scheme for the management of convulsive status epilepticus is outlined below.

Step-By-Step Management of Convulsive Status Epilepticus

I.   Ensure adequate cardiorespiratory function, insert an oral airway, give oxygen.

II.   Insert IV line. Measure blood count, electrolytes, blood urea nitrogen, glucose, calcium, magnesium, AED levels where applicable, and toxicology screen. Send arterial blood for pH, pCO_2, and HCO_3.

III.   Start IV line with normal saline. Give 50 mg of 50% glucose and 100 mg of thiamine.

IV.   Give IV lorazepam, 0.1–0.2 mg/kg at 2 mg per minute (maximum adult dose 8 mg).

V.   Give IV fosphenytoin, 20 mg phenytoin equivalents/kg at 150 mg phenytoin equivalents per minute. (If fosphenytoin unavailable, give phenytoin, 20 mg/kg at no more than 50 mg per minute, diluted in 100 ml of normal saline.)

VI.   If seizures persist, give additional IV fosphenytoin, 10 mg phenytoin equivalents/kg at same rate as before (or phenytoin, 10 mg/kg at same rate as before, if fosphenytoin unavailable).

VII. If seizures persist, give IV midazolam, 0.2 mg/kg load followed by 0.1–0.4 mg/kg per hour infusion.

VIII. If seizures persist, give IV phenobarbital, 20 mg/kg at 100 mg per minute.

IX.   If seizures persist, induce barbiturate coma or initiate very high-dose phenobarbital therapy.

All of the agents used in treating status epilepticus have the potential to suppress respiration and reduce blood pressure. These parameters must be followed closely, and patients may require intubation with mechanical ventilation or blood pressure support. Arrhythmias can also occur with IV administration of phenytoin, so cardiac monitoring is necessary.

Many of the adverse effects of IV phenytoin occur because it is relatively insoluble in water and the vehicle in which it is administered can cause hypotension. Fosphenytoin, a water-soluble prodrug that is rapidly and completely converted to phenytoin, was developed to avoid these problems. Compared to phenytoin, fosphenytoin produces less pain at the injection site, has lower risk of serious consequences from extravasation, and causes fewer instances of hypotension or other cardiovascular complications. Doses are expressed in "mg phenytoin equivalents" or "mg PE" which is the amount of phenytoin that will be produced by conversion.

B. Seizures and Pregnancy

Seizure disorders pose some difficult management issues for women who want to have children. All AEDs have teratogenic potential, but seizures themselves also pose a risk to the fetus. The risk to the fetus from uncontrolled convulsive seizures probably outweighs the risk of any of the AEDs. Many neurologists avoid valproic acid in women of child-bearing age because neural tube defects may be more common with this drug than with other AEDs, but there is no convincing evidence that any one AED is safer than the others. Fortunately, the absolute magnitude of risk with any of these agents is low, and the vast majority of women give birth to perfectly healthy children. Patients should be encouraged to discuss any planned pregnancies with their neurologist prior to conception. If the patient has been seizure-free, it may be possible to withdraw AEDs. If not, single-drug treatment at the lowest possible dose should be the objective. Free levels of drugs should be documented before conception. Drug levels may fall as the pregnancy progresses, but the free fraction typically falls less. At regular intervals, the medication dosage should be adjusted as necessary to keep the free level the same as the prepregnancy free level. Some protection can be provided against congenital anomalies by prescribing folic acid before conception and during the first trimester. A deficiency of vitamin K–dependent clotting factors may produce a bleeding diathesis in the first 24 hours of life, so oral vitamin K should be administered to the mother for one month before the expected date of delivery, and the infant should receive an intramuscular injection of 1 mg of vitamin K at birth.

C. Refractory Seizures

A small proportion of patients with seizures fail to respond even when optimally managed. In these circumstances the treating physician should review the following points: Is the original diagnosis of epilepsy accurate? If the diagnosis still stands, was the correct type of epilepsy identified and were the appropriate AEDs used? If so, is the patient truly compliant as determined by adequate AED levels? Were the medications pushed to the highest doses the patient could tolerate? Were combination regimens attempted? Does the patient's lifestyle require modification? Patients who continue to be refractory to medical management should be referred to a major epilepsy center where experimental AEDs or epilepsy surgery may be available.

VI. Discussion of Case Histories

Case 1. Seven-year-old boy with absence seizures.
This history is typical of absence (petit mal) seizures. The provocation of the attacks by hyperventilation is also characteristic. Other entities to be considered in the differential diagnosis would be complex partial seizures (which can also be associated with motionless staring with no

other symptoms, but are less readily provoked by hyperventilation), an attention deficit disorder, or some other form of behavioral disturbance. The EEG findings were bursts of generalized 3-Hz spike-and-wave activity occurring spontaneously and provoked by hyperventilation. In view of the normal neurologic examination and the generalized nature of the child's EEG discharges, no imaging studies are indicated. The treatment of choice is ethosuximide, introduced slowly and built up to a dose of 500–750 mg per day. The drug is well tolerated and eliminates both the seizure activity and the EEG discharges in almost all cases. The outlook for normal neurologic and intellectual development in a patient such as this is excellent.

Case 2. Young woman with partial seizure disorder.

This young woman has seizures that by history are initially simple partial, progress to complex partial, and then progress to secondarily generalized tonic-clonic seizures. Her seizures are probably a result of the prolonged complicated febrile convulsions when she was age 15 months. Unless they were obtained previously, she should have EEG studies looking for focal slowing and interictal epileptiform activity and a brain MRI scan looking for a structural cause of her seizures. In this instance the brain MRI should be delayed until after delivery. A search for a toxic-metabolic cause of seizures is unnecessary given the long history.

Teratogenic effects of AEDs occur during the first trimester. Because this patient was first seen during her second trimester, it would be prudent to continue drug therapy at the current dose. The patient should be seen frequently during the remainder of her pregnancy. Free levels of phenytoin should be checked regularly. The dose should be adjusted to maintain a stable free level, and in the last month of pregnancy the patient should take oral vitamin K.

After delivery, if antiepileptic doses have been increased during the pregnancy, they should be reduced to prepregnancy doses by the first month postpartum. The mother must strive to obtain sufficient sleep, as sleep deprivation is a common precipitant of seizures. An MRI scan should be obtained, as mentioned above. Regular follow-up under the supervision of a neurologist should be arranged and the patient encouraged to discuss future planned pregnancies so that folate can be prescribed and AED withdrawal can be considered before future conceptions.

Case 3. Middle-aged woman in convulsive status epilepticus.

The emergency room physicians' diagnosis of convulsive status epilepticus is correct. The four tonic-clonic seizures in this patient with failure to return to normal consciousness in between certainly satisfies the definition of status epilepticus. Emergency management of the patient should follow the scheme outlined in Part V. Even if seizures cease rapidly, all patients who have just been treated for status epilepticus should be admitted to an intensive care unit for at least 24 hours of close observation. An epileptic disorder presenting de novo as status epilepticus requires immediate investigation. In this patient, the likelihood of finding significant underlying problems is high, especially given the history of headaches for the past week. An MRI scan in this patient revealed multiple areas of signal abnormality that enhanced with contrast. The patient proved to have multiple small cerebral metastases from a primary tumor that was never identified.

6

Neuromuscular Disorders

Mark B. Bromberg and Douglas J. Gelb

I. Case Histories

Case 1. A 45-year-old woman reports that about 3 months ago, she began having trouble standing up from low chairs, and the problem has progressed to the point where she now must use her arms to push off from any chair. She recently started having difficulty holding up her arms to set her hair. Her weakness is symmetric. Her head and neck muscles are strong, and she has no shortness of breath. She does not have pain or sensory disturbance. There is no family history of neurologic disorders. She has no relevant past medical history and is taking no medication.

On examination, she has normal mental status and cranial nerve function. Muscle bulk and tone are normal. Neck flexor strength is grade 4 on the 5-point Medical Research Council scale. Shoulder abduction is grade 4+ and hip flexion is grade 3+, in a symmetric distribution. She must be helped to a standing position and cannot perform a deep knee bend. Tendon reflexes, plantar responses, and sensory examination are normal.

Questions:

1. Does this localize to the peripheral nervous system? If so, is the problem at the level of nerve, neuromuscular junction, or muscle?

2.   What tests would you order to confirm the suspected localization? Is this likely to be a treatable condition?

Case 2. A 55-year-old man describes double vision, mild limb weakness, and rapid fatigability with routine activities. He first noted double vision 6 months ago. It resolved after several days but reappeared
2 weeks ago, and at the same time he began having trouble climbing
stairs. His endurance has decreased markedly, to the point where he
now must rest after walking a short distance. He has no pain or sensory loss. Past and family medical histories are unremarkable for neurologic disorders. He takes no medications.

On examination, he has normal mental status and cranial nerve function except for weakness in the distribution of the right cranial nerves
III and VI, mild right ptosis, and bilateral eye closure weakness. There
is normal strength of shoulder abduction and hip flexion at first, but
prominent fatigue after several repetitions of muscle activation. Tendon
reflexes, plantar responses, and sensory examination are normal.

Questions:

1.   What are the important differences between this and the first
case? Is the lesion at the same site?

2.   What tests, if any, would distinguish between the two conditions?

3.   How should this patient be managed?

Case 3. A 60-year-old man fell 1 year ago and fractured his left ankle.
After the cast was removed, he noted weakness and atrophy of his calf.
Prolonged physical therapy did not help. Six months ago he began having trouble unscrewing jar caps and turning keys, and when he tried
hard he would get muscle cramps. He is constantly fatigued and has
lost 30 pounds. His wife says she "can see his muscles working."

On examination, the patient has normal mental status and cranial
nerves. He is thin and has frequent muscle twitching (fasciculations).
The intrinsic muscles of both hands are atrophic, and atrophy is also
prominent in anterior and posterior muscles in the left leg. A clasp-
knife phenomenon (spasticity) is evident with passive manipulation of
all limbs. Strength is mildly reduced everywhere but markedly reduced

in distal upper extremity muscles, and he has a flail left foot. Deep tendon reflexes are hyperactive, and he has a right extensor plantar (Babinski) response. Sensory examination is normal.

Questions:

1. How does this pattern of weakness differ from the patterns in Cases 1 and 2?

2. Where does this localize in the nervous system?

3. How should this patient be managed?

Case 4. A 45-year-old woman has difficulty walking and numbness of her legs. She was active until 6 months ago when she noted tingling in her toes that progressed over several weeks to include much of her legs. Her fingers have recently developed a similar tingling. She notes difficulty standing from a chair and complains of unsteadiness in walking. She recalls that 1 year ago she had similar problems but to a lesser degree. They resolved without seeking medical consultation.

On examination, she has normal mental status and cranial nerves. There is mild weakness of distal muscles in the upper extremity and mild weakness of proximal and distal muscles in the lower extremity. Tendon reflexes are absent. Her gait is very unsteady, and she cannot walk with her eyes closed. Vibratory perception is absent in the feet and reduced at the fingers.

Questions:

1. What components of the nervous system are involved? How do they differ from those in Case 3?

2. How would electrodiagnostic tests help distinguish between Cases 3 and 4?

3. How should this patient be managed?

II. Background Information

The peripheral nervous system can be divided into the autonomic and somatic nervous systems. The somatic system is further subdivided into sensory and motor nerves. Motor nerves activate muscles through the neuromuscular junction. The autonomic, somatic sensory, and somatic motor nerves are physically intermingled at some levels of the nervous system and separated at others, but it is generally useful to conceptualize them as distinct pathways. Each can be associated with a variety of symptoms.

Lesions of the autonomic system can produce dysfunction of practically any visceral organ. Some of the more prominent symptoms include postural hypotension, sphincter dysfunction, impotence, and sweating abnormalities. Lesions of sensory pathways can produce pain, a positive symptom, or a spectrum of negative symptoms. In increasing order of severity, these negative symptoms are paresthesias (sensations typically likened to "pins and needles"), hypesthesia (reduced sensation), and anesthesia (absence of sensation). Lesions of the peripheral motor system can also produce both negative symptoms (e.g., weakness and muscle atrophy) and positive symptoms (e.g., fasciculations and muscle cramps).

III. Approach to Neuromuscular Diseases

Neuromuscular diseases are a consideration whenever a patient's symptoms are limited to weakness, numbness/paresthesia, or both. Unlike the central nervous system, where a single structural lesion may produce widespread effects because of disruption of ascending and descending fiber tracts, a single structural lesion in the peripheral nervous system produces symptoms in a narrowly localized region of one limb. Many diseases affect the peripheral nervous system diffusely, however, producing multiple lesion sites. For these diseases, it is impossible to speak of localization to a single lesion site. While the localization approach described in Chapter 1 is still valid for multifocal and diffuse diseases, the process is complicated and tedious. Instead, these diseases are best described by characterizing which components of the peripheral nervous system are affected. For example, some diseases affect peripheral nerves and not muscles, while other diseases do the converse. To diagnose neuromuscular disease and develop a management strategy, four steps are necessary:

1. Identify the components of the peripheral nervous system that are involved (see Parts IV and V of this chapter).

2. Determine the specific condition (see Part VI of this chapter).

3.   Determine the likelihood of **autonomic instability** or **respiratory failure**. These are the only two complications of neuromuscular disease that represent **true emergencies** (see Part VII of this chapter).

4.   Assess the progression of the patient's condition. The rate of progression of many neuromuscular diseases can accelerate rapidly and unexpectedly. If the patient has a condition that can affect respiratory muscles or autonomic stability, and if there has been recent progression, the patient should generally be admitted to a hospital for observation and treatment until it is clear that the condition has stabilized. Elective intubation and other management issues are discussed in Part VII.

IV. Anatomic Localization

Disorders of the neuromuscular system can be viewed in a proximal-to-distal anatomic pattern, with different clinical syndromes corresponding to each level of peripheral nervous system involvement. Of course, before trying to localize a patient's condition within the peripheral nervous system, the possibility of a central disorder should be considered. Findings on the neurologic examination that help to distinguish between central and peripheral lesions are discussed in Chapters 1 and 2.

The most proximal lesion sites in the peripheral nervous system are the anterior horn cells, which are affected in **motor neuron diseases,** including amyotrophic lateral sclerosis (ALS). The principal clues that suggest a motor neuron disease are (1) motor symptoms and signs (both positive and negative) in the absence of sensory abnormalities and (2) a patchy distribution, often asymmetric, with no obvious pattern of proximal versus distal muscle involvement.

Lesions affecting dorsal and ventral roots, or the spinal roots that they form, are called **radiculopathies.** There are a variety of patterns of involvement and causes of radiculopathy. Structural causes, such as herniated vertebral disks, usually affect a single nerve root on one side. They are associated with pain in the distribution of the affected root and less commonly with numbness and weakness in that distribution. Metabolic diseases, such as diabetes mellitus, can affect multiple roots, causing a polyradiculopathy; it may be mild and asymptomatic or signaled by severe back pain. Patients with radiculopathies usually have both sensory and motor symptoms, though one or the other may predominate. Thus, in patients with both sensory and motor symptoms in whom the distribution of symptoms and signs is consistent with the known distribution of one or more nerve roots, radiculopathy is likely.

Before forming peripheral nerves, fibers exiting the nerve roots undergo a complex crossing and regrouping to form the brachial plexus and lumbosacral plexus. Common causes of **plexopathies** are cancer, radiation therapy, metabolic disorders such as diabetes mellitus, or trauma. There are also idiopathic plexopathies, much more common in the brachial plexus than in the lumbosacral plexus. Although the cause is not known, they are thought to be autoimmune. When patients have symptoms and signs that would suggest a polyradiculopathy but the pattern does not conform to the distribution of any individual nerve root or combination of nerve roots, nor to the distribution of any combination of peripheral nerves, plexopathy is likely.

Moving another step distally, peripheral nerve lesions take the form of **polyneuropathies** when involvement is diffuse or **mononeuropathies** when a single nerve is involved. Polyneuropathies frequently affect both sensory and motor nerves, though there are exceptions that involve only one type of nerve. For sensory nerves there is both a peripheral and a central branch, and both may be affected. Most polyneuropathies affect the longest nerves in the body earliest, and symptoms and signs occur in the feet first and progress proximally. When signs and symptoms reach approximately knee level, nerves to the fingers become involved. These neuropathies are usually symmetric.

The next step in the proximal-to-distal progression is the neuromuscular junction. In **disorders of the neuromuscular junction**, the most prominent weakness typically occurs in proximal muscles. For obvious reasons, there are no sensory symptoms.

Finally, there are primary disorders of muscle that include **dystrophies**, **congenital myopathies**, and acquired disorders such as **polymyositis** and **inclusion body myositis**. As with disorders of the neuromuscular junction, primary muscle disorders typically result in a proximal distribution of weakness. Weakness of distal musculature is uncommon. With some exceptions (such as myotonic dystrophy and facioscapulohumeral dystrophy), primary muscle diseases usually spare muscles innervated by cranial nerves, so symptoms like diplopia, dysarthria, and dysphagia are rare—in contrast to myasthenia gravis, the most common neuromuscular junction disease.

Additional information obtained from the history may be useful. The manner of onset, time course of changes, distribution within the body, factors that exacerbate or ameliorate symptoms, and family history are important.

V. Electrodiagnostic and Other Laboratory Studies

The tests that are most consistently helpful in the diagnosis of peripheral nervous system disorders are electrodiagnostic studies. These consist of nerve conduction studies, tests of neuromuscular junction transmission, and the needle electromyogram (EMG). These tests can be considered an extension of the clinical neurologic examination. Nerve conduction studies assess conduction along peripheral nerves. Both sensory and motor nerves are studied. Measurements include the amplitude of the response (which reflects the number of nerve fibers present) and conduction velocity (which is a function of the myelin sheath around nerve fibers). Thus, nerve conduction studies help determine if a nerve disorder reflects primary axonal loss or demyelination. The integrity of the neuromuscular junction can be assessed by repeated stimulation of the motor nerve: A normal neuromuscular junction has adequate reserve to ensure that each stimulus will result in an action potential in the muscle fiber, whereas synaptic transmission sometimes fails when there is a neuromuscular junction disorder. There are characteristic patterns of failure that identify postsynaptic defects such as myasthenia gravis and presynaptic defects such as the Lambert-Eaton myasthenic syndrome. The third component of an electrodiagnostic evaluation is the needle EMG, which records the electrical activity of muscle fibers preceding muscle contraction. Needle EMG is very sensitive to denervation and can be used to distinguish between neuropathic changes in muscle (due to primary nerve damage such as radiculopathy, motor neuron disease, or polyneuropathy) and myopathic changes (due to primary muscle disorders).

Nerve and muscle biopsies are supplementary diagnostic tests. The sural nerve at the ankle is most commonly examined. A nerve biopsy can be useful in determining whether the underlying nerve pathology is primary axon damage or primary demyelination, or it may provide evidence of a vasculitis affecting the small arterioles supplying the nerve. Muscle biopsies help distinguish between dystrophies, congenital myopathies, metabolic myopathies, and inflammatory myopathies. Common muscle biopsy sites are vastus lateralis and biceps brachii muscles. Another informative test is determination of the serum creatine kinase (CK) level. This enzyme is found in highest concentration in skeletal muscle, and an elevated serum level can be an indication of muscle damage. Acetylcholine receptor antibodies in the serum can be assayed in patients being evaluated for myasthenia gravis. These are fairly sensitive and very specific. For a focal process, such as a mononeuropathy, plexopathy, or radiculopathy, imaging studies of the affected structure can be helpful.

VI. Specific Neuromuscular Diseases

Many of the diseases that affect the peripheral nervous system at various levels have already been mentioned. This section provides further descriptions of the clinical course of some of these conditions and discusses their management.

A. Motor Neuron Diseases

Although there are diseases (especially in infants and children) that exclusively involve lower motor neurons (LMNs), and there are other conditions that exclusively involve upper motor neurons (UMNs), the most common form of motor neuron disease in adults is ALS, which involves both LMNs and UMNs. The pattern of involvement is variable, however, with LMN involvement predominating in some patients and UMN involvement predominating in others. Even in an individual patient, the pattern of involvement may change over time. For example, a patient may initially present with primarily LMN involvement and only later develop UMN symptoms and signs.

As noted in Chapter 2, weakness, spasticity, hyperreflexia, and the Babinski sign are all features of UMN involvement. LMN involvement is manifested by weakness and atrophy of the affected muscles. Fasciculations occur in all individuals, including healthy control subjects, but they are more profuse and continuous when there is extensive damage to lower motor neurons, so they commonly occur in patients with ALS. Cramps are also common in denervated muscles. These are often most distressful to the patient when lying in bed, and they may interfere with sleep.

ALS may begin at any adult age but it is more common with increasing age. As the disease progresses (and sometimes at the outset), involvement of bulbar muscles is common, resulting in dysarthria and dysphagia. For some reason, extraocular muscles are not affected, nor is there bladder or bowel incontinence from sphincter muscle weakness. The rate of progression varies significantly between patients. Although many patients rapidly become disabled and die within several years, others may experience much more gradual progression over 10 years or more.

The cause of motor neuron disease is not known, and there is no known cure. Most cases of motor neuron disease are sporadic, but familial forms also exist. Some cases of familial ALS are associated with mutations in the gene for superoxide dismutase (an antioxidant enzyme), suggesting that oxidative stress may contribute to neuronal death even in sporadic forms of the disease. Another line of evidence suggests that glutamate toxicity may play a role in the pathogenesis of ALS. Glutamate is the principal excitatory neurotransmitter in the nervous system, including motor neurons, but excess levels of glutamate are toxic to neurons. Riluzole, a drug that modulates glutamatergic neurotransmission, results in a modest prolongation of survival in patients with ALS. Several trials of other experimental medications, including nerve growth factors, are in progress. In the meantime, the main focus of treatment is supportive care. Thus, it is imperative that all potentially treatable conditions be excluded before making the diagnosis of motor neuron disease. In particular, structural causes of the UMN and LMN abnormalities must be considered. The most common source of confusion is degenerative disease of the cervical spine, which may produce UMN signs in the lower extremities on the basis of spinal cord compression and LMN signs in the upper extremities because of compression of multiple cervical nerve roots. The diagnosis can usually be clarified using the distribution of findings, the presence or absence of sensory abnormalities, and the results of imaging studies and electrodiagnostic tests, but occasionally the situation remains unclear.

B. Nerve Root Disorders (Radiculopathies)

The most common cause of radiculopathy is degenerative disease of the spinal column, involving the vertebral bodies, the facet joints, or the disks. The nerve roots may also be compressed by other structural lesions, including tumors and abscesses. The diagnostic and management considerations for these structural causes of radiculopathy are discussed in Chapter 15.

Nerve roots may also be involved by many of the same processes that produce neuropathies, including vasculitis, metabolic abnormalities, and inflammatory demyelination. Usually the radiculopathy and neuropathy coexist; the evaluation and management will be discussed below (see Section D). On occasion, the radiculopathy occurs without a significant neuropathy; this is most often seen in diabetic patients, especially in the thoracic nerve roots. Such patients should be evaluated for a structural cause (especially neoplastic) before concluding that the radiculopathy is due to metabolic disease.

Herpes zoster produces a radiculopathy that may be excruciatingly painful; it is usually straightforward to diagnose because of the accompanying skin lesions, but they are occasionally absent. Patients are treated with an antiviral medication and symptomatic pain treatment. Further details are provided in Chapter 10. Lyme disease and cytomegalovirus both may produce a polyradiculopathy; treatment is directed at the underlying infection.

C. Plexus Disorders (Plexopathies)

The common causes of plexus disease have already been discussed. For some reason, diabetes affects the lumbosacral plexus much more frequently than the brachial plexus, whereas the converse is true of autoimmune plexopathies. Diagnosis of a plexus disorder rests on establishing relevant details of the history (e.g., a history of radiation therapy or recent immunization), electrodiagnostic tests to confirm the localization, and—if the cause is not clear from the history—imaging the plexus to exclude a structural lesion. Treatment is directed at the underlying cause; only supportive therapy (mainly pain control and physical therapy) is available for idiopathic plexopathies.

D. Peripheral Nerve Disorders (Neuropathies)

Patients with peripheral nerve disorders may have an isolated abnormality of a single peripheral nerve (mononeuropathy), a combination of several mononeuropathies (mononeuropathy multiplex; Figure 6-1), or a more generalized process involving peripheral nerves (polyneuropathy; Figure 6-2). Using the terminology defined in Chapter 3, polyneuropathy is a diffuse process, whereas mononeuropathy multiplex is multifocal.

The most common cause of mononeuropathy is compression, especially at a site where the nerve is particularly confined and subject to trauma (such as the median nerve at the carpal tunnel, the ulnar nerve at the elbow, or the peroneal nerve at the knee). In typical cases, no diagnostic testing may be necessary; when there are atypical features, electrodiagnostic studies usually clarify the diagnosis. When the nerve is compressed at an unusual site, imaging studies may be necessary. Compression mononeuropathies (also called entrapment

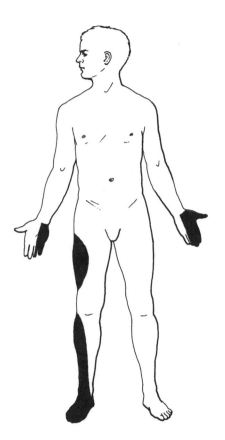

MONONEUROPATHY MULTIPLEX

Figure 6-1. The regions of sensory involvement in a patient with mononeuropathy multiplex. This is a multifocal process affecting several discrete peripheral nerves (in this case, the left median nerve, right ulnar nerve, right lateral cutaneous nerve of the thigh, and right peroneal nerve). The involved areas are not confluent or symmetric.

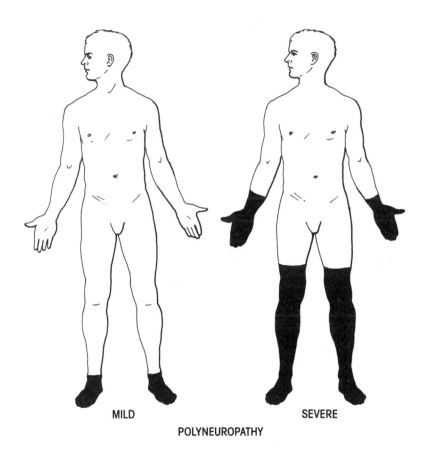

MILD   SEVERE

POLYNEUROPATHY

Figure 6-2. *"Stocking-glove" distribution of sensory loss typical of polyneu-ropathy. This is a diffuse process in which involvement is confluent and sym-metric. With mild disease (the left-hand figure) only the distal lower extremities are involved. With more severe disease (the right-hand figure) there is proximal extension in the lower extremities and the distal upper extremities are also involved.*

mononeuropathies) often respond to stabilization of the joint with a splint or protection with a pad. When they do not respond, the nerve is sometimes surgically exposed and decompressed or moved to a less vulnerable site.

Unlike peripheral nerves elsewhere in the body, cranial nerves are generally well insulated from external pressure, so compression injury to cranial nerves is usually due to pressure from within the nervous system itself. Mass lesions such as tumors or aneurysms or even tortuosities in the vertebral or basilar arteries can compress cranial nerves directly. Cranial nerves may also be compressed as a result of increased intracranial pressure caused by distant mass lesions. A lesion of cranial nerve III due to transtentorial herniation is the most prominent example. Analogously, trauma can damage cranial nerves either directly or by producing shear injury. Cranial nerves I and IV are at particular risk for shear injury. Isolated cranial nerve palsies often result from ischemic disease of penetrating arteries, especially in patients with diabetes or hypertension. Inflammatory disease, both infectious and noninfectious, can cause cranial neuropathies. Neoplastic spread to the meninges can do the same.

Bell's palsy, or idiopathic facial nerve palsy, deserves special mention because it usually has a benign course, in contrast to stroke (with which it is sometimes confused). There is evidence that Herpes simplex or varicella-zoster viruses are responsible for most cases of Bell's palsy. The distinctive feature of Bell's palsy is a LMN pattern of facial weakness, including the forehead muscles (see Chapter 2). There is often associated pain, especially in the ear, and there may be changes in hearing or taste. Patients may also have sensory complaints. Almost all patients recover to some extent within 3 months, and the recovery is complete in 55–85% of patients. Complete facial weakness at the peak of the episode (present in roughly one-half the patients), non-ear pain, and older age are associated with a poorer prognosis. The literature suggests that a brief burst of steroids may improve outcome, but this has never been convincingly demonstrated.

Patients who have multiple cranial neuropathies without involvement of the brainstem parenchyma itself should be evaluated for inflammatory diseases or carcinomatous involvement of the meninges (see Chapter 10). Patients who have multiple mononeuropathies in the limbs may simply have several entrapment mononeuropathies, especially if they engage in activities that involve forceful, repetitive movements. Obese patients have an increased risk of developing compression mononeuropathies, and so do patients with diabetes or thyroid disease. In the absence of these factors, however, or when mononeuropathies occur at sites where entrapment is unusual, the most likely cause of mononeuropathy multiplex is vasculitis. Another possible cause is hereditary neuropathy with liability to pressure palsies, which should be considered even when there is no apparent family history.

When mononeuropathy multiplex is severe, the nerve involvement can become confluent, resembling polyneuropathy. In such cases, the most reliable way to distinguish mononeuropathy multiplex from polyneuropathy is to inquire about the onset of the disease. Mononeuropathy multiplex affects first one nerve and then another in an unpredictable sequence, whereas polyneuropathy affects nerves in a systematic pattern that is evident throughout the course of the disease. The typical pattern of polyneuropathy is that the longest nerves in the body are affected first, and progressively shorter nerves become involved as the condition progresses, resulting in a "stocking-glove" distribution of symptoms. Some polyneuropathies may exhibit variations or deviate from this pattern. In some cases, only myelinated nerves are affected; in others, only unmyelinated nerves are involved. In one case (leprosy), it is said that the coldest (i.e., the most exposed) nerves are involved! In general, if the pattern of nerve involvement cannot be expressed in a rule that makes some physiologic sense, a polyneuropathy is unlikely. For example, it is hard to imagine a plausible rule that would permit involvement of the right median nerve but not the left, or of the left median and radial nerves but not the left ulnar nerve. These would be examples of mononeuropathy multiplex, not polyneuropathy. In time, however, patients with either of these patterns of nerve involvement from mononeuropathy multiplex might progress to have involvement of the median, ulnar, and radial nerves bilaterally, at which point the pattern of nerve involvement would resemble that seen with a polyneuropathy (assuming similar involvement in the lower extremities). Only by taking a detailed history of the onset and progression of the symptoms could the distinction be made.

There are many causes of polyneuropathy. A frequently used mnemonic is DANG THERAPIST:

D   iabetes
A   lcohol
N   utritional (vitamins B_{12}, B_1 [thiamine], B_6, and E)
G   uillain-Barré (acute inflammatory demyelinating polyradiculoneuropathy [AIDP])

T   oxic (lead, arsenic, other metals, many medications)

HE reditary (see below)

R   ecurrent (chronic inflammatory demyelinating polyradiculoneuropathy [CIDP])

A   myloid

P   orphyria

I   nfectious (leprosy, human immunodeficiency virus [HIV],
Lyme, diphtheria, mononucleosis)

S   ystemic (uremia, hypothyroidism, lupus, Sjögren's, Wegener's)

T   umors (paraneoplastic; also CIDP associated with myeloma)

The first two diagnoses in this list merit special comment. Diabetes is the most common cause of polyneuropathy in the United States, and probably the world. There are several patterns of diabetic polyneurop-athy, including a painless loss of sensation with weakness (resulting in unnoticed foot injury and ulcers) and a painful loss of distal leg sensa-tion. Alcohol has traditionally been considered to be another common cause of neuropathy, but it appears that the neuropathy associated with alcohol use may be primarily related to malnutrition. Patients with neuropathy who have a history of alcohol use should be evalu-ated for other potential causes of neuropathy, rather than attributing their condition to alcohol.

In trying to narrow the differential diagnosis in an individual patient, it is obviously helpful to take a detailed history to see whether there is any other evidence that the patient has one of the conditions mentioned in the mnemonic. The pattern of nerve involvement can also be helpful, since different "rules" are followed by different causes of polyneuropa-thy, as already mentioned. For example, pure sensory neuropathies may be associated with paraneoplastic syndromes or connective tissue disor-ders, such as Sjögren's syndrome. Pure sensory neuropathies are uncom-mon, however. Although patients with mild polyneuropathy often report only sensory symptoms and they are unaware of mild weakness, weakness is evident on clinical testing or electrophysiologic testing.

The differential diagnosis of a polyneuropathy may also be nar-rowed by determining whether the process is demyelinating or axonal. Demyelinating neuropathies primarily affect the myelin sheath, resulting in slowed conduction in myelinated nerves. Axonal neuropathies primarily involve the axon processes themselves; both myelinated and unmyelinated fibers are affected. Demyelinating and axonal neuropathies can usually be distinguished based on the results of nerve conduction studies: Demyelinating neuropathies result in abnormal nerve conduction velocities with relatively normal amplitudes, while axonal neuropathies produce the opposite pattern. Most metabolic and systemic diseases produce axonal polyneuropathies. The most common demyelinating polyneuropathies are characterized by inflammation of the myelin sheath and are called inflammatory demyelinating polyradiculoneuropathies. Involvement of myelin occurs both proximally at the root and distally along peripheral nerves. Examples include acute forms (**AIDP**, the most common cause of the clinical condition known as **Guillain-Barré syndrome**) and chronic forms such as **CIDP**. The weakness peaks within 4 weeks in patients with AIDP, whereas the characteristic course of CIDP is slowly progressive or relapsing and remitting.

Hereditary neuropathies are usually very slowly progressive and may go unnoticed in affected family members. The most common forms of hereditary neuropathy fall into the general category of hereditary motor sensory neuropathy, or Charcot-Marie-Tooth (CMT) disease (based on the names of the first clinical observers). CMT disease encompasses a group of neuropathies that are distinguished, in part, on the basis of clinical and electrodiagnostic criteria (such as whether nerve conduction velocities are slow or normal). Further distinction of different forms of CMT is based on the identification of different mutations in genes coding for proteins in myelin, including myelin protein zero, an integral protein in the myelin membrane, and peripheral myelin protein 22.

Treatment of neuropathies depends on the underlying cause. For diabetic neuropathy, the only available treatment at this time is tight glucose control. AIDP and CIDP are believed to include a humorally mediated component and respond to both plasma exchange and intravenous immunoglobulin. Prednisone is also effective for CIDP, but not for AIDP. There are no specific treatments for hereditary neuropathies.

E. Neuromuscular Junction Disorders

Defects of neuromuscular transmission include presynaptic terminal disorders such as botulism and the Lambert-Eaton myasthenic syndrome, and postsynaptic disorders such as myasthenia gravis. Myasthenia gravis is much more common than Lambert-Eaton myasthenic syndrome, and other disorders of the neuromuscular junction (e.g., botulism) are extremely rare. One characteristic feature of myasthenia gravis is fatigability: With repeated muscle use, more neuromuscular junctions fail to transmit impulses, and weakness rapidly becomes apparent as a sense of fatigue. Transmission improves with disuse or rest. The Lambert-Eaton myasthenic syndrome and botulism also produce impaired transmission in autonomic ganglia, causing symptoms such as dry mouth and impotence. Although the reasons are not clear, neuromuscular junction transmission abnormalities in botulism and myasthenia gravis frequently affect a combination of extraocular and lid levator muscles, while these muscles are less involved in the Lambert-Eaton myasthenic syndrome. Detailed electrodiagnostic testing can also reveal clear differences between the various disorders of the neuromuscular junction.

There are two approaches to treating myasthenia gravis: Symptomatic treatment with acetylcholinesterase inhibitors and treatment directed at the presumed pathogenesis of the disease with immunosuppressive agents. Acetylcholinesterase inhibitors, such as the oral drug pyridostigmine (Mestinon), slow the enzymatic degradation of acetylcholine. Acetylcholinesterase inhibition forms the basis of the intravenous edrophonium (Tensilon) test for myasthenia gravis, in which a patient is given a single dose of this short-acting drug to see if weakness briefly improves. Although pyridostigmine can be very effective, it does not treat the underlying pathology, which is thought to be an autoimmune antibody-mediated attack on the postsynaptic receptor or neighboring muscle membrane. For this reason, immunosuppressive medications (such as prednisone or azathioprine) are used. Alternative treatments include administration of intravenous immunoglobulin or removal of the offending antibodies by plasma exchange. This is a procedure in which units of whole blood are removed from the body and separated into the red cell and plasma fractions. The red cells are reinfused, while the plasma with the antibodies is discarded. This also may be very effective but does not address antibody production. In severe myasthenia gravis, a combination of all of these treatment modalities is used. A supplemental therapeutic approach is to remove the thymus gland surgically. The exact role of the thymus in myasthenia is unclear, but it probably has a role in initiating the production of autoimmune antibodies. Myasthenia gravis is associated with thymoma in some patients, so a computed tomography scan of the thorax is generally included in the initial diagnostic evaluation.

F. Muscle Disorders (Myopathies)

As with neuropathies, the differential diagnosis for myopathy is very broad, including hereditary, metabolic, infectious, and inflammatory disorders. Some of the traditional categories and distinctions have started to erode in recent years as a result of advances in molecular biology, but in general, the hereditary conditions are called muscular dystrophies. These most often present early in life, but some forms only become symptomatic in middle age or later. The progression is gradual.

Metabolic myopathies may result from biochemical defects that interfere with the mobilization of energy sources (typically, abnormalities of glycogen metabolism or of lipid metabolism). Certain of these defects result in normal function most of the time (presumably because the muscles can use glucose normally) but cramping after prolonged exercise (when glucose supplies are exhausted and alternative energy sources must be used). Some of the other defects produce unremitting weakness, and in these cases the disease may be progressive. Disorders that interfere with the ability of mitochondria to generate usable energy for cellular processes also produce myopathies. Other metabolic myopathies result from endocrine disorders, including hypothyroidism, hyperthyroidism, hyperparathyroidism, and Cushing's syndrome. Exogenous steroid therapy is a frequent cause of myopathy. Chronic alcohol use may also produce a myopathy.

Polymyositis is the prototypical inflammatory myopathy. As with other myopathies, there is a gradual course, typically over weeks to months. Muscle pain occurs more commonly than with other myopathies, but the disease is painless in a significant proportion of patients. Some patients have an associated skin rash, typically on the face and hands, called *dermatomyositis*. About 10–20% of adult patients with dermatomyositis have a systemic malignancy. In contrast, the incidence of systemic malignancy in patients with polymyositis is no higher than in the general population. While serum CK levels and EMG are typically abnormal in polymyositis, the results usually do not distinguish between this disorder and other primary muscle diseases. The best test for making this distinction is the muscle biopsy.

A muscle biopsy is especially important for distinguishing polymyositis from inclusion body myositis (IBM), another inflammatory myopathy that is being recognized with increasing frequency. In addition to inflammation, the biopsy shows vacuolar inclusions in muscle fibers. One clinical clue that a patient may have IBM rather than polymyositis is a distinctive pattern of weakness, with prominent involvement of forearm flexor muscles and knee extensor muscles. Dysphagia is also common in IBM, and there is mild involvement of facial muscles more often than in polymyositis. IBM is a disease of adults, with symptoms usually beginning in the sixth decade, and it affects men more often than women. It is slowly progressive.

There is no known treatment for inclusion body myositis. Polymyositis responds to prednisone, although relapses sometimes occur when a prednisone taper is attempted, necessitating long-term steroid use that can itself cause myopathy as well as many other side effects including diabetes mellitus, osteoporosis, high blood pressure, promotion of cataracts, and bleeding gastric ulcers. Evidence suggests that steroids may also slow the rate of progression in patients with some muscular dystrophies, though the mechanism is not known and the benefits must be weighed against the potential for long-term complications. There are no specific therapies for muscular dystrophies or congenital myopathies. Metabolic myopathies are addressed by treating the underlying disease when possible.

VII. Symptomatic Treatment

It should be apparent from the discussion so far that specific treatments are available for some neuromuscular diseases (such as myasthenia gravis and polymyositis) but not for others (such as motor neuron disease, IBM, and muscular dystrophy). Either way, treatment directed at symptoms rather than at the underlying disease process may be beneficial.

A. *Emergency Measures*

As noted in Part III, any patient who has a rapidly progressive condition with the potential to affect muscles of respiration should be admitted for observation until it is clear that the clinical situation is stable. These patients should be monitored with daily (and sometimes more frequent) bedside respiratory testing of forced vital capacity (FVC) and negative inspiratory force. Patients whose FVC falls below 10–12 ml/kg require elective intubation. Patients with a rapidly deteriorating negative inspiratory force or FVC should be intubated even sooner, when the FVC falls to 15 ml/kg.

When a patient has a condition that can produce autonomic insufficiency (particularly AIDP), continuous electrocardiogram monitoring and frequent assessment of vital signs are necessary until the clinical situation has stabilized. Significant hypotension and arrhythmias should be treated with medications as needed; in some cases, temporary or permanent cardiac pacing may be required.

B. Non-Urgent Measures: Motor Symptoms

Whether or not there is a treatment for the underlying cause of a patient's weakness, efforts should be made to prevent unnecessary deterioration and to take full advantage of the strength that remains. Physical therapists can teach patients exercises to this effect, and occupational therapists can recommend facilitative devices and environmental modifications to improve function. A formal swallowing evaluation by a speech pathologist may be indicated for patients with dysphagia; depending on the results, simple swallowing strategies may be adequate for some patients, while others may require a temporary or permanent feeding tube. Strategies are also available for patients with dysarthria.

Patients with progressive, irreversible diseases such as motor neuron disease should be encouraged at a relatively early stage in their illness to consider whether they want to be intubated when their respiratory function fails. They should express their wishes clearly to family members, preferably by taking formal legal measures such as writing a living will or designating a durable power of attorney for medical issues.

C. Non-Urgent Measures: Sensory Symptoms

Neuropathic pain often responds to symptomatic treatment with tricyclic antidepressant medications or certain antiepileptic drugs, notably carbamazepine, gabapentin, and phenytoin. The necessary doses are often much lower than those required to treat depression or seizures. Because these medications have many potential side effects and the treatment will not change the underlying condition, patients should be started at low doses and titrated up slowly. An alternative treatment is capsaicin cream, a medication that depletes substance P. It often produces initial irritation, so some advocate applying a topical lidocaine preparation before applying the capsaicin.

There is no reliable treatment for numbness or paresthesias, but if the patient reports significant discomfort, tricyclic antidepressants or gabapentin may be tried.

VIII. Discussion of Case Histories

Cases 1 and 2.

In Cases 1 and 2, the absence of sensory symptoms suggests a primary muscle disease, a neuromuscular junction disorder, or a disease exclusively of motor neurons. In both patients, the limb weakness appears to involve mainly proximal musculature, which is typical of a primary muscle disease or a neuromuscular junction disease (but not motor neuron disease). The prominence of diplopia in the second patient makes a defect in neuromuscular junction transmission most likely, and the fatigability is characteristic of myasthenia gravis. Case 1 is an example of polymyositis, a primary disorder of muscle.

The course of myasthenia gravis fluctuates, accounting for the initial episode of diplopia in Case 2. Primary muscle disease, such as polymyositis, does not fluctuate in this manner.

In both cases, nerve conduction studies were normal for both sensory and motor nerves. This provided additional evidence that these patients did not have a disorder of the peripheral nerves. The first electrodiagnostic difference noted between the two cases was in tests of neuromuscular transmission, with signs of failure in Case 2. In particular, the findings were consistent with those seen in myasthenia gravis and ruled out the other main diagnostic consideration, Lambert-Eaton myasthenic syndrome. This patient was treated with pyridostigmine, with marked improvement. His symptoms did not resolve, however, and prednisone was eventually added.

In Case 1, the EMG was consistent with myopathic damage, but it is difficult to distinguish by EMG between several of the primary muscle diseases, including inflammatory muscle disease (polymyositis and IBM), muscular dystrophy, and congenital myopathy. The best test to distinguish among the primary muscle diseases is muscle biopsy, which in this case showed characteristic findings of polymyositis. This patient was treated with steroids, and her symptoms gradually resolved. The steroids were successfully tapered.

Cases 3 and 4.

In both Case 3 and Case 4 there is evidence of LMN dysfunction such as weakness, fasciculations, and atrophy in Case 3, and weakness with areflexia in Case 4. In Case 4, there is also sensory disturbance, so the site of pathology must be at the level of nerve roots, plexus, or peripheral nerves. This patient's sensory symptoms fit a "stocking-glove" distribution, as is typically seen in a peripheral polyneuropathy, but she has both distal and proximal weakness, which would be unusual early in the course of a polyneuropathy. In most neuropathies, the longest nerves in the body are affected first, and the disability progresses from distal to proximal. In contrast, when there is a polyradicular component, roots going to proximal muscles as well as distal muscles are affected, causing proximal and distal weakness. Thus, the pattern of this patient's symptoms suggests a combined polyradiculopathy and polyneuropathy. The patient in Case 3 has no sensory problems and thus represents an example of motor neuron disease. In addition to the LMN involvement, this patient also has signs of UMN involvement, with spasticity, brisk reflexes, and an extensor plantar response. This pattern of both UMN and LMN involvement is seen in ALS. LMN loss is widespread in ALS, resulting in diffuse atrophy that can explain the weight loss and the general level of fatigue. The initial fall could have been the result of leg weakness unrecognized by the patient at the time.

Electrodiagnostic studies confirmed these impressions. The patient in Case 4 had a nerve conduction study that showed markedly reduced conduction velocity implying an element of demyelination. Based on these results, together with the clinical history and the findings on physical examination, the diagnosis of CIDP was made. In this case, an initial episode remitted spontaneously, while the recurrence took place over 6 months. This woman refused a course of steroids but accepted treatment with intravenous immunoglobulin, and her symptoms stabilized.

The patient in Case 3 had normal nerve conduction studies, but needle EMG showed widespread denervation, consistent with the clinical diagnosis of motor neuron disease. He received physical therapy and appropriate counseling and was treated with riluzole. His weakness continued to progress, and he developed an aspiration pneumonia 18 months later. His respiratory status declined precipitously, and in accordance with his previously expressed wishes, he was not intubated or resuscitated.

7

Dementing Illnesses

Linda M. Selwa and Douglas J. Gelb

I. Case Histories

Case 1. A 72-year-old woman with a history of hypertension has been brought to the emergency room by her daughter, who says, "She's been getting worse for 6 months, but I hoped it wouldn't come to this." Her decline began with stomach troubles, which prompted her first visit to a doctor in years, and ranitidine (Zantac) was prescribed. She was started on methyldopa (Aldomet) because her blood pressure was noted to be high, and when her blood pressure failed to normalize, the dose was increased. She began calling her daughter late at night to complain that she couldn't sleep and that she was scared to be alone. She was given a prescription for flurazepam (Dalmane) to treat her insomnia. Her gait became unsteady, and she fell and hurt her hip 1 week ago. She has been taking pain medicine ever since. When her daughter went to check on her late this afternoon, she was lying in bed and the sheets were soaked with urine. She did not recognize her daughter at first, and when she did, asked her, "Who are all those little men with you?"

On examination, the patient is alert but agitated and inattentive. Her speech is fluent, but often tangential or irrelevant. She follows simple commands but becomes irritated with complicated ones. She is disoriented to time and thinks she has been brought to "the precinct house." She states her name correctly, except that she gives her maiden name rather than her married name. She recalls two of four objects after 4 minutes and can spell "world" forward but not backward. When asked to name the president, she becomes angry. She can name all five of her siblings but can't remember where they each live. The rest of her examination is normal, except that her reflexes are slightly brisker on the right than on the left. She has a high serum white blood cell count, pyuria, normal electrolytes, and normal renal and hepatic function. A head CT scan and lumbar puncture are normal.

Questions:

1. Is this woman likely to have Alzheimer's disease?

2. How would you evaluate her in the emergency room?

3. What underlying illnesses are possible?

4. How would you direct her subsequent evaluation and treatment?

Case 2. An 81-year-old man came to see his family doctor because his wife "thought he needed to be checked." The patient reported that nothing was wrong with him and that his wife had always been overly protective. His wife reminded him that he had had trouble driving recently, getting lost on several familiar streets, and that at a recent reunion, he had been unable to recall friends. She said they had gotten an accountant 2 years ago because he felt the finances were "just too complex" and several bills had gone unpaid. She noted that her husband was not taking his usual care in dressing. The patient responded that she "was making mountains out of anthills." He said that she would do better to worry about the recent burglary in their house. When his wife asked, "What burglary?" the patient said he had not wanted to worry her, but ever since they returned from a recent trip, "things were missing" around the house and new scratches had appeared on their antique furniture. He had concluded that the home was burglarized and might still be "under watch."

Except for a long history of gout and an ulcer many years ago, the patient has no history of medical problems. He takes no medications. His general physical examination is normal. He is very outgoing and speaks fluently, frequently joking about his age. He makes frequent paraphasic errors (i.e., he uses incorrect words) and sometimes makes up his own words. He cannot recall any of three simple objects and says "that was much too long ago." He is aware of the clinic name but not the town and says it is "fallish" in 1982 or 1992. He cannot name the current president, but when told the answer, he says, "I knew that. I thought you asked if I had ever met him." He is unable to name two of his five children. He has significant difficulty drawing a clock. The remainder of his examination is normal.

Questions:

1. Does this man have Alzheimer's disease?

2. What tests would be appropriate in his evaluation?

3. What other questions about his daily life would be important in management?

4. Would it be appropriate to discuss a durable power of attorney?

Case 3. A 64-year-old woman was brought in for evaluation because she had been "acting strangely" for several months. Six months ago, she lost a significant amount of vision in her right eye and was told she had a "stroke in the eye." Since then, she had complained of headaches and seemed to have a gradually progressive memory problem. She had been intermittently sleepy, was often confused about her location, and did inappropriate things that were "out of character," including urinating in bed and not dressing properly. At times, she appeared to function perfectly normally but at other times seemed delusional.

At the time of evaluation, she had a low-grade fever and complained of headache. Her general physical examination was normal. She was alert at times but at other times tended to doze off. She had fluent speech, with normal comprehension, repetition, and naming abilities. She could spell "world" but had difficulty spelling it backwards. She could only recall two of four objects at 5 minutes. She was disoriented to place but could readily report all of her seven grandchildren's ages and middle names. She could name the president, mayor, and secretary of state. She demonstrated an appropriate level of abstraction in interpreting similarities and differences, but her judgment seemed impaired. Except for visual acuity of 20/50 in the right eye, there were no other abnormalities. She had a high peripheral white blood cell count, erythrocyte sedimentation rate (ESR) of 74, and normal electrolytes. Urinalysis revealed a urinary tract infection (UTI). Head CT and lumbar puncture were normal except for minimally elevated cerebrospinal fluid (CSF) protein of 60.

Questions:

    1. Is this woman likely to have Alzheimer's disease?

    2. What further evaluation is necessary?

    3. What is the best plan for follow-up and treatment?

II. Approach to Dementing Illnesses

Patients with symptoms of cognitive impairment should be evaluated systematically by addressing the following questions:

    A. Are the patient's symptoms truly abnormal?

    B. Does the patient have memory deficits exclusively, or are other cognitive functions impaired also?

    C. Is the problem progressive?

    D. Does the patient have a potentially reversible cause of progressive dementia?

    E. Do the patient's history, examination, and test results suggest a specific primary dementing illness, especially Alzheimer's disease, multi-infarct dementia, or dementia with Lewy bodies?

    The following discussion expands on each of these questions and their significance.

A. Is It Abnormal?

As public awareness of Alzheimer's disease has grown, it has become more common for patients or their family members to express concern to physicians about declining memory. This concern is especially common with older patients, but even young adults frequently worry about the fact that they have trouble thinking of words or remembering facts. People who have watched close associates or family members struggle with Alzheimer's disease may be especially concerned when they perceive themselves having similar difficulties. They become very self-conscious, as any slight mistake serves to confirm their worst fears. The physician's task is to identify those patients in whom there is a legitimate suspicion of dementia and reassure the rest.

A detailed description of specific incidents can be helpful in this regard. Patients who are concerned about an occasional lost bill or missed appointment are often just anxious. Anxiety and self-consciousness can exacerbate commonplace difficulty in retrieving information, such as inability to produce the name of a casual acquaintance. In contrast, when patients report problems with routine cooking or other chores at home, when they have episodes of disorientation while driving in areas that should be familiar, or when employers or colleagues at work express concern about their job performance, a thorough evaluation is necessary.

It is sometimes maintained that patients with dementing illnesses are oblivious to their problem, so patients who are worried that they might have dementia probably don't. This rule is not reliable. On the other hand, if a patient is able to provide a detailed account of the circumstances in which memory lapses have occurred, and the specific details that were forgotten at the time, a dementing illness is unlikely. When the patient acknowledges memory problems but must turn to family members to provide examples, the memory loss is probably significant.

B. Is It Dementia?

Dementia is defined as an acquired impairment of memory and at least one other cognitive function, without clouding of the sensorium or underlying psychiatric disease. This definition explicitly excludes some important categories of disease, which must be considered before concluding that a patient has dementia.

Delirium is defined as an acute confusional state characterized by clouded, reduced, or shifting attention and often associated with sensory misperceptions and disturbed thinking. These patients usually have a toxic or metabolic problem, and their evaluation is described in Chapter 11.

Differentiation between dementia and depression may be extremely difficult at times. A "chicken and egg" problem arises: Demented patients often are (understandably) depressed, while patients with primary depression may have so much slowing of their thought and speech and such limited motivation that they appear demented. This has been called the "pseudodementia" of depression. If a patient has vegetative signs, such as changes in eating or sleeping patterns, or if the symptoms had an obvious precipitant such as the death of a spouse, depression is a major consideration. Dementia can also be associated with changes in eating or sleeping, however, and cognitive symptoms may go unnoticed until the death of a spouse who had previously been "covering for" the patient's deficits. Various diagnostic tests have been suggested for differentiating dementia and depression, but none is completely reliable. At times, an empiric trial of antidepressant medication is necessary.

A particularly difficult diagnostic challenge arises when patients and their family members report that they have observed no change in thinking or behavior beyond the memory problem. In some of these patients, more generalized impairment becomes evident in response to direct questioning: Have there been mistakes in writing checks, balancing the checkbook, paying bills (beyond simply forgetting to pay them), preparing taxes, or figuring change at stores? Has the patient been getting lost in previously familiar places? Does he or she have difficulty understanding complicated instructions? Have there been problems with routine household tasks such as using a dishwasher or mowing the lawn? Does the patient seem to have trouble seeing things, even with optimal corrective lenses? The mental status examination and formal neuropsychologic testing can also help elicit nonmemory deficits.

A patient in whom a thorough history and careful testing reveal only memory deficits, with no evidence of other cognitive impairment, does not have dementia. This condition has been referred to by a variety of terms, including "isolated memory impairment," "age-associated memory impairment," and "mild cognitive impairment." Patients with this profile form a heterogeneous group. In longitudinal studies, about 50% of these patients develop dementia within 5 years. Of the remainder, some probably develop dementia over an even longer time-frame, but others never do. Some of these patients may represent one extreme of the mild memory loss that occurs with normal aging, and others may have a pathologic process that is completely distinct from the established dementing illnesses. Either way, these patients are often able to compensate for their memory loss by following highly structured routines, keeping meticulous notes, and using other memory aids. Although this can still be a very distressing condition, it is far less debilitating than advanced dementia. Unfortunately, there is no way to predict with certainty which patients with this clinical presentation will persist in having a pure memory problem and which patients will ultimately develop dementia. Patients must be informed of both possibilities and followed over time.

Striking loss of short-term and long-term memory with preserved immediate recall and relatively preserved remote memory occurs in Korsakoff's syndrome, a condition most common in chronic alcoholics. A similar pattern of deficits can result from bilateral temporal lobe damage due to anoxia, encephalitis (especially herpes simplex), head trauma, or bilateral surgical procedures. In all of these conditions, other cognitive functions remain intact, so these are not dementing illnesses.

C. Is It Progressive?

A wide variety of neurologic insults, such as head trauma, meningoencephalitis, and subarachnoid hemorrhage, may cause a significant deterioration in cognitive function that subsequently remains stable or improves. These nonprogressive dementias do not present the same diagnostic or management issues as the progressive dementias and are not to be considered further here.

D. Is There a Potentially Reversible Cause?

Dementia is a clinical syndrome, not a specific disease. Many different diseases can produce dementia. The four most common causes are Alzheimer's disease, dementia with Lewy bodies, frontotemporal dementia, and a multi-infarct state. Unfortunately, there is no reliable diagnostic test for any of these diagnoses. While a reasonably accurate diagnosis can usually be established from historic information and examination findings, it is also important to exclude any other reasonably common cause of dementia for which a specific diagnostic test is available, focusing especially on the causes for which treatment is available.

A careful history and thorough physical examination can identify many of the situations in which dementia is just one component of a more generalized disease process, such as Parkinson's disease, tertiary syphilis, or hypothyroidism. A structural imaging study of the brain should be obtained, looking for hydrocephalus or mass lesions (such as primary or metastic brain tumors, abscesses, or subdural hematomas). An imaging study is also helpful in determining the likelihood of a multi-infarct state. Blood should be screened for thyroid disease and deficiency of vitamin B_{12} or folate. Serum FTA (fluorescent treponemal antibody) or MHA-TP (microhemagglutination–*Treponema pallidum*) should be sent to screen for neurosyphilis (VDRL and RPR [rapid plasma reagin] are not sufficient in this context, because they convert back to normal in a substantial fraction of patients with late stages of syphilis). If the dementia has progressed rapidly, the evaluation should include HIV testing and spinal fluid analysis for chronic meningitis or other inflammatory conditions. Systemic inflammatory diseases such as systemic lupus erythematosus or temporal arteritis may present with dementia, and an ESR can be used as a screen. Hematologic diseases, systemic infections, and disorders of electrolytes, glucose, renal, or hepatic function are unlikely to be the underlying cause of dementia without producing delirium or obvious systemic symptoms. Even so, screening for these conditions is important because dementia from any cause may be exacerbated by systemic illness, and treatment of the systemic disease may result in significant improvement of cognitive function even when the underlying dementing illness is irreversible. Furthermore, a demented patient may fail to report symptoms that would otherwise make a systemic illness obvious.

To summarize, a standard battery of tests to screen for potentially reversible causes of dementia would include the following:

serum   Electrolytes, blood urea nitrogen, creatinine, glucose, calcium, liver enzymes, complete blood cell count, differential, ESR, vitamin B_{12}, folate, thyroid-stimulating hormone, and FTA or MHA-TP.
urine   Urinalysis.
imaging   Head CT or MRI.

Patients and families should be warned in advance that the yield from this investigation is likely to be low, because Alzheimer's disease, dementia with Lewy bodies, frontotemporal dementia, and multi-infarct dementia are far more common than all of the remaining causes of dementia combined. Structural causes of dementia are particularly unlikely if no focal abnormalities are evident on examination. There are occasional examples of patients with nonfocal examinations who are found to have slowly growing tumors or bilateral subdural hematomas (where the bilateral focal findings "cancel each other out"), but these are rare.

E. Which Diagnosis Is Most Likely?

Because there are no completely reliable diagnostic tests for the most common primary dementing illnesses, the diagnosis is based on how closely a patient's history, examination, and test results match the typical pattern of one of these conditions. Definitive diagnosis usually requires neuropathologic confirmation, but clinical features permit an accurate diagnosis during life in most patients. Physicians should be open with patients and families about the likely diagnosis or diagnoses. Although physicians sometimes avoid using terms like **dementia** or **Alzheimer's disease** because they are reluctant to frighten or depress patients, they should realize that the possibility will not come as a surprise to most patients and families.

III. Primary Dementing Illnesses

A. Alzheimer's Disease

1. Epidemiology, pathology, and etiology

Alzheimer's disease is the most common cause of progressive dementia in adults. Its prevalence rises exponentially with age after age 65 years. In one survey of community residents, Alzheimer's disease affected 3% of individuals between the ages of 65 and 74 years, 18.7% of individuals aged 75–84 years, and 47% of individuals over age 85 years. Familial Alzheimer's disease (FAD), with an autosomal dominant pattern of inheritance, accounts for about 10% of cases of Alzheimer's disease. There is no straightforward hereditary pattern in the remaining 90% of patients, although genetic factors do play a role.

The cause of Alzheimer's disease remains unknown, despite extensive investigation. The characteristic pathologic features are "plaques" of dystrophic neurites around a central core of beta amyloid and "tangles" of paired helical filaments in the cytoplasm of neuronal cell bodies. Additional plaque-like deposits have been identified using antibodies that bind to a novel protein extracted from paired helical filaments. Cell loss is most prominent in the temporal and parietal lobes. A number of neurochemical abnormalities have been described, including loss of choline acetyltransferase in neurons with cell bodies in the nucleus basalis of Meynert.

The role of beta amyloid in the pathogenesis of Alzheimer's disease remains unclear. Beta amyloid is a part of a larger protein, called beta amyloid precursor protein (APP), which is present in normal brain cells. In some families with FAD the disease is linked to mutations in the APP gene (located on chromosome 21), providing strong evidence that APP has a role in the pathogenesis of Alzheimer's disease in these families. Additional evidence is supplied by transgenic mice that express APP mutations and show behavioral and neuropathologic features analogous to human Alzheimer's disease. Although abnormal APP may be sufficient to trigger the development of Alzheimer's disease, it may not be a necessary condition—mutations in the APP gene account for only 5–10% of FAD cases and less than 1% of all cases of Alzheimer's disease. Most of the mutations that have been identified in FAD occur on chromosome 14 and involve the gene for a protein that has been dubbed presenilin-1. Mutations in a highly homologous gene on chromosome 1, called the presenilin-2 gene, have also been linked to FAD. About 50% of cases of FAD have mutations in genes that have not yet been identified. It may be that all these mutations in some way affect amyloid or some other final common pathway, or it may be that there are multiple independent pathophysiologic processes that can lead to Alzheimer's disease.

The genes for APP and the presenilins are deterministic: All individuals who inherit the defective gene will develop Alzheimer's disease unless they die of some other disease first. Susceptibility genes for Alzheimer's disease—genes associated with an increased likelihood of developing the disease, but not a 100% correlation—have also been identified. The strongest association is with the gene for apolipoprotein E (ApoE). There are three common alleles of the ApoE gene: E2, E3, and E4. The frequency of the E4 allele in patients with late-onset sporadic Alzheimer's disease is approximately double the frequency found in control groups. Moreover, in this group of patients, the age of onset of Alzheimer's disease correlates with the number of E4 alleles, such that the average age of symptom onset is considerably lower in homozygotes for E4 than in heterozygotes, and highest of all in patients with no copies of the E4 allele. Even so, some homozygotes never develop the disease, and a significant fraction of patients with Alzheimer's disease have no E4 allele. Other genes that may be associated with a higher risk of Alzheimer's disease include the HLA-A2 gene and low-density lipoprotein–related protein gene. It remains unclear how ApoE and other genes influence pathogenesis and how these factors interact with amyloid and the presenilins.

2. Clinical features

Although patients with Alzheimer's disease have widespread cognitive deficits, not all cognitive functions are affected equally. There is no "typical" pattern of deficits. Some patients have nearly preserved language function and social skills that allow them to compensate for their memory deficits, which are only evident with explicit testing. Others have dramatic word-finding difficulty but they are still able to handle their finances. Some become irritable and argumentative while others become placid. There are countless variations. Even so, memory loss is typically the first symptom noted in Alzheimer's disease, and it remains the most prominent symptom throughout the early course of the disease (if not longer). Indeed, if some other cognitive dysfunction (such as a language disturbance, "frontal lobe deficits," or a problem with visuospatial perception) is the principal abnormality, conditions such as frontotemporal dementia or focal cortical degeneration should be considered.

Patients with typical clinical features of Alzheimer's disease and no evidence for any other cause of dementia even after systematic screening tests are classified as having **probable Alzheimer's disease;** this is the highest degree of diagnostic certainty that can be achieved while the patient is alive. Patients with atypical clinical features (such as an abnormal gait early in the course, or predominance of a focal cognitive deficit) and patients in whom another potential cause of dementia is present are classified as having **possible Alzheimer's disease.** When patients meet all the clinical criteria for probable Alzheimer's disease *and* autopsy findings are typical of Alzheimer's disease, they are classified as having **definite Alzheimer's disease.** Depending on the neuropathologic criteria applied, 64–86% of patients who meet the clinical criteria for probable Alzheimer's disease and who later come to autopsy prove to have definite Alzheimer's disease.

For most patients with Alzheimer's disease, dementia is the only neurologic abnormality present early in the course of the disease, but additional abnormalities commonly develop over time. Parkinsonian features (specifically bradykinesia and rigidity) are especially common and are present in a substantial proportion of patients at the time of their initial evaluation. This can lead to diagnostic uncertainty, because 25–40% of patients with Parkinson's disease develop dementia, and dementia with Lewy bodies is also characterized by a combination of cognitive impairment and parkinsonism. Indeed, the neuropathologic features of these conditions also overlap. In general, patients whose parkinsonian features are less prominent and developed later than their cognitive deficits usually have Alzheimer's disease, but exceptions occur.

Myoclonus is also common in advanced Alzheimer's disease, but it is rarely present at the onset of cognitive impairment. Seizures occur in up to 10% of patients, especially late in the course. Complex partial seizures can be quite subtle in demented patients, so this possibility should be considered whenever episodes of unresponsiveness are reported. Patients with Alzheimer's disease may also develop spasticity, dysarthria, and dysphagia. Incontinence occasionally occurs early in the course but is much more common later, and it is often one of the most difficult issues caretakers confront. Another difficult management problem is posed by psychiatric manifestations. When these are prominent early in the course of the disease, an alternative diagnosis—especially dementia with Lewy bodies or fronto-temporal dementia—should be considered, but psychiatric symptoms eventually occur in about 50% of patients with Alzheimer's disease. Delusions, agitation, and depression are common. Hallucinations are less common but also occur. Wandering behavior and sleep disturbances can also present management challenges.

The course of Alzheimer's disease is extremely variable, so it is very difficult to predict exactly when individual patients will lose specific functions or how long they will live. The average length of survival after the onset of symptoms is 8–10 years. Patients with Alzheimer's disease have a shorter life expectancy than age-matched controls. Some studies have indicated that the best guide to prognosis is the rate at which deterioration has occurred to date; other studies indicate that the current degree of severity is the best predictor. In any case, family members should be aware that the disease is invariably progressive: At some point, patients will have to restrict their activities, allowing others to handle finances, cook, or do home repairs. Patients will eventually develop deficits in reading, reasoning, or visual perception that make it unsafe for them to drive. At later stages, the ability to maintain personal hygiene is lost, and patients may become progressively more agitated to the point of violence or progressively more withdrawn to the point of akinesia. They will eventually lose the ability to recognize even spouses and children. Death usually results from infection, most often due to aspiration pneumonia or urosepsis.

3. Diagnostic tests

The principal role for brain imaging studies in diagnosing Alzheimer's disease is to exclude other potential causes of progressive dementia. The reading of "atrophy" on a CT or magnetic resonance imaging scan is not standardized, and it can occur without any clinical evidence of dementia, just as dementia patients may have normal brain volume. Functional imaging studies (positron emission tomography, single photon emission computed tomography) show a typical pattern of reduced temporo-parietal metabolism and blood flow in patients with probable Alzheimer's disease, but the sensitivity and specificity of these results have not been established, especially in patients with early or equivocal dementia. Despite the strong association between ApoE genotype and the risk of developing Alzheimer's disease, at least 35–50% of patients with Alzheimer's disease carry no E4 alleles. It has been suggested that the presence of an E4 allele is specific for Alzheimer's disease in patients who meet clinical criteria for probable Alzheimer's disease, but this result requires verification in a wide range of clinical settings. The cerebrospinal fluid of patients with Alzheimer's disease contains higher than normal levels of the microtubule-associated protein tau and lower than normal levels of the amyloid protein extending to position 42 (Aβ42), but the sensitivity and specificity of these results (individually or in combination) have yet to be established in a population of patients with dementia of diverse etiologies. Elevated cerebrospinal fluid levels of neuronal thread protein, as well as other serologic tests, radiologic tests, skin tests, and pupillary reaction measurements, have also been proposed to have diagnostic utility, but no test has yet been demonstrated to have sufficient sensitivity or specificity to be useful clinically.

4. Treatment

Two cholinesterase inhibitors, donepezil (Aricept) and tetrahydroaminoacridine (tacrine hydrochloride, Cognex), are currently approved and available for treatment of patients with Alzheimer's disease. They both produce a modest, but statistically significant, improvement on neuropsychologic measures and on clinician and family ratings of symptom severity. The amount of improvement is equivalent to the amount an average patient deteriorates in 6 months, so the effect of treatment can be likened to "setting the clock back" by 6 months. Treatment does not stop progression or even slow it down. The duration of the beneficial effect is unknown—the longest period of follow-up in any study was 30 weeks—but the effect is probably temporary because the drugs are not directed at the underlying cause of disease. The two medications appear to produce a similar degree of improvement. Because of a more favorable side-effect profile and dosing schedule, donepezil has largely supplanted tacrine. Another cholinesterase inhibitor that has also been shown to produce modest cognitive improvement in Alzheimer's disease, rivastigmine (Exelon), has been approved for release, and other cholinesterase inhibitors are at various stages of development and review.

Antioxidants may have a beneficial effect in patients with Alzheimer's disease, based on a study in which patients were randomized to receive either alpha-tocopherol (vitamin E), selegiline, both, or neither.

The placebo group reached the primary outcome states (nursing home placement and death) more quickly than the other three groups. These results must be interpreted with caution, for several reasons. First, there was no significant difference between the groups with respect to scores on cognitive tests. Second, even the difference between groups on the primary outcome measures was only evident after a post-hoc statistical correction for baseline level of function. Third, the combination of vitamin E and selegiline was no more effective than either agent alone. Finally, the degree to which vitamin E crosses the blood-brain barrier has been questioned, raising the possibility that any benefit that it produces might simply be due to its systemic effects. Despite these reservations, vitamin E is fairly safe and well tolerated at the doses used in the study (1,000 IU twice a day), so it is reasonable for patients to take it. There is less reason to prescribe selegiline, because it has more potential side-effects and confers no added benefit.

Some studies have suggested that gingko extracts may be beneficial in Alzheimer's disease, but the evidence to date is not persuasive. A variety of other classes of agents, including muscarinic and nicotinic agonists, serotonergics, glycinergics, noradrenergics, calcium channel blockers, metabolic enhancers, and nerve growth factors, are still under investigation.

Epidemiologic studies indicate that postmenopausal estrogen replacement therapy may be associated with a reduced risk of developing Alzheimer's disease, and chronic users of nonsteroidal anti-inflammatory drugs may also have a lower risk of developing Alzheimer's disease than other individuals. All of the evidence to date comes from nonrandomized population analyses, so although the findings may signify that these medications have a protective effect, another possibility is that these medications are typically used by patients who for some reason already have a lower than average risk of developing Alzheimer's disease. Whether or not these agents have a protective effect, controlled trials have demonstrated no benefit for estrogen or prednisone in patients who already *have* Alzheimer's disease.

The current standard for managing patients with Alzheimer's disease consists of donepezil (with or without vitamin E) together with symptomatic treatment. This includes antipsychotic agents or antiepileptic drugs for agitation, and antidepressants and antibiotics as necessary. "Sundowning" and sleep disorders sometimes respond to light therapy. Safety issues are very important, and access to stoves, power tools, driving, and even unsupervised walks should be individually discussed and monitored. Measures to ease the burden on caregivers are also critical. Families should be advised of community resources such as senior apartment complexes, home health aides, day care activities, visiting nurses, temporary respite programs, and (for more debilitated patients) full-time nursing care or nursing home placement. The availability of these resources depends on the community and the family's financial situation and insurance coverage, and families may wish to consult a social worker. Patients should be encouraged to issue advance directives while they are still competent. Advance directives are documents expressing patients' wishes regarding medical, legal, and financial decisions. The two most common forms of advance directives are the living will and power of attorney. In a living will, a patient expresses specific preferences regarding specific situations (such as when the patient would want to be put on mechanical ventilation, if ever). With power of attorney, the patient designates an individual who will be responsible for making these decisions for the patient. Neither a living will nor a power of attorney can be issued unless the patient is legally competent, and neither one can take effect until the patient has become incompetent.

B. Dementia with Lewy Bodies

Lewy bodies are eosinophilic intracytoplasmic neuronal inclusions that were first described in the substantia nigra and other subcortical locations in patients with Parkinson's disease (see Chapter 8). It is now recognized that widespread cortical Lewy bodies can be identified at autopsy in many patients with dementia, and dementia with Lewy bodies is considered to be the second most common degenerative dementia of the elderly. Retrospective studies of the medical records of patients with these neuropathologic findings identified a number of clinical characteristics that seemed to distinguish these patients from patients with Alzheimer's disease. The three most helpful were parkinsonian motor features early in the course of the disease, prominent psychiatric manifestations (especially visual hallucinations) early in the course, and fluctuations in cognitive function. In subsequent prospective studies these characteristics were reported to predict with a high rate of accuracy which patients would have widespread cortical Lewy bodies. Nevertheless, there is considerable overlap between dementia with Lewy bodies, Alzheimer's disease, and Parkinson's disease with respect to both clinical and neuropathologic features. Classification systems and pathophysiologic theories are still evolving.

There have been no clinical trials to date of management strategies directed specifically at dementia with Lewy bodies. The parkinsonian motor signs sometimes respond to the same medications used to treat Parkinson's disease. It is not known whether donepezil is effective for the dementia that occurs in this condition, but it is probably worth trying, especially because it is difficult to be confident of the diagnosis. The same symptomatic treatment modalities used for Alzheimer's disease also apply to dementia with Lewy bodies, except that extreme sensitivity to antipsychotic agents has been reported, so these medications should be used with caution.

C. Frontotemporal Dementia

In contrast to Alzheimer's disease, which preferentially involves the temporal and parietal lobes, some degenerative disorders have a predilection for the frontal and temporal lobes. Fronto-temporal dementia is now thought to constitute 10–15% of all cases of dementia. These disorders have a younger age of onset than Alzheimer's disease or multi-infarct dementia. The most common clinical presentation is a profound alteration in personality and behavior, which can manifest either as inertia and withdrawal or as social disinhibition. Speech output is usually attenuated. Memory is relatively preserved initially. Some cases are characterized by progressive aphasia with otherwise intact cognitive function.

The clinical syndrome of frontotemporal dementia encompasses a heterogeneous group of disorders, with neuropathologic findings that overlap the traditional diagnoses of Pick's disease and corticobasal ganglionic degeneration. About one-half of the cases are familial, usually with an autosomal dominant inheritance pattern. More than a dozen families have been identified with syndromes linked to a particular region of chromosome 17, and there is evidence that these mutations alter the ability of tau proteins to bind microtubules.

Frontotemporal dementia is steadily progressive, but the decline can be rapid or slow. There is no specific treatment. Behavioral management is often the most prominent practical issue.

D. Multi-Infarct Dementia

There is general agreement that dementia can result from the accumulated effects of multiple strokes, each of which in isolation would be insufficient to produce dementia and could even be completely asymptomatic. There is not much agreement about anything else concerning this condition. How big must the strokes be? How many are required? Are specific locations important? Is the diagnosis likely if the patient and family members cannot recall a single episode of focal neurologic deficits or abrupt deterioration? How specific are white matter abnormalities on magnetic resonance imaging that are typically considered to represent ischemic disease? There is not even a consensus on terminology; the terms *vascular dementia, ischemic vascular dementia, multi-infarct dementia, leukoaraiosis,* and *Binswanger's disease* are used interchangeably by some authors, whereas other authors impart specific and distinct meaning to some of these terms and discourage the use of some of the other terms altogether. In fact, different consensus groups meeting to clarify the situation each chose different terms for the diagnosis and produced somewhat different diagnostic criteria. Even so, all investigators agree that certain factors increase the likelihood that a patient's dementia is due to vascular disease: a history of recognized strokes, focal abnormalities on the neurologic examination, a history of stroke risk factors, abrupt onset of dementia, stepwise progression, and brain imaging studies that suggest multiple ischemic lesions.

The course of multi-infarct dementia is even less predictable than the course of Alzheimer's disease. The average life expectancy after symptom onset is 6–8 years. In principle, progression can be halted completely if future strokes can be prevented, so these patients are candidates for all of the primary and secondary stroke prevention measures discussed in Chapter 4. One difficult issue that can arise is whether carotid stenosis should be considered symptomatic or asymptomatic in a patient with multi-infarct dementia but no history of discrete episodes of focal neurologic deficits. As discussed in Chapter 4, endarterectomy is an effective treatment for severe stenosis in both symptomatic and asymptomatic patients, but the results are far more compelling for symptomatic patients. Patients who are thought to have multi-infarct dementia on the basis of penetrating artery disease would fall into the category of asymptomatic carotid stenosis. In this situation the patients' overall physical condition and coexisting medical problems may be the most important factors in deciding whether to perform an endarterectomy.

Other than stroke prevention, only symptomatic therapy is available, and the same considerations that apply to Alzheimer's disease in that regard are relevant to patients with multi-infarct dementia.

E. Normal-Pressure Hydrocephalus

Patients with obstruction to ventricular outflow accumulate CSF at increased pressure in all portions of the ventricular system proximal to the obstruction. This condition, called obstructive hydrocephalus, is associated with cognitive deterioration, gait disturbance, and incontinence, together with symptoms and signs of increased intracranial pressure. Treatment is directed at removing the obstruction, if possible, and draining the enlarged ventricular system.

Normal-pressure hydrocephalus (NPH) is an analogous syndrome, except that the ventricular enlargement occurs without an increase in intracranial pressure, and there is no structural obstruction to outflow. Some of these patients have a history of previous meningeal irritation (e.g., from meningitis or subarachnoid hemorrhage), presumably resulting in impaired CSF absorption at the level of the arachnoid granulations. In other patients no cause can be identified. In any event, NPH is a syndrome characterized by the clinical triad of dementia, gait disturbance, and incontinence; enlargement of the ventricular system on brain imaging studies; and clinical improvement in response to ventricular shunting procedures.

Unfortunately, the entire syndrome rarely presents in a clear-cut fashion. Some patients have one or two components of the clinical triad, but not all three. Some patients have sulcal enlargement that is at least as prominent as the ventricular enlargement, suggesting that the primary problem is brain atrophy, not hydrocephalus. Moreover, the clinical triad is not necessarily specific (e.g., patients with Alzheimer's disease can develop gait abnormalities because of parkinsonian features or spasticity, and incontinence is common late in the disease). Ultimately, the important question is which patients are likely to respond to shunting. Many different clinical rules have been suggested. For example, some investigators have found that shunting is most likely to be beneficial in patients for whom dementia was not the presenting symptom. Others have found that the longer symptoms have been present, the less likely a shunt will produce improvement. Unfortunately, for every rule that has been proposed, there are also studies finding it to be an unreliable guide to shunt response. This has led to a search for a useful diagnostic test. Cisternography, blood flow studies, CSF pressure monitoring, CSF infusion tests, and high-volume lumbar punctures have all been proposed as indicators of likelihood of response to shunting. None of these tests has proved to be consistently reliable.

The clinician is therefore compelled to make a judgment call when some features suggest NPH but others do not. In such situations, shunting is often worth a try (assuming the patient and family agree, after all the relevant issues have been explained). The procedure is fairly benign (the main complications are infection and subdural hematoma), and although dramatic improvement is uncommon, even a slight chance of significant functional recovery may be worth the risk of the procedure.

F. Creutzfeldt-Jakob Disease

Creutzfeldt-Jakob disease (CJD) is a rare condition characterized by rapidly progressive dementia (with a mean survival time of 5 months), myoclonus, and ataxia. Most patients (80%) are ages 50–70 years. The majority of patients demonstrate a characteristic abnormality on EEG, periodic complexes occurring about once a second. The typical neuropathologic findings are widespread neuronal loss and vacuolation, producing a spongy appearance; this condition is also called *subacute spongiform encephalopathy.*

The disease is usually sporadic, but about 5–10% of cases are familial, and there have been rare cases of transmission via corneal transplants, contaminated surgical instruments, implanted EEG electrodes, and growth hormone (derived from pooled pituitary tissue). The transmissible agent has been called a *prion*; it is a proteinaceous particle that contains little or no nucleic acid. A closely related protein having the exact same sequence of amino acids but a different post-translational structure and hence different physical properties occurs in normal human brain. Familial forms of CJD and related diseases show genetic linkage to point mutations in the gene that codes for this protein.

A new variant of CJD was described in Great Britain in the mid-1990s, with a younger age of onset, prominent psychiatric manifestations, no periodic complexes on EEG, and some distinctive neuropathologic features. Prion glycosylation patterns in these patients resemble those seen in cattle affected by an epidemic of bovine spongiform encephalopathy that erupted in the late 1980s. The implications of this development are still unclear. A number of prion-related transmissible spongiform encephalopathies of animals have been recognized for years, with no previous suggestion of transmission to humans.

Even though CJD is rare, it should be considered when a patient presents with very rapid progression of dementia, or with prominent myoclonus or ataxia early in the disease. An EEG may be diagnostic. Elevated levels of a normal brain protein known as 14-3-3 protein are found in the CSF of 96% of patients with sporadic CJD. The levels are also elevated in patients with other acute neurologic disease such as herpes simplex encephalitis or recent stroke, but in the proper clinical setting this test can be useful. There is no known treatment for CJD, but if the diagnosis can be established, important prognostic information can be delivered to the family.

G. Other Neurologic Diseases That Produce Dementia

Dementia is common in Parkinson's disease, as discussed earlier. A number of other movement disorders typically produce dementia. Several of these are discussed in Chapter 8. Dementia can also occur with some forms of muscular dystrophy, some myopathies, amyotrophic lateral sclerosis, some epileptic syndromes, and multiple sclerosis. In most cases, the diagnosis is apparent from the constellation of neurologic abnormalities, and management is dictated by the underlying disease process.

IV. Discussion of Case Histories

Case 1. This woman's presentation suggests a toxic delirium, rather than dementia. She is irritable, inattentive, and disoriented. She was apparently hallucinating when her daughter found her. Dementia cannot be diagnosed in the setting of a clouded sensorium.

Patients with delirium most often have a toxic or metabolic problem. Initial evaluation should include electrolytes, a search for underlying infection, and a drug screen to evaluate for narcotics or other contributing agents. In this woman's case, a combination of medications is likely to be at fault, or at least to exacerbate any underlying problem. Geriatric patients are very susceptible to the cognitive effects of a number of drugs, including narcotics, H_2-blockers, anticholinergics, tricyclic antidepressants, and phenothiazines. They are quite sensitive to benzodiazepines, particularly those with longer half-lives, like flurazepam. In addition to her other troubles this woman had a UTI, which can cause fairly severe confusion in the elderly.

Once the acute delirium has subsided, one must bear in mind that many of those who present with delirium do have underlying central nervous system disease. If this patient had any residual cognitive deficits after simplifying her medication regimen and treating her UTI, an MRI scan of the brain would be appropriate in view of her asymmetric reflexes and history of hypertension. Baseline neuropsychometric testing might be helpful in monitoring for future progression.

Comment: All of the patient's medications were stopped and she was managed with calcium channel blockers and nonsteroidals. Her UTI was treated with a single dose of trimethoprim/sulfamethoxazole. Her mental status cleared completely, and no further tests were performed. She continued to have normal cognitive function at her subsequent clinic visits.

Case 2. This man has a typical history of moderately advanced Alzheimer's disease. He has a prominent memory disturbance with associated language disturbance, visuospatial deficits, and delusions. Social skills remain relatively intact. Formal neuropsychometric testing might be useful to demonstrate to him that there is objective evidence of cognitive impairment and that his wife is not just "making mountains out of anthills." Such testing could also identify his areas of relative strength. An imaging study is important to look for structural lesions, but these are unlikely given his history and a nonfocal examination. This patient should have the standard laboratory tests to look for a potentially reversible cause of dementia. Hearing should also be assessed to see if it is contributing to problems understanding spoken language.

Other issues that must be addressed in patients with progressive dementia include safety, behavior problems, and family support. The patient's driving ability needs reassessment. Consideration should be given to whether he should operate tools, cook, or handle any financial matters. The wife's ability to care for the patient and meet her own needs in this situation should be tactfully assessed and support offered. The patient and family should be educated about the illness, and advance directives should be discussed.

Case 3. As with the patient in Case 1, this woman's presentation suggests a subacute delirium rather than dementia. The salient features are intermittent sleepiness, disorientation, and poor processing of new material, with intact higher cognitive functions. Again, the clouded sensorium precludes the diagnosis of dementia. As with any patient who has delirium, primary considerations are metabolic abnormalities (especially drug-related) and infectious or inflammatory processes. Of particular concern in this woman is the history and examination finding of unilateral visual loss. A focal finding makes a metabolic problem less likely and should prompt vigorous evaluation for some other explanation. The lumbar puncture and head CT were thus completely appropriate tests, as chronic meningitis (especially cryptococcal) or abscess was a realistic concern.

Comment: In this woman, symptoms did not resolve after treatment of her UTI and repeat ESR 10 days later was 70. Because of her persistent headaches and history of visual loss, temporal artery biopsies were performed and showed temporal arteritis. After treatment with steroids, mental status and headaches improved and she resumed an entirely independent life. Temporal arteritis is discussed further in Chapters 12 and 13.

8

Movement Disorders

Linda M. Selwa and Douglas J. Gelb

I. Case Histories

Case 1. A 70-year-old woman comes to see you for "shakiness" in one hand that began approximately 6 months ago. She also complains bitterly about "getting older" and losing a lot of her previous energy and motivation. She no longer attends conferences that once occupied much of her time and energy, and she has limited her gardening activities significantly this year. She takes no medications. Her general physical examination is normal. She presents her history clearly and concisely and responds appropriately to questions and commands. Her cranial nerves are normal except for a rather expressionless face, with no clear facial weakness. She has a slight stoop, but there is no postural instability. Her stride is normal. She has decreased arm swing on the left, and she turns en bloc in four steps. Her finger movements are slow but normally coordinated. She has a prominent rest tremor in the left arm that improves with volitional movement. There is some cogwheel rigidity on the left. She has normal strength, reflexes, and sensation.

Questions:

1. What would you tell this woman about her diagnosis?

2. What potential complications should be addressed at this stage?

3. What therapy is appropriate?

Case 2. A 59-year-old woman with diabetes presents with complaints of "stiffness, slowness," and unilateral tremor for the last 3 months. She has fallen twice, but says that she just tripped. She has been experiencing abdominal bloating and weight loss. Her diabetes has been difficult to manage, and she is also troubled by numbness in her feet. The patient wonders whether her "foot problem" may be causing some of her unsteadiness. Medications include thyroid hormone replacement, insulin, metoclopramide (Reglan), and diltiazem (Cardizem). On examination, she has normal mental status and cranial nerves, though her face is expressionless. Her gait is festinating and slow, with reduced arm swing. There is mild postural instability. She has marked bradykinesia, rigidity, and a mild bilateral rest tremor. There is full strength in all muscle groups. Her reflexes are normal in the upper extremities and at the knees but can only be elicited at the ankles with reinforcement. Except for some mild reduction of vibration sense at the toes bilaterally, she has normal sensation throughout.

Questions:

1. How would you proceed with the evaluation?

2. Does she need evaluation for peripheral polyneuropathy?

3. What is the most appropriate treatment for this woman?

II. Background Information

A. Definitions

action tremor: a tremor that is most prominent on voluntary contraction of a muscle; this encompasses both postural tremor and kinetic tremor. The term *action tremor* is currently discouraged because of potential ambiguity.

akinesia: lack of voluntary movements.

athetosis: low, sinuous writhing of the distal parts of limbs.

ballism: violent, large-amplitude, involuntary flinging movements of the proximal parts of limbs.

bradykinesia: reduced speed and spontaneity of voluntary movements.

chorea: rapid, jerky involuntary movements appearing irregularly and unpredictably in various body parts.

cogwheeling: ratchet-like, rhythmic interruptions in resistance to passive manipulation.

dyskinesia: any abnormal involuntary movement.

dystonia: involuntary, sustained muscle contractions often having a preferred direction, resulting in maintenance of an abnormal posture or repetitive twisting movements.

festination: an involuntary tendency for steps to accelerate and decrease in amplitude.

intention tremor: this term is currently discouraged because of potential ambiguity but classically refers to a movement tremor that is most prominent on approaching the target of a goal-directed movement (i.e., a terminal movement tremor).

kinetic tremor: tremor that is accentuated with goal-directed movement of a limb. Kinetic tremor can be subdivided into *initial tremor* (occurring predominantly at the initiation of movement), *transition tremor* (predominantly during the movement), or *terminal tremor* (predominantly at the termination of movement); see also *intention tremor.*

myoclonus: rapid shock-like muscle jerks similar to chorea, but more discrete (less likely to blend into one another) and more likely to be localized.

postural tremor: a tremor that is most prominent when the body part is maintained in a nonresting posture (such as keeping the arms extended parallel to the floor), less prominent when the body part is completely relaxed.

rest tremor: tremor that is most prominent when the body part is in complete repose and fully supported against gravity, less prominent with movement or maintenance of a posture (also called *resting tremor*).

rigidity: increased resistance to passive manipulation throughout the range of movement, equal in flexors and extensors.

task-specific tremor: kinetic tremor present during certain tasks, such as writing, but absent during other activities.

tics: abrupt, transient, stereotypical, coordinated movements or vocalizations that can often be voluntarily suppressed but at the expense of a buildup of inner tension that is relieved when the suppression is removed.

tremor: involuntary rhythmic oscillation of a body part, produced by either alternating or synchronous contractions of reciprocally innervated antagonist muscles.

B. Classification of Movement Disorders

The term **movement disorder** refers to a heterogeneous group of conditions that result in abnormal form or timing of voluntary movement in individuals with normal strength, sensation, and cerebellar function. These disorders are closely associated with dysfunction of the basal ganglia, which can be thought of as a brain system devoted to the implementation of motor plans developed in the cortex. The basal ganglia consist of the striatum (the caudate and putamen), the globus pallidus, the substantia nigra, and the subthalamic nucleus. Movement disorders can be grouped into four general categories.

Hyperkinetic movement disorders are characterized by involuntary movements that intrude into the normal flow of motor acts. Examples include chorea, athetosis, and ballism, which may all represent points on a spectrum of clinical manifestations of the same underlying pathophysiologic mechanism. These movements correlate with dysfunction within the striatum or the subthalamic nucleus. They are suppressed by dopamine antagonists and exacerbated by dopamine agonists. Tics are also classified as hyperkinetic movement disorders.

Parkinsonism is characterized by bradykinesia, rigidity, and rest tremor. It correlates with disruption of striatal dopaminergic transmission, improves with dopamine agonist treatment, and worsens in response to dopamine antagonists.

Dystonia is marked by twisting and repetitive movements or sustained abnormal postures, often with a preferred direction. It is classified as **focal** (involving specific, localized muscle groups), **segmental** (involving two or more contiguous areas of the body), **multifocal** (involving two or more noncontiguous areas), **hemidystonia** (involving one side of the body), or **generalized** (involving the entire body). The neuroanatomic substrate is not known, although some evidence implicates the putamen. No drug consistently improves or exacerbates dystonia.

Postural and kinetic tremors may be due to abnormalities of cerebellar outflow to the thalamus.

III. Approach to Movement Disorders

Appropriate management of a patient with a movement disorder depends on the answers to two questions:

1. How can the patient's movements be characterized?

2. Are there accompanying abnormalities?

A comparison of these features to the patterns typically observed in established movement disorders usually permits an accurate diagnosis.

IV. Specific Movement Disorders

A. *Parkinson's Disease*

1. Clinical features

The cardinal signs of Parkinson's disease are bradykinesia, rest tremor, rigidity, and (eventually) postural instability. These combine to produce characteristic manifestations. One is festination, a tendency toward decreased amplitude and increased frequency when carrying out a sustained motor activity. In the typical parkinsonian gait, for example, the steps get smaller and smaller and faster and faster until the patient is practically walking in place. Another example is micrographia, or small handwriting, which gets progressively smaller toward the end of a writing sample. The motor control of speech is also subject to this phenomenon: Patients typically speak at low volumes, growing progressively softer and faster as they continue to speak. This type of dysarthria is classified as hypokinetic. Another typical manifestation is reduced facial expression and blinking rate (a "masked face"). As a result of the postural instability and rigidity, patients tend to turn en bloc when walking; rather than pivot 180 degrees in a single step, they make many small angular adjustments while standing in one place. Patients often have particular difficulty initiating movement, appearing totally "frozen," but after intense effort they set themselves in motion and then proceed to carry out the movement almost normally. Sometimes their initiation of movement can be facilitated by placing an obstacle in their way; it can be quite striking to watch a patient fixed in one spot suddenly begin walking normally when asked to step over the examiner's foot. Before long, however, the steps become smaller and faster, and the patient often gets stuck again. A similar phenomenon is described in a sudden emergency, such as a fire, in which patients have even been observed to run.

The characteristic tremor of Parkinson's disease is a rest tremor, becoming less prominent with voluntary movement. It has a frequency of 4 Hz, and in the hands there is classically a "pill-rolling" character. A low amplitude action tremor of 7–8 Hz also occurs in Parkinson's disease. An individual patient may have either type of tremor or both. Both kinds of tremor may fluctuate dramatically from one moment to the next, independent of medication regimen.

The signs often begin in a single limb, gradually progressing to involve the other limb on the same side, and eventually to the other side of the body. A commonly used scale for grading the severity of motor dysfunction is the one developed by Hoehn and Yahr: stage 1 = unilateral disease, stage 2 = bilateral disease without impairment of balance, stage 3 = bilateral disease with some postural instability but physically independent, stage 4 = severe disability but able to walk or stand unassisted, stage 5 = wheelchair-bound or bedridden without assistance.

Approximately 25–40% of patients with Parkinson's disease develop dementia. As discussed in Chapter 7, this can sometimes make it difficult to distinguish Parkinson's disease from dementia with Lewy bodies or Alzheimer's disease with parkinsonian features. Patients with Parkinson's disease may also experience delusions or hallucinations. These are often related to drug therapy but can also occur independently. Depression is also common in patients with Parkinson's disease. It appears to be a direct manifestation of the underlying neuropathologic changes, rather than a purely reactive depression, but debate continues on the subject.

2. Epidemiology, pathology, and etiology

The incidence of Parkinson's disease rises sharply with age; prevalence has been estimated at 0.02% in those under age 50 years and 1.1% in subjects over age 80 years. Parkinson's disease appears to be somewhat more common in men than in women and more common in whites than in other racial groups. Genetic transmission is rare, but a few pedigrees have been described with familial Parkinson's disease or parkinsonism.

Pathologically, Parkinson's disease is characterized by *Lewy bodies*—acidophilic cytoplasmic inclusions with a dense core and peripheral halo. Lewy bodies are most commonly found in the substantia nigra and in the locus ceruleus. Diffuse neuronal loss is observed in the pigmented nucleus of the substantia nigra with an associated deficit of dopamine production in the nigrostriatal pathway.

The cause of Parkinson's disease is unknown. Various lines of evidence have suggested a role for genetic factors, mitochondrial abnormalities, or environmental factors (including viral infections). Parkinsonism was linked to a mutation in the alpha-synuclein gene in one family.

3. Differential diagnosis

There is no diagnostic test for Parkinson's disease. Even when the diagnosis is made by experienced clinicians, it is confirmed at autopsy in only 75% of patients. Nonetheless, the diagnosis is usually straightforward based on the presence of typical clinical features, a substantial and sustained response to dopaminergic therapy, and the exclusion of several similar illnesses.

Drug-induced parkinsonism is the condition that most closely mimics Parkinson's disease. It must be carefully considered in all cases, particularly when symptom onset is acute or subacute. Early withdrawal of the offending agent is important. Parkinsonism is a frequent side effect of neuroleptic medications, including phenothiazines and butyrophenones (and similar drugs such as metoclopramide). Reserpine and related antihypertensives may produce parkinsonism; it can also occur after manganese poisoning or exposure to carbon monoxide.

A clinical picture resembling Parkinson's disease can occur in multi-infarct disease or even rarely after a single subcortical stroke. There are also several syndromes, sometimes known as "Parkinson's plus" disorders, in which parkinsonism accompanies other neurologic abnormalities. The clinical and neuropathologic findings that distinguish these illnesses are reviewed below (see Section H). Although some of these patients have a positive response to dopaminergic therapy, many do not, and in those who do the response may be only partial and temporary.

The most common diagnostic question that arises in the context of Parkinson's disease is whether a patient simply has essential tremor. This condition is discussed further in the next section (see Section B). Classically, the tremor has different characteristics from the tremor of Parkinson's disease, but patients with Parkinson's disease do not always exhibit the "classic" tremor, so differentiation from essential tremor on this basis is sometimes difficult. The most reliable way to distinguish the two disorders is on the basis of accompanying rigidity or bradykinesia, but these may be quite subtle, especially early in the course. At times, a patient must be observed for months to years before the diagnosis is clear.

4. Treatment

Dopamine replacement is the cornerstone of therapy. Sinemet is a combination of L-dopa, which crosses the blood-brain barrier and is converted to dopamine within neurons, and carbidopa, which blocks peripheral dopa decarboxylase, minimizing systemic side effects and increasing the amount of L-dopa entering the brain. A long-acting preparation is available. Treatment with L-dopa is generally started once there is some evidence of postural instability; some investigators feel that starting replacement early leads to more motor fluctuations later in the course. Selegiline (Deprenyl) is a monoamine oxidase (MAO) inhibitor that, when used in early stages of Parkinson's disease, postpones the need to initiate dopamine therapy. It is still not clear whether it slows the progression of Parkinson's disease or has a purely symptomatic benefit.

Other useful medications include amantadine (Symmetrel) and dopamine receptor agonists, which may help modulate motor fluctuations. The currently available dopamine agonists—bromocriptine (Parlodel), pergolide (Permax), pramipexole (Mirapex), and ropinirole (Requip)—have different affinity profiles for the five known dopamine receptors, but it is not clear how these differences influence their relative efficacy and toxicity. In some cases, these drugs can reduce the required Sinemet dose after dyskinesias become prominent. Another strategy for reducing the required Sinemet dose and prolonging the response to each dose (thereby possibly modulating motor fluctuations) is to add tolcapone (Tasmar) or entacopone (Comtan). These medications inhibit dopamine breakdown by the enzyme catechol-O-methyl transferase (COMT). Anticholinergic medications are mainly valuable for treatment of rest tremor. All of these drugs (dopamine agonists, COMT inhibitors, and anticholinergic agents) can produce hallucinations and excessive daytime somnolence.

For severely affected patients who can no longer be managed effectively with medications, several surgical options are available. Ablative procedures, including pallidotomy and thalamotomy, are intended to counteract an imbalance in the circuit connecting basal ganglia, thalamus, and cortex. Implantation of a stimulating electrode in the thalamus, globus pallidus, or substantia nigra is another way to achieve this goal without producing a permanent anatomic lesion. Transplantation of fetal adrenal tissue is still experimental.

5. Potential complications

Even with optimal management, patients' motor function generally worsens gradually. The most common problem encountered is fluctuation between "on" times when mobility is good and "off" times when mobility is poor. Many patients begin to experience dyskinesias in cycles related to their medication regimen as storage sites for the dopamine diminish. The dyskinesias may be biphasic, coinciding with both peak and trough dopamine levels. At the same time, the response to dopamine becomes briefer and less reliable. Patients often fall more as the illness progresses, and dysarthria and dysphagia can result in significant disability late in the disease. Slowed gastric emptying and reduced intestinal motility are common symptoms leading to anorexia and weight loss.

6. Prognosis

Dopamine replacement has made a dramatic difference in patients' longevity since the 1960s. Patients who would once have suffered early disability and death now have a life expectancy that is not significantly different from others in their age group. Nonetheless, symptoms progress even with optimal therapy, and some patients become severely disabled.

B. Essential Tremor

Essential tremor is a common movement disorder without clearly defined pathophysiology. The only finding is a postural and terminal kinetic tremor most prominent in the upper extremities. The tremor is commonly unilateral at the onset, with progression to involve the other side over 2 or 3 years. There is often an associated head tremor, and at times this is the presenting symptom or even the only symptom. There may also be an associated voice tremor, which is less likely to occur in isolation. The frequency of essential tremor ranges from 4–12 Hz, with wide fluctuations in amplitude. These patients do not have rigidity, postural instability, or bradykinesia. Many cases are familial. Generally, symptoms are mild and associated with only minor progression over decades, but in some cases the condition is disabling enough to interfere with writing, dressing, and eating. This tremor often responds briefly but dramatically to ethanol consumption, which may be a useful diagnostic feature.

Beta-blockers are the most helpful therapy. Primidone, anticholinergics, benzodiazepines, and perhaps acetazolamide are also beneficial in some cases. For severe, refractory essential tremor, surgical implantation of a deep brain stimulator in the thalamus produces dramatic improvement in approximately 85% of patients. There has been no controlled study directly comparing thalamic stimulation to thalamotomy, but potential advantages of deep brain stimulation include a lower risk of hemorrhage, the ability to customize stimulus parameters, and reversibility.

C. Huntington's Disease

Huntington's disease is an autosomal dominant condition characterized by progressive chorea and dementia typically beginning in the late third and fourth decade of life. The cognitive disturbances begin as personality changes and evolve to severe memory dysfunction and global intellectual decline. The chorea is often difficult to detect early in the illness. When it is relatively infrequent, patients can often incorporate the chorea into normal voluntary actions; for example, they may quickly reach up to smooth their hair as soon as an involuntary twitch begins. The chorea grows progressively more severe over time, and patients often manifest varying degrees of athetosis, dystonia, or parkinsonism. Slowed saccadic eye movements and slowed distal fine motor skills can usually be detected on examination even before the involuntary movements become apparent. Dysarthria and dysphagia are prominent throughout the course. Gait abnormalities are extremely common and eventually become disabling. Depression is also very common, and other psychiatric disorders may also occur. The diagnosis of Huntington's disease is based on the presence of the characteristic movement disorder in an individual with a positive family history; psychiatric or behavioral abnormalities without an accompanying movement disorder are not specific. For patients who have the typical clinical manifestations of Huntington's disease but no family history, testing for the Huntington's mutation may be diagnostic.

In approximately 10% of patients with Huntington's disease, clinical symptoms begin before age 20 years; this juvenile form is often characterized by prominent parkinsonism rather than chorea. Juvenile onset is more common in patients who inherited the disease from their father.

The pathogenesis of Huntington's disease remains unknown. The genetic abnormality responsible for Huntington's disease is an expanded, unstable trinucleotide repeat on the short arm of chromosome 4, but the mechanisms by which this defect leads to symptoms have not yet been elucidated. Pathologic examination reveals marked atrophy with loss of selective subsets of cells in the striatum, particularly at the head of the caudate. Some neuronal loss is also described in the globus pallidus and thalamus. Characteristic changes in neurotransmitters and receptors (especially GABA [gamma-aminobutyric acid], benzodiazepine, acetylcholine, and excitatory amino acids) have been described.

Therapy is primarily supportive. Phenothiazines are used to modify chorea or behavioral disorders. Other mood-stabilizing agents can be helpful. Swallowing problems and gait difficulty should be addressed with education and therapy. Dysphagia, immobility, and dementia usually lead to death in 15–20 years.

Difficult psychosocial and ethical issues arise from the ability to screen for a genetic condition that does not produce clinical manifestations until midlife and for which only limited symptomatic treatment is available. Individuals at risk for Huntington's disease should receive extensive counseling before they decide whether to be tested. Even if they decide not to be tested, genetic counseling is essential.

D. Tardive Dyskinesia

As many as 20% of patients treated with neuroleptic agents develop hyperkinetic movement disorders, especially dyskinetic movements or dystonic postures. These often appear late in the course of therapy; the incidence increases in proportion to the duration of exposure and is highest in the elderly. The most common dyskinesias are repetitive, stereotyped oro-bucco-lingual movements, but in many patients, the trunk and distal extremities are involved as well. The pathophysiologic mechanism is uncertain but may be related to supersensitivity of postsynaptic striatal dopamine receptors or GABA-ergic striatal dysfunction. Treatment consists of eliminating neuroleptics if possible or titrating to the lowest doses needed to control psychotic symptoms. Dyskinesias may or may not resolve after discontinuation of the offending agents; improvement may take weeks to months. For disabling persistent movements, benzodiazepines, reserpine, or tetrabenazine can be useful.

E. Dystonias

Dystonia may be a feature of almost every condition discussed in this chapter (as well as a number of other neurologic diseases and systemic problems), but it may also occur as an isolated problem. Although any pattern of muscle activity may be seen, the most common examples of dystonia in adults are the focal syndromes of torticollis, blepharospasm, and writer's cramp. In torticollis, the patient's head may be turned to one side, flexed, extended, tilted, or any combination of these movements. It may be maintained in a fixed position, or there may be superimposed jerking movements or tremor. In blepharospasm, there is involuntary, bilateral eye closure, often exacerbated by bright light or other environmental stimuli. In writer's cramp, the hand assumes an involuntary, often twisted posture when the patient attempts to write. Many analogous task-specific dystonias also exist. In addition to the inconvenience and embarrassment resulting from these conditions, the sustained muscle contractions often cause considerable pain. The severity of focal dystonia typically fluctuates widely and can be influenced both by the patient's emotional state and environmental stimuli. The underlying pathogenesis of focal dystonia is not known. Until recently, focal dystonias were often assumed to be psychogenic, and the differentiation between an organic focal dystonia and a psychiatric condition is still difficult at times—especially since many psychiatric patients are treated with neuroleptic medications, which can themselves produce dystonia. Hemidystonia implies structural damage in the contralateral hemisphere.

Dystonia that begins in adulthood is usually focal or segmental, whereas approximately 50% of cases of childhood-onset dystonia are generalized. Early-onset generalized dystonia is called *idiopathic torsion dystonia* (formerly termed *dystonia musculorum deformans*). It usually begins in one body region and spreads to the rest of the body over 1–10 years. Idiopathic torsion dystonia is inherited as an autosomal dominant trait with reduced penetrance; it has been mapped to chromosome 9, and carrier testing is possible in some families. There is a rare form of childhood-onset generalized dystonia accompanied by parkinsonism and hyperreflexia that worsens as the day progresses and improves with sleep. Patients with this condition have a dramatic and sustained response to L-dopa.

Many classes of pharmacotherapy have been used to treat dystonia, most often anticholinergic agents but also dopamine agonists, dopamine antagonists, benzodiazepines, catecholamine agonists, and catecholamine antagonists. None of these agents has been effective for more than a handful of patients. Focal dystonias can be treated with local injections of minute quantities of botulinum toxin to weaken the overactive muscles. Although this approach fails to address the abnormal motor programming responsible for the disorder, it can produce significant symptomatic relief. The effect is temporary, so the injections must be repeated every few months. Botulinum toxin injections can at best provide regional relief to patients with idiopathic torsion dystonia, who eventually develop severe disability in most cases.

F. Wilson's Disease

Wilson's disease is an autosomal recessive disorder of copper metabolism characterized by progressive, but often reversible, tremor, dystonia, dysarthria, dysphagia, cognitive deterioration, and psychiatric symptoms. These manifestations may occur in any combination and in any temporal sequence. The tremor may be a rest tremor, a postural tremor, or a kinetic tremor. Clinically significant hepatic involvement is common, and other organ systems may also be affected. In general, patients who present with liver abnormalities usually do so between the ages of 8 and 16 years, whereas those who present with neurologic symptoms usually do so after puberty.

Histopathologic examination reveals excess copper deposition in the liver and throughout the brain, with prominent degeneration of the putamen, globus pallidus, brainstem nuclei, and even white matter. Copper deposition in the cornea leads to the characteristic Kayser-Fleischer ring of hyperpigmentation around the limbus; this physical finding is present in practically all patients with neurologic manifestations, but it may be subtle and only evident on slit-lamp examination in early cases.

The underlying defect in copper metabolism is not fully understood. Normal copper intake is approximately 1 mg per day, but the normal copper requirement is only approximately 0.75 mg per day. In normal individuals, copper is absorbed in the upper intestine and transported to the liver, where the excess is secreted in the bile and packaged in some way that prevents reabsorption in the gastrointestinal tract, resulting in excretion in the stool. Biliary secretion of ceruloplasmin, a glycoprotein that binds and transports copper, is presumed to be a component of this process, but the details are not known. Wilson's disease results from a mutation in a gene on chromosome 13 that codes for a copper-binding, membrane-associated adenosine triphosphatase. Although the mechanism remains obscure, this mutation interferes with the excretion of copper into the bile, producing a positive copper balance that over time leads to an accumulation of copper, at first in the liver but eventually in other organs, including the brain. For some reason, serum levels of ceruloplasmin are low in most patients with Wilson's disease, but this appears to be a secondary phenomenon. In fact, ceruloplasmin levels are normal in up to 15% of patients with the disease and low in 10–20% of asymptomatic carriers. Even so, a serum ceruloplasmin level is a fairly good screening test for Wilson's disease. Increased copper in a 24-hour urine collection is probably more reliable, but a little more involved. A slit-lamp examination for Kayser-Fleischer rings can be a critical step in establishing the diagnosis. Total levels of serum copper are of little value, but elevated levels of free serum copper can be helpful. A liver biopsy to determine hepatic copper content is the single most reliable test for Wilson's disease.

Without treatment, the disease was once uniformly fatal. Patients are now treated with penicillamine, a chelating agent, or tetrathiomolybdate, which impairs intestinal absorption of copper and also forms complexes with copper in the blood. Penicillamine has traditionally been the mainstay of treatment, but it is associated with a high incidence of adverse effects, including neurologic deterioration at the onset of treatment in 25–50% of patients. Tetrathiomolybdate is generally well tolerated, and the therapeutic results have been impressive, but it is still an experimental agent. Alternative medications include zinc, which also blocks intestinal absorption of copper, and trientine, another chelating agent. Therapy must be continued permanently; zinc is often used as maintenance therapy after initial treatment with one of the other medications. Orthotopic liver transplantation is currently reserved for patients with severe hepatic failure.

G. Gilles de la Tourette's Syndrome

Tourette's syndrome is the most flagrant of a spectrum of tic disorders. Evidence suggests that it is much more common than previously appreciated, but most cases are mild and do not come to medical attention. It is inherited in an autosomal dominant pattern with incomplete and sex-specific penetrance (males more commonly affected than females). Polygenic factors may play a role. In addition to recurrent motor tics involving multiple muscle groups, there are frequent vocal tics such as grunting, barking, humming, or clearing of the throat. The most dramatic symptom is coprolalia, the involuntary utterance of obscenities, which occurs in up to two-thirds of patients. Obsessive-compulsive disorder and attention deficit-hyperactivity disorder each occur in approximately 50% of patients. These associated behavioral problems are usually more disabling than the tics themselves. The cause of Tourette's syndrome is not known. Most patients with mild tics can avoid the use of medications. Tics tend to become less severe over time and may resolve. For moderate or severe tics, haloperidol, pimozide, or other neuroleptic medications are often very effective. Clonidine and clonazepam have also been effective in some patients.

H. Multisystem Degenerations

A number of neurologic diseases are characterized by symptoms that overlap several of the traditional diagnostic categories, leading to considerable diagnostic confusion. Some of these conditions are hereditary, and advances in molecular genetics are demonstrating unexpected relationships between some disorders previously thought to be distinct, while suggesting that other conditions might be more heterogeneous than previously suspected. Much uncertainty remains, and it is best to consider these conditions in terms of broad diagnostic categories.

1. Spinocerebellar degenerations (including Friedreich's ataxia)

A number of diseases affect varying combinations of ascending and descending pathways in the spinal cord, including spinocerebellar tracts, corticospinal tracts, and posterior columns. Peripheral nerves and dorsal root ganglia may also be involved. The most common and best characterized example of this group of disorders is Friedreich's ataxia. This is an autosomal recessive disorder characterized by progressive limb and gait ataxia with onset before age 25 years, absent tendon reflexes in the lower extremities, and axonal sensory peripheral neuropathy. Dysarthria, extensor plantar responses, scoliosis, pes cavus, and cardiomyopathy are frequently associated findings and eventually develop in most patients. Less frequent complications include optic atrophy, deafness, and diabetes mellitus. Pathologic hallmarks are demyelination and degeneration in the posterior column, pyramidal and spinocerebellar tracts of the spinal cord, and cell loss and demyelination in the dorsal root ganglia and peripheral nerves. Disability usually occurs within 15 years, but survival can continue into the 40s or even 60s in some cases.

Friedreich's ataxia is caused by a triplet repeat expansion on chromosome 9, within a gene that appears to code for a mitochondrial protein. The pathophysiologic consequences of this mutation are not yet understood. Triplet repeat expansions in other genes on other chromosomes have been identified in a number of other spinocerebellar ataxias. Some of these mutations produce a fairly wide spectrum of clinical phenotypes. Symptomatic treatment is the main focus of management for all of these disorders.

2. Olivopontocerebellar atrophy

Olivopontocerebellar atrophy (OPCA) is characterized by gradually progressive truncal and limb ataxia, generally associated with spasticity and occasionally including cranial neuropathies, retinal degenerations, or involuntary movements. There are sporadic, autosomal dominant, and autosomal recessive forms of this disorder. All are characterized pathologically by progressive neuronal loss in the inferior olives, ventral pons, and cerebellar cortex. Examination findings include striking truncal and appendicular ataxia. In some cases, hyperreflexia, supranuclear ophthalmoplegia, lower cranial neuropathies, tremor, and even peripheral neuropathy have been reported late in the disease. Dementia occurs in roughly 20% of patients and is often mild. Steady progression is the rule, but it often takes place slowly over years to decades. Treatment is symptomatic.

Clinical differentiation between hereditary OPCA and spinocerebellar degeneration is often difficult, and molecular genetic studies suggest that some of the distinctions may be artificial. Patients who have clinical features of OPCA together with parkinsonism or autonomic dysfunction are classified as having multiple system atrophy.

3. Parkinson's plus syndromes

There are several syndromes that consist of parkinsonism in association with additional neurologic abnormalities. Progressive supranuclear palsy (PSP) is the most distinctive of these syndromes. The earliest symptoms often resemble typical Parkinson's disease, but patients eventually develop characteristic eye movement abnormalities. The initial abnormality is often a downgaze palsy. Patients next develop an upgaze palsy and then difficulty with voluntary horizontal gaze. Oculocephalic reflexes are intact, indicating that the gaze palsy is supranuclear (see Chapter 2). Other features that help distinguish PSP from Parkinson's disease are that in PSP, tremor is less common, prominent gait disturbances and falling occur earlier in the illness, and a response to levodopa is less common. Neck dystonia and axial (trunk and head) rigidity are often present in PSP. Dysphagia develops early in the course and can be a severely limiting feature, and dysarthria is also prominent. There has been debate about how common cognitive deficits are in PSP. Although the initial descriptions of the disease highlighted cognitive impairment as one of the salient features of PSP, subsequent authors noted that many of the deficits could be explained on the basis of the patients' bradykinesia, dysarthria, and impaired oculomotor control. Even so, there do appear to be independent cognitive deficits that are often quite subtle. Communication is generally disrupted much more by the dysarthria than by the dementia.

A trial of Sinemet is usually warranted, because some patients experience significant benefit, at least transiently. Positive results have been reported in occasional patients with dopamine agonists, tricyclic antidepressant agents, or methysergide, but most patients do not respond to these medications. Regardless of treatment, patients usually continue to deteriorate and ultimately lose the ability to walk. Most of them eventually require a feeding tube to prevent aspiration and provide adequate nutrition. Patients progress to disability and death in an average of 6 years.

Striatonigral degeneration is a condition characterized by parkinsonism without prominent tremor. It progresses more rapidly than Parkinson's disease but more slowly than PSP. It is poorly responsive to dopaminergic agents.

Dementia with Lewy bodies results in cognitive deficits, behavioral abnormalities, and parkinsonism (see Chapter 7). These symptoms can develop in any order.

Corticobasal ganglionic degeneration is distinguished by marked asymmetry in the motor dysfunction, at least initially. In addition to parkinsonism (primarily rigidity and bradykinesia), these patients often have dystonic posturing and apraxia on one side of their body, leading at times to an "alien limb" phenomenon in which patients report that the limb seems to float about their body independent of voluntary control. As mentioned in Chapter 7, histopathologic characteristics of this condition overlap those seen in patients with frontotemporal dementia. Dopaminergic treatment helps some of these patients.

4. Multiple system atrophy

One distinctive form of Parkinson's plus syndrome is characterized by prominent autonomic nervous system abnormalities in addition to parkinsonism; it used to be known as Shy-Drager syndrome. Autonomic disturbances can also occur in patients with OPCA. Moreover, some patients manifest both parkinsonism and cerebellar dysfunction, with or without autonomic impairment. Thus, parkinsonism, cerebellar dysfunction, and autonomic impairment can occur separately or in any combination, and the term **multiple system atrophy** is applied to patients who have any two (or all three) of these features. They may also have spasticity, cranial nerve abnormalities, anterior horn cell dysfunction, or peripheral polyneuropathy in any combination. The clinical findings and presentation vary widely, but the course is gradually progressive. The diagnosis may not be apparent until enough symptoms have developed. L-dopa itself can cause orthostatic hypotension, so if a patient previously diagnosed with Parkinson's disease begins to develop severe orthostatic hypotension, multiple system atrophy should only be diagnosed if the orthostatic hypotension persists after withdrawing L-dopa or if the patient develops other signs of autonomic dysfunction.

Pathologic changes include widespread neuronal loss in the striatum, brainstem, cerebellum, and spinal cord nuclei. For those patients who have parkinsonism, the response to dopaminergic therapy is unpredictable. Treatment is symptomatic. Supportive therapy for gait disturbance or dysphagia may be helpful. Orthostatic hypotension is generally treated with mineralocorticoids such as fludrocortisone (Florinef) and support stockings; indomethacin is sometimes helpful. Beta-adrenergic antagonists (e.g., propranolol, pindolol) and alpha-adrenergic agonists (e.g., clonidine, midodrine) may also be tried. Syncope is often difficult to treat and is a factor in the relatively poor prognosis; mean survival is 6–8 years.

V. Discussion of Case Histories

Case 1. This patient has typical stage 1 Parkinson's disease. She may be frightened by this diagnosis, especially since Parkinson's disease was not easily treated when she was younger. It is therefore important to make sure she understands that the disease is readily treatable but that it will require continuing attention. In stage 1 disease, treatment with selegiline alone would be recommended.

She also relates symptoms that suggest she may be depressed. Her eating and sleeping habits, as well as her mood, need to be assessed. Depression is a common complication of Parkinson's disease, and it is often inadequately addressed because so many of the features could potentially be due to the Parkinson's disease itself. It is also important to perform at least some preliminary evaluation of memory function. If a mental status examination indicates any problems, formal evaluation of intellectual function and affect might provide a baseline to help assess any future decline.

Comment: This patient did very well on selegiline and antidepressants.

Case 2. In this patient, the progression has been fairly rapid, and the patient already has bilateral parkinsonian findings on examination after only 3 months of symptoms. These atypical features suggest that the patient may not have idiopathic Parkinson's disease. This case illustrates the common phenomenon of drug-induced parkinsonism. The patient's bradykinesia and tremor began almost immediately after starting metoclopramide (Reglan). All the usual symptoms of Parkinson's disease can be induced by even relatively brief exposure to this medication, and a careful history is critical in diagnosis. The first diagnostic maneuver is to stop Reglan. Continuing the medication and treating with anticholinergics or dopamine is inappropriate. Symptoms may take several weeks or more to subside, so follow-up evaluations will be necessary.

Regarding the patient's complaint of foot numbness: The examination findings of hyporeflexia at the ankles and reduced vibration sense at the toes are consistent with peripheral polyneuropathy, a common complication of diabetes. Because her feet are not painful, the findings are mild, and there is a likely explanation, there is no need for further evaluation at this point. It is unlikely that the polyneuropathy is contributing significantly to her gait disturbance, as she has normal distal strength and joint position sense.

Comment: This patient's motor symptoms disappeared within 3 weeks of stopping metoclopramide. She continued to have numbness in her feet, but this symptom did not bother her once it was explained to her.

Sleep Disorders

I. Case Histories

Case 1. A 55-year-old man who is followed in the hypertension clinic mentions to his doctor that he was in an accident last week, but luckily, nobody got hurt. He says he must have "fallen asleep at the wheel"—it happens to him every so often. He doesn't understand why he should be sleepy, because he goes to bed at 10 PM every night and sleeps through the night until he gets up at 7 AM the next morning. His wife confirms this but adds that she really couldn't say whether he is asleep that entire time because she sleeps in a different room to avoid his snoring.

The patient's general examination is notable for his hypertension, mild obesity, and a large neck. His neurologic examination is normal.

Questions:

1. What diagnoses should be considered?

2. What investigations are necessary?

3. How should this patient be managed?

Case 2. A 45-year-old man asks his family doctor to give him a prescription for Prozac. He believes he is depressed, and has heard good things about this medicine. He explains that he has no energy, can't concentrate, and is tired all the time. He can never seem to fall asleep at night. In fact, he can hardly even lie in bed for any length of time, because of a constant unpleasant sensation in his legs "like worms are crawling over them," causing an almost irresistible urge to move the legs. This feeling only goes away when he is moving his legs or walking. He prefers standing, anyway, because he often gets epigastric pain when he lies down. He wonders if he is going crazy.

Questions:

1. What diagnoses should be considered?

2. What investigations are necessary?

3. Should fluoxetine (Prozac) be prescribed?

4. What other treatment options are available?

Case 3. A 4-year-old girl has been brought to the pediatric emergency room at 2 AM by her parents, who say that at 1 AM they were awakened by her frantic screaming. They rushed to her room and saw that she was agitated, sweating profusely, and breathing rapidly, and her pulse was racing. They were unable to calm her. She returned to normal over the next few minutes and seemed unaware that anything was wrong. She now seems to be normal except that she is sleepy. Two similar episodes occurred 1 month ago, but the family had just moved to a new city at the time and the girl's parents had attributed the episodes to the unfamiliar surroundings and the stress of adjusting to a new day care situation.

Questions:

1. What diagnoses should be considered?

2. What investigations are necessary?

3. What treatment should be given?

II. Definitions

dyssomnia: a disorder resulting in insomnia or excessive daytime sleepiness (or both).

hypersomnia: excessive daytime somnolence.

insomnia: the subjective impression of inadequate sleep.

parasomnia: an abnormal movement or behavior that occurs during sleep or is brought on by sleep.

III. Approach to Sleep Disorders

Diagnosis of sleep disorders depends on accurate characterization of patients' complaints. There are only three kinds of complaints regarding sleep: trouble staying awake (hypersomnia), trouble sleeping (insomnia), and abnormal sensations or behavior during sleep (parasomnias). These complaints often go together. For example, people who have trouble staying awake may nap excessively during the day and then have trouble falling asleep at night. Some people who have trouble falling asleep at bedtime are not fully rested the following day, so they have trouble staying awake. People who have abnormal behavior during sleep may fail to get the required amount of normal sleep and have trouble staying awake the following day.

Two types of sleep study are commonly used to supplement the clinical diagnosis of sleep disorders. A **polysomnogram** is an all-night recording of eye movements, EEG (central and occipital leads), electrocardiogram, EMG (chin and anterior tibialis leads), ear oximetry, airflow at the nose and mouth, and thoracic and abdominal wall motion. The testing sometimes includes video and additional EEG monitoring, or other physiologic assessments such as esophageal pH, end-tidal pCO_2, or intrathoracic pressure. A **Multiple Sleep Latency Test** (MSLT) is a measure of daytime sleepiness. A subject is asked to take four or five brief naps at 2-hour intervals on the day after an adequate night's sleep. The time necessary to fall asleep is measured for each of these naps, and EEG, EMG, and eye movements are monitored.

There are two principal stages of sleep that alternate at about 90-minute intervals in the normal adult. **Rapid eye movement** (REM) sleep can be characterized as a period when the brain is active and the body is paralyzed, whereas in **nonrapid eye movement** (NREM) sleep, the brain is less active but the body can move. Most dreams occur during REM sleep. On the polysomnogram, REM sleep is characterized by EMG suppression, irregular low-voltage activity on EEG, and rapid eye movements. The eye movements sometimes correspond to dream content. NREM sleep is characterized by normal resting EMG, progressive slowing of EEG activity, and no rapid eye movements.

When normal subjects first fall asleep, they progress through four stages of NREM sleep that are differentiated on the basis of EEG characteristics. Stages 3 and 4 are often called slow wave sleep or delta sleep because they are characterized by high-amplitude slow waves (also called delta waves) on EEG. Delta sleep may last from a few minutes to an hour, depending on the subject's age, and the subject then reverts to stage 2 sleep. Shortly after this, the first REM sleep period begins. This lasts approximately 15–20 minutes and is followed by another NREM cycle. This alternation between REM and NREM continues throughout the night, but after the first third of the night stages 3 and 4 are less apparent so that NREM sleep consists primarily of stage 2 sleep, with brief periods of stage 1 sleep. The periods of REM sleep grow longer as the night continues.

IV. Trouble Staying Awake

Excessive daytime somnolence (hypersomnia) can be obvious or subtle. At one extreme, patients with chronic, severe hypersomnia can have "sleep attacks," in which they fall asleep even during activities where a nap is clearly inappropriate. The sleep attacks usually last about 15 minutes, at which point patients awaken feeling refreshed. They are not overwhelmed by sleepiness again for 1–2 hours. At the other extreme, patients may not even appreciate that they are sleepy. They may be more aware of the consequences of hypersomnia, including loss of energy, fatigue, headaches, lack of initiative, memory lapses, difficulty concentrating, and short temper. Indeed, in many instances, the barrier to diagnosis results from a failure to recognize that there is a problem with sleep in the first place. Patients with symptoms that could be manifestations of hypersomnia should be asked directed questions to determine if they have an underlying sleep disturbance. Once hypersomnia has been identified, the most common causes—insufficient sleep, sleep apnea, and narcolepsy—are often easily recognized based on historic features.

A. Insufficient Sleep

Sleepiness is to be expected in the setting of sleep deprivation. The demands of modern life lead many people to allot themselves inadequate time for sleep at night. As a consequence, they suffer from unrecognized, self-imposed sleep deprivation. This problem is so common that many people consider it normal to be drowsy or even fall asleep during the day, especially in unstimulating situations or after a big lunch. This is not normal behavior for fully rested individuals, however. This problem is managed by educating the patient about healthy sleep habits ("sleep hygiene").

B. Sleep Apnea

Sleep apnea is a condition in which patients periodically stop breathing while asleep. Central sleep apnea results from abnormal central nervous system control of respiration, which can be caused by a variety of processes. Much more commonly, sleep apnea is caused by temporary obstruction of the upper airway; in fact, obstructive sleep apnea is the most common medical cause of excessive daytime somnolence.

Even in normal subjects, the pharyngeal muscles that maintain airway patency relax during sleep. There is normally enough residual volume in the airway to permit airflow, but in patients with obstructive sleep apnea, the muscle relaxation results in complete or nearly complete occlusion of the airway. For airflow to be restored, the pharyngeal muscles must be activated, and this requires partial awakening. Sleep cannot be fully restorative when it is disrupted repeatedly throughout the night by these episodes of apnea and partial arousal, and the result is excessive somnolence during the day. Some patients with increased upper airway resistance during sleep do not experience episodes of apnea but still exhibit either decreased ventilation or increased respiratory effort with a similar disruption of restorative sleep.

The cornerstone of this diagnosis is a history of apneic episodes during sleep. Patients are not aware of the episodes because they are brief and arousal is only partial, so the history usually must be obtained from the bed partner. Patients characteristically snore loudly, punctuated with bouts of interrupted breathing that often terminate with snorts or gasps. The diagnosis is also supported by the presence of any conditions that can predispose to obstructive sleep apnea by causing upper airway narrowing. These include enlarged tonsils, adenoids, soft palate, uvula, or tongue, obesity (causing fat deposition around the upper airway), facial and mandibular deformities, malignant infiltration of the soft tissue of the neck, and laryngeal muscle weakness. Polysomnography is used to confirm the diagnosis of sleep apnea and to quantify the severity in terms of number of apneic episodes per hour, degree of blood oxygen desaturation, and the presence of any significant cardiac arrhythmias.

Sleep apnea can result in hypersomnia not only for the patient but also for the bed partner and sometimes other family members who suffer disrupted sleep because of the loud snoring. In addition, chronic obstructive sleep apnea is associated with an increased risk of systemic hypertension, cardiac arrhythmias, sudden death, myocardial infarction, stroke, and motor vehicle accidents. Successful treatment of the sleep apnea can reduce the risk of at least some of those conditions.

The most effective treatment of obstructive sleep apnea (short of tracheostomy) is nasal continuous positive airway pressure (CPAP). This raises the pressure in the oropharynx, and thus in the upper airway, reversing the pressure gradient across the wall of the airway and propping it open. This treatment is beneficial in 80–90% of patients; the main reasons for treatment failure are poor compliance (because the patient finds the nightly use of a mask over the nose uncomfortable or unappealing) and nasal obstruction. Other treatment options include weight loss for overweight patients (usually easier said than done), uvulopalatopharyngoplasty (which is helpful in about one-half the patients, but it is difficult to predict which half), surgical correction of other abnormalities that obstruct the airway (e.g., tonsillectomy or correction of facial and mandibular deformities), and medications. The most commonly used medication is protriptyline (Vivactil), which produces partial benefit in 30–50% of patients with mild disease.

C. Narcolepsy

Narcolepsy is a syndrome consisting of excessive daytime somnolence and disordered regulation of REM sleep, resulting in intrusion of components of REM sleep into NREM sleep and the waking state. It usually begins in teenage years. There are four cardinal symptoms:

1. **Chronic excessive daytime somnolence.** Unlike other forms of somnolence, the sleepiness that occurs in narcolepsy cannot be relieved by any amount of normal sleep.

2. **Cataplexy** is a sudden loss of postural tone that occurs while the patient is awake but is otherwise identical to the atonia that occurs during REM sleep. The atonia may involve only a single muscle group, resulting in subtle manifestations such as slight buckling of

the knees, drooping of the head or jaw, ptosis, or even just a subjective feeling of weakness, or it may be generalized and lead to complete bodily collapse and paralysis. Consciousness is preserved before, during, and after the attack, although some patients pass directly from the attack into REM sleep. Attacks are precipitated by strong emotion, particularly laughter.

3. Sleep paralysis, like cataplexy, consists of atonia identical to that of REM sleep. It occurs at the onset of sleep or on awakening. The patient is conscious or half-awake but unable to move. This is often accompanied by intense fear and a sense of being unable to breathe.

4. Hypnagogic (or hypnopompic) hallucinations are vivid auditory or visual dream-like experiences that occur at the onset of sleep (or on awakening).

The diagnosis of narcolepsy is straightforward when the age of onset is typical and all four cardinal symptoms are present. Some patients experience only some of the symptoms, however. Moreover, while cataplexy almost never occurs outside the setting of narcolepsy, the other three symptoms can be seen with any condition that causes sleep deprivation or disruption. The MSLT is used to support the diagnosis: A narcoleptic patient characteristically has a mean sleep latency of 5 minutes or less, whereas rested normal individuals require an average of more than 10 minutes to fall asleep. The MSLT also provides a measure of the tendency to enter REM sleep prematurely, without the normal progression through stages 1–4 of NREM sleep. Any period of REM sleep that occurs in the first 15 minutes of sleep is noted and referred to as a sleep-onset REM period. The occurrence of two or more sleep-onset REM periods is highly suggestive of narcolepsy. In ambiguous cases, HLA typing is sometimes helpful. More than 95% of Asian and Caucasian patients with narcolepsy have the HLA-DR1501 and HLA-DQB1-0602 antigens. The usefulness of this testing is limited, however, because these antigens can also be present in normal subjects, and there are well-documented cases of narcolepsy in individuals without the antigens.

Narcolepsy is treated primarily with stimulant medications, especially dextroamphetamine (Dexedrine) or methylphenidate (Ritalin). Modafinil (Provigil), an agent that affects alpha$_1$-adrenergic tone, has alerting properties and appears to have less problematic side effects than amphetamines. Cataplectic attacks respond to tricyclic antidepressants such as imipramine (Tofranil) and protriptyline (Vivactil). Improved sleep hygiene and scheduled therapeutic naps may be useful adjuncts to pharmacotherapy.

D. Other Causes of Hypersomnolence

Excessive sleepiness may be caused by many medications, including sedative-hypnotics, antiepileptic drugs, antihypertensives, antidepressants, and antihistamines. Withdrawal from stimulants may also result in hypersomnolence. Many metabolic abnormalities can also cause sleepiness, or more often, obtundation or stupor. These include hepatic encephalopathy, uremic encephalopathy, hyperglycemia, hypoglycemia, hypercalcemia, and (severe) hypothyroidism. Other causes include meningitis, encephalitis, chronic subdural hematoma, and the post-traumatic syndrome.

V. Trouble Sleeping

Many different physiologic and psychologic factors can interfere with sleep, and many patients with insomnia have more than one of these factors. The goal is to identify the contributing factors and treat the ones for which therapy is available. There are three main patterns of insomnia: Sleep-onset delay (trouble falling asleep), early morning arousal (trouble staying asleep), and sleep fragmentation (repeated awakenings).

A. Sleep-Onset Delay

1. Psychophysiologic insomnia

People who are trying to fall asleep are relatively free of distractions. They tend to focus on any residual unpleasant thoughts, emotions, or sensations, especially if they are anxious. This makes it difficult for them to relax and fall asleep, which, in turn, makes them more anxious, leading to even greater delay in falling asleep and frequent arousals. On subsequent nights, the anxiety about falling asleep may be enough to provoke this cycle, even after the original unpleasant situation has resolved. Over time, patients may develop a conditioned association between their bed and unsuccessful sleep; they often find that they sleep better outside the bedroom. *Psychophysiologic* insomnia is the term used for this cycle of conditioned behavior, regardless of the original cause (and even when no specific cause can be identified).

Psychophysiologic insomnia is most often due to anxiety related to life stressors. Depression is another common cause. Any conditions that are associated with physical discomfort can also contribute. One example is **restless legs syndrome,** a condition that occurs almost exclusively when lying down or sitting and is characterized by deep paresthesias and crawling sensations in the calves and legs with a compulsion to move the legs. Paresthesias resulting from carpal tunnel syndrome, other mononeuropathies, and polyneuropathy can be equally disturbing.

Physical illnesses are less common precipitants of psychophysiologic insomnia than psychologic conditions, but they are important in some patients. Dyspnea and orthopnea can interfere with sleep onset or lead to frequent arousals. Patients with significant mobility problems often have difficulty falling asleep or staying asleep because of minor discomforts that would ordinarily be overcome by slight shifts in position. Hyperthyroidism and Cushing's disease can compromise the initiation of sleep, and so can such medications as steroids, dopaminergic agents, xanthine derivatives (including caffeine and theophylline), and adrenergic agonists.

Most patients can be treated with behavioral interventions (together with treatment of any underlying conditions that are identified). Patients should be instructed to set a fixed time for retiring and awakening, eliminate daytime naps, refrain from caffeine after noon, avoid exercise or anxiety-provoking activities after dinner, and sleep in a dark, quiet, comfortable room. Patients should also be encouraged to associate the bed primarily with sleep; all reading, TV watching, and eating should be done elsewhere. If they are lying in bed unable to fall asleep, they should leave the room and do something relaxing, returning to bed when they feel sleepy. In fact, it may be useful to restrict the total length of time they spend in bed (and prohibit any naps). This will make them sleepier, increasing the likelihood that when they do go to bed they will fall asleep readily and sleep continuously. Once this goal is achieved, the duration of time allowed for sleep can be gradually lengthened.

In some situations, sedative-hypnotic medications are an appropriate adjunct to therapy, but there is some potential for drug dependence. These agents are typically most helpful when applied for a limited number of nights.

2. Delayed sleep phase syndrome

Some people are able to fall asleep readily and sleep for normal periods of time but do so at the "wrong times." These people have sleep-wake schedule disturbances. The most common example is delayed sleep phase syndrome. Patients with this condition do not feel sleepy at bedtime, so they stay up until 3 AM or later. They then sleep for a normal interval if allowed to do so, but if the demands of work or school require them to awaken at 8 AM or earlier they become chronically sleepy, especially in the mornings. These patients usually compensate by sleeping late on weekends. In some cases, they can adjust their work schedules to accommodate their sleep patterns, but this is not practical for most patients. One approach to treatment is to awaken patients early in the morning and expose them to bright light for at least an hour. This leads them to fall asleep earlier in the night, so that being awakened early on subsequent mornings eventually becomes less onerous. Sustained benefit requires continued strict adherence to a regular sleep schedule.

B. Early Morning Arousal

1. Psychiatric and psychologic causes

Depression is the most common cause of early morning awakening in older patients. Depression is also associated with a shortened REM sleep latency, reduced slow-wave NREM sleep, and variable disturbance of sleep onset. Alcohol also disrupts sleep in the latter part of the night. This can result in a cycle whereby patients treat their own insomnia with alcohol (because it helps induce drowsiness); they then experience early morning awakening, resulting in more daytime sleepiness, so they take more alcohol on subsequent nights.

2. Psychophysiologic factors

Just as psychophysiologic factors can result in a cycle exacerbating sleep-onset delay, they can also increase the tendency to awaken early, producing greater daytime sleepiness, leading to more anxiety, resulting in even greater tendency to awaken early, and so forth. The behavioral interventions used to treat psychophysiologic insomnia are the same whether it manifests as sleep-onset delay or early morning awakening.

3. Advanced sleep phase syndrome

The advanced sleep phase syndrome is a sleep-wake schedule disturbance analogous to the delayed sleep phase syndrome, except that these patients fall asleep too early. This condition is very rare.

C. Sleep Fragmentation

Sleep that is frequently interrupted is not sufficiently restorative. Interruptions may result from sleep apnea (see Part IV of this chapter) or from medical conditions such as nocturia, orthopnea, or gastroesophageal reflux. Cluster headaches typically occur during REM sleep and awaken patients. Sleep fragmentation may even result from the need to awaken to take prescribed medications. Endocrine disorders and medications (especially corticosteroids and dopaminergic agents) can also produce this problem.

Any of these conditions may initiate the same kind of psychophysiologic cycle that leads to delayed sleep onset or early morning awakening. The same behavioral interventions are indicated, together with treatment directed at the underlying conditions.

D. Sleep State Misperception

Occasional patients complain of unrelenting insomnia but are found to have no objective abnormalities on sleep studies. This uncommon condition is called *pseudoinsomnia*, or *sleep state misperception*. It may be caused by a failure to perceive sleep, or it may represent hypochondrosis or another psychiatric disturbance. Of course, it is always possible that existing techniques are simply not adequate to demonstrate the underlying abnormality.

VI. Abnormal Behavior During Sleep

Most of the undesirable movements or behaviors that occur during sleep are associated with NREM sleep, probably because the atonia of REM sleep prevents most movements and behaviors of any kind, desirable or undesirable. In fact, when parasomnias occur during REM sleep, they are usually associated with disruption of the normal atonia.

A. NREM Sleep Parasomnias

1. Night terrors

Night terrors occur primarily in children but occasionally in adults. The child suddenly arouses from slow-wave sleep, screams, and manifests intense anxiety and autonomic activation (e.g., dilated pupils, perspiration, tachycardia, tachypnea, and piloerection). The child cannot be awakened or consoled but calms down after several minutes and returns to sleep. There is usually amnesia for the event, although there may be a vague recollection of a frightful image or mood. In contrast to typical dreams or nightmares, there is no sense of a coherent theme or "plot." Reassurance is often the only treatment necessary, but imipramine or diazepam can be used for particularly frequent events.

2. Sleepwalking and sleep talking

Sleepwalking and sleep talking disorders often overlap with night terrors and are thought to have a similar mechanism. All three conditions may represent a disorder of arousal from slow-wave sleep resulting in episodes of only partial awakening. Although any of these disorders may be exacerbated by anxiety and psychosocial stress, they are usually not associated with severe psychopathology.

Sleepwalking (somnambulism) involves complex behaviors that can include sitting up in bed, walking, dressing, eating, voiding, and even driving a car. Sleepwalkers can avoid objects, but coordination is poor. Most episodes last a few seconds to a few minutes. This condition is fairly common in childhood, but most children grow out of it between ages 7 and 14 years. No treatment is usually necessary except for reassurance. Safety restraints on doors, windows, and stairways may be required. When episodes are frequent, patients may be treated with bedtime diazepam. Sleep talking is analogous to sleepwalking; speech is often incoherent or elementary.

3. Enuresis

Enuresis (bedwetting) is involuntary micturition during sleep in an individual who has control of the bladder while awake. Enuresis may be a symptom of underlying urogenital disease or another medical problem, but it is usually idiopathic. In many patients, it probably represents delayed maturation; at age 5 years, about 15% of boys and 10% of girls have episodes of enuresis, which usually disappear by late childhood or adolescence. Psychologic factors or family dynamics sometimes play a role. For frequent episodes, children may be treated with behavioral techniques, with tricyclic antidepressants at low doses, or with deamino-8-D-arginine vasopressin (DDAVP).

4. Periodic movements of sleep

Periodic movements of sleep are characterized by stereotyped, periodic movements of the legs, typically resulting in dorsiflexion of the ankle and small toes, with flexion of the knee and hip, sometimes producing a "kicking" movement. These are the same muscles involved in the "triple flexion" response (see Chapter 2), but the movement is slower. These movements occur in "trains" during sleep. Similar movements may accompany arousals from sleep apnea, so it is important to exclude that diagnosis. Some patients with periodic movements of sleep have restless legs syndrome (see Part V of this chapter) when awake, but most do not. In contrast, 80–90% of all patients with restless legs syndrome also have periodic movements of sleep. Periodic movements of sleep are usually treated with bedtime levodopa, dopamine agonists, clonazepam, or gabapentin. These medications can also be used to treat restless legs syndrome.

5. Miscellaneous

Bruxism (tooth grinding) affects 10–15% of the population. It may contribute to periodontal disease and temporomandibular joint dysfunction. Rhythmic movement disorder is the label given to a group of uncommon parasomnias in which patients have stereotyped, repetitive movements such as banging of the head or rocking of the body, just before sleep onset and continuing into light sleep. This typically occurs in normal infants or toddlers and usually resolves in the second or third year of life.

B. REM Sleep Parasomnias

1. REM sleep behavior disorder

REM sleep behavior disorder is a condition in which the atonia that normally accompanies REM sleep breaks down and patients "act out" parts of dreams. Motor activity is often vigorous enough to cause injury to patients or their bed partners. Most patients are elderly, and the condition is usually idiopathic, but there may be an underlying neurologic disorder in up to one-third of patients. It is sometimes difficult to distinguish this condition from nocturnal seizures on the basis of the history, and polysomnography is very helpful in this regard. Patients are usually treated successfully with clonazepam.

2. Nightmares

Nightmares are particularly vivid and disturbing dreams that often are associated with arousal from REM sleep. In contrast to night terrors, there is hardly any autonomic arousal, patients are readily awakened, and the patients can remember the dream, which usually has a story element. Chronic nightmares are often psychiatric in origin. Post-traumatic stress disorder is a common cause.

3. Miscellaneous

Cluster headaches typically occur during REM sleep and are sometimes included in discussions of parasomnias. Further details are presented in Chapter 12. Penile erections are normal in REM sleep and very rarely they are painful enough to disrupt sleep.

VII. Discussion of Case Histories

Case 1. This patient has hypersomnia. Falling asleep at the wheel outside the setting of sleep deprivation is never normal. It is unlikely that this man is suffering from insufficient sleep since he allocates 9 hours for sleep each night. One important consideration would be a medication effect, as antihypertensive agents can be associated with hypersomnia. The most likely diagnosis, however, is obstructive sleep apnea. The history of snoring severe enough to prompt his wife to sleep in another room is the strongest reason to suspect the diagnosis. His obesity and big neck both could contribute to upper airway narrowing. Hypertension is present in about 40% of patients at the time of diagnosis. The patient should be asked when he developed his hypersomnia, when he began snoring, and when he started gaining weight. He does not describe any of the features that might suggest narcolepsy, although it would be important to inquire about them explicitly.

This man should be referred for polysomnography (especially because his wife cannot reliably say whether he is experiencing apneic episodes during sleep). If frequent episodes of apnea are documented, the study should be repeated with a trial of CPAP to see if the patient is likely to respond to this treatment. He should also be encouraged to lose weight, and his antihypertensive regimen should be investigated to be sure it is not contributing to his problem. He should be warned not to drive alone until his hypersomnia has been adequately diagnosed and treated.

Case 2. This man is correct that many of his symptoms can be features of depression. Depression and sleep disorders have many common features, however. It is often difficult to determine which problem is primary and which is secondary. In this case, the biggest clue that the delayed sleep onset might have a cause other than depression is the patient's report that he is unable to lie down for a prolonged period of time. The specific symptoms he describes are characteristic of restless legs syndrome. In addition, he notes epigastric discomfort when he is lying down, suggesting that he may also have gastroesophageal reflux. Both of these conditions can interfere with sleep onset, setting up a cycle of anxiety and insomnia as described in Part V. Moreover, restless legs syndrome is almost always associated with periodic leg movements of sleep, which can produce sleep fragmentation and lead to further insomnia.

The diagnosis of restless legs syndrome is based on the history. Patients should be evaluated for iron deficiency and uremia, both of which are associated with this disorder. This patient should be treated with levodopa/carbidopa (Sinemet) or a dopamine agonist such as bromocriptine (Parlodel), pergolide (Permax), pramipexole (Mirapex), or ropinirole (Requip). He should also receive appropriate treatment for gastroesophageal reflux; diagnostic studies are necessary only if his symptoms fail to respond.

Most likely, this patient has already established a pattern of psychophysiologic insomnia that will persist even after treatment of his reflux and restless legs syndrome. He will need education about proper sleep hygiene, and he may require the kinds of behavioral interventions described in Part V. Only if depressive symptoms persist despite all these measures should treatment of depression be considered. Even then, fluoxetine (Prozac) would probably be contraindicated because it can cause insomnia.

Case 3. The description of this girl's episode is classic for night terrors. The previous episodes may indeed have been exacerbated by the stress of a new home and day care environment, but the family should be informed that there is no evidence that this condition is caused by underlying psychologic disease. No additional investigations are necessary, and no treatment is indicated at this point other than good sleep hygiene and safety measures to prevent injury. The girl and her parents should be reassured that she does not have a serious disease, and she will probably outgrow these episodes, but they may recur during stressful intervals.

10

Multifocal Central Nervous System Disorders

I. Case Histories

Case 1. A 29-year-old right-handed woman with a history of IV drug abuse has come to the emergency room because of the acute onset of inability to speak. Two days earlier, she had noticed weakness of the left arm after injecting heroin there and concluded that she must have "hit a nerve." She has been experiencing fevers, chills, and sweats for the past week, and feels tired all the time. Her general examination is notable for a temperature of 39°C and petechiae on both legs. Neurologic examination reveals almost no verbal output, nearly normal comprehension, and left hemiparesis and sensory loss to all modalities (face worse than arm worse than leg). Hyperreflexia exists throughout the left arm and leg, and a Babinski sign is present on the left.

Questions:

1. Where's the lesion?

2. What diagnoses should be considered?

3. What diagnostic tests would be helpful?

4. How should this patient be managed?

Case 2. A 35-year-old man has made an appointment with his family doctor because for the past 3 weeks, his left foot has had a tendency to drag after the third mile of his daily 5-mile run. Two years ago, he had a similar problem with the right foot, but he had twisted that ankle a week earlier, and when the symptoms resolved over the next month, he thought nothing more of them. His only other neurologic symptom had been partial loss of vision in the left eye 8 months ago. This had developed gradually over 5 days and resolved at almost the same rate; he had attributed it to the stress of a divorce and a new job.

His general physical examination is normal. He has normal mental status. An afferent pupillary defect exists on the left, but his cranial nerves are otherwise normal. He has moderate weakness of left ankle dorsiflexion and walks with a mild foot drop on the left, but his motor examination is otherwise normal. Hyperreflexia is found at the left knee and ankle, and there is a Babinski sign on the left. Sensation is intact to all modalities.

Questions:

1.   Where's the lesion?

2.   What diagnoses should be considered?

3.   What diagnostic tests would be helpful?

4.   How should this patient be managed?

Case 3. A 67-year-old woman has come to the emergency room because of the second episode of Bell's palsy within 6 months. The first episode resulted in only mild weakness of the right face, so she was not treated. She has improved only minimally in the interim. The second episode began yesterday morning when she noted a tendency to drool out of the left side of her mouth, and she awoke this morning with complete inability to move the left side of her face. She has also noted that her voice is more hoarse than it used to be, and she thinks the hearing in her right ear is deteriorating. In addition, she reports that 2 weeks ago, she developed pain in her lower back on the right; for the last week, it has radiated into her right posterior thigh, leg, and little toe.

Her general physical examination is unremarkable. Neurologic examination confirms bilateral facial weakness (including forehead muscles) worse on the left, hearing loss in the right ear, reduced movement of the left side of the palate, and absent gag reflex on the left side. She has slight weakness of right ankle plantar flexion, but the motor examination is otherwise normal. She has no right ankle jerk, but all other reflexes are normal and symmetric. The sensory examination is normal.

Questions:

1. Where's the lesion?

2. What diagnoses should be considered?

3. What diagnostic tests would be helpful?

4. How should this patient be managed?

II. Approach to Multifocal Disorders

There is something elegant about localizing all of a patient's symptoms and signs to a single lesion site. Nature is not always elegant, however. Many processes affect the nervous system diffusely; most neuromuscular diseases, dementing illnesses, movement disorders, and sleep disorders fall into this category, as do many systemic illnesses. Still, even these diffuse conditions possess some pattern and symmetry. In fact, the particular pattern of involvement is generally the basis for making a diagnosis.

For multifocal conditions, in contrast, the neurologic presentation is characterized primarily by the lack of pattern. Fortunately, there are only a few conditions like this, so the diagnosis is often straightforward. In other words, the lack of pattern is itself a revealing pattern. The classic multifocal disease is multiple sclerosis (MS). Other inflammatory diseases and neoplastic processes can also produce multifocal manifestations. The time course and epidemiologic factors help to distinguish among these possibilities (see Chapter 3).

There are two broad categories of multifocal disorders. Some diseases propagate in random directions from a single focus, which is typical of infections and neoplastic diseases. Other processes are intrinsically multifocal. Most diseases in this category (including MS) are inflammatory but not infectious.

III. Focal Diseases with Multifocal Propagation

A. Metastatic Cancer

Approximately 25% of patients with systemic cancer develop central nervous system (CNS) metastases, and in more than two-thirds of these patients, the metastases are symptomatic. The spinal cord may be involved by direct metastasis, or, more commonly, by epidural compression from a bony metastasis, as discussed in Chapter 15. Brain metastasis is particularly likely in patients with melanoma or testicular cancer, approximately one-half of whom have an intracranial tumor found at autopsy. Approximately one-third of patients with lung cancer and 15% of patients with breast or kidney cancer have intracranial metastases at autopsy. Because lung cancer and breast cancer are common, they are the most likely sites of primary tumor in patients with brain metastases. The next most common primary tumors are gastrointestinal, genitourinary tract, and malignant melanoma, in that order.

Diagnosis of brain metastases is based on the clinical reasoning described in Chapter 3: chronically progressive focal lesions are likely to be neoplastic, and when there is a history of a primary malignancy elsewhere in the body, CNS metastasis is the prime consideration. The preferred diagnostic test is an MRI scan of the brain. A metastasis typically appears on MRI or CT scans as a well-demarcated, contrast-enhancing, spherical lesion with surrounding edema. This appearance is not specific, however, and a biopsy is sometimes necessary to establish the diagnosis, even in patients with a known primary cancer. The presence of multiple lesions with characteristic features increases the likelihood of metastases.

When the systemic cancer is controlled and only a single brain metastasis exists, it should be surgically resected if possible, followed by radiation therapy. Not only does this provide a definitive pathologic diagnosis of the brain lesion, but it also prolongs survival and reduces the risk of local recurrence compared with radiation therapy alone. Even when two or three metastatic lesions are present, resection may be appropriate if the lesions are surgically accessible. The more lesions that exist, however, the less feasible surgical resection becomes. In such cases, radiation therapy is the main treatment option (although the largest lesion is sometimes resected for palliation). Chemotherapy may also be effective in treating some brain metastases.

Approximately 15% of patients with brain metastases have no other symptoms of malignancy at the time their CNS lesions are discovered.

These patients require a thorough search for the primary neoplasm so that it can be treated appropriately. Furthermore, if the primary cancer can be found, and multiple brain lesions with typical characteristics of metastasis are present, there is no need for biopsy or surgical resection. Special emphasis should be placed on the search for a pulmonary neoplasm, because it is the most common primary tumor in patients with metastatic CNS disease, and other primary tumors often metastasize to the lung before spreading to the rest of the body. The evaluation should therefore include a chest x-ray, sputum samples for cytology, and (if the diagnosis is still unknown) a CT scan of the chest. These patients also require rectal examinations, and stool should be screened for occult blood. Men require careful testicular and prostate examinations, and women need careful breast examinations. If this evaluation is not productive, an abdominal CT scan (for occult renal carcinoma) should be obtained. The yield of upper and lower gastrointestinal series is too low to make them worthwhile in this setting. If the diagnosis remains obscure, stereotactic brain biopsy (or surgical resection when there is only one lesion) is necessary.

Even before the diagnosis is established, many patients require treatment for the mass effect produced by the edema surrounding the metastases. Dexamethasone usually produces dramatic reduction in brain edema and clinical symptoms. The optimal dose is not known. A common approach is to give 10 mg IV initially, followed by 4 mg every 6 hours, increasing the dose if no clinical improvement is observed. When the mass effect is so great that there is a risk of cerebral herniation, hyperventilation and osmotic diuresis may also be necessary (see Chapter 11).

Seizures occur in approximately 25% of patients with brain metastases and are treated with anticonvulsants according to standard principles (see Chapter 5). For patients who have not yet seized, prophylactic antiepileptic drugs are usually not recommended, except for patients with metastatic melanoma, which has a high incidence of hemorrhage.

In 5–10% of patients with cancer, there is clinical evidence of spread to the meninges. This spread has been given a variety of labels, including leptomeningeal metastasis, carcinomatous meningitis, or meningeal carcinomatosis. It can occur with almost any cancer but is most commonly associated with hematologic malignancies, melanoma, and cancer of the breast or lung. Meningeal carcinomatosis can present in several ways. It can cause meningeal irritation, producing a syndrome resembling meningitis. Patients may present with symptoms of hydrocephalus when the cancer cells block CSF outflow. Tumor cells in the meningeal spaces may also compress nerve roots or cranial nerves as they leave the neuraxis, resulting in multiple cranial neuropathies or polyradiculopathies. The diagnosis is usually made by cytologic examination of the CSF. Individual samples may be negative, so patients may require three or more lumbar punctures before the diagnosis is established. Intrathecal chemotherapy combined with radiation therapy helps to prolong life, but even with optimal treatment, life expectancy is 6 months.

Cancers also can metastasize more distally in the peripheral nervous system. The brachial plexus and the lumbosacral plexus can be invaded by tumor cells, and this is the first symptom of cancer in some patients. Individual peripheral nerves or muscles can also be sites of metastasis, but this is less common. Focal metastases in the peripheral nervous system are usually treated with radiation therapy.

Tumors can also cause remote effects without metastasizing; these manifestations are called *paraneoplastic syndromes* and are usually diffuse rather than multifocal. Examples include cerebellar degeneration, various forms of polyneuropathy (pure sensory neuropathy is the most specific), Lambert-Eaton myasthenic syndrome, dermatomyositis, and encephalopathy. Paraneoplastic syndromes appear to be caused by autoimmune phenomena; different syndromes are associated with specific abnormal antibodies. In more than one-half of the patients with paraneoplastic syndromes, neurologic symptoms precede other manifestations of cancer; therefore, prompt diagnosis may permit the underlying cancer to be identified and treated earlier than would have been possible otherwise.

B. Central Nervous System Infections

Infectious agents can reach the CNS either by direct spread (e.g., from the sinuses or the inner ear) or via the bloodstream. When infections reach the CNS, the resulting damage can be focal (e.g., an abscess or a focal myelitis), multifocal (multiple abscesses or multiple discrete sites of nervous system involvement), or diffuse (meningitis or encephalitis). The approach to focal and multifocal infectious processes is presented in this section. Diffuse meningitis is discussed in Chapter 12. Encephalitis is usually due to a viral infection, and treatment is primarily supportive care (except for herpesviruses, which are discussed later in this section).

1. Abscesses

An *abscess* is a localized area of suppuration and necrosis that forms when an appropriate organism reaches a relatively hypoxic region of the body where host defenses are inadequate to eradicate the infection. Initially, the region of inflammation is poorly demarcated, but over the course of 2 or 3 weeks, a well-defined fibrous capsule forms. CNS abscesses can be caused by anaerobic bacteria, aerobic bacteria, fungi, or parasites.

In many ways, CNS abscesses are analogous to metastatic tumors in the CNS. Both processes produce mass lesions. The time course is characteristically subacute for abscesses and chronic for metastases, but this distinction is not always reliable. Abscesses and metastases are often indistinguishable radiographically: Both characteristically appear as contrast-enhancing lesions with surrounding edema, and the area of enhancement often produces a ring around the lesion. The likely diagnosis can sometimes be established by examining spinal fluid (cytopathology for metastases, cultures for abscesses), but the yield is often low, and a risk of brain herniation exists when a lumbar puncture is performed on a patient in whom a focal mass lesion has produced a significant elevation of intracranial pressure. For abscesses and metastases, a presumptive diagnosis can sometimes be made by identifying similar lesions elsewhere in the body, but definitive diagnosis usually requires direct tissue examination (i.e., biopsy or surgical resection). The optimal treatment of a solitary CNS abscess is either resection or stereotactic CT-guided aspiration in conjunction with systemic antibiotics. The same approach applies when several large lesions are surgically accessible. When multiple abscesses are present, systemic antibiotic therapy is the cornerstone of treatment, although the largest lesions may still be aspirated or (less often) excised. The choice of antibiotics depends on the underlying organism. Thus, when surgical resection is not an option, biopsy of one of the lesions may be desirable. When biopsy is not possible, patients are treated empirically, typically with penicillin or a third-generation cephalosporin (cefotaxime or ceftriaxone) in combination with metronidazole. Chloramphenicol also provides good coverage and CNS penetration but carries a greater risk of toxicity. When there are reasons to suspect a particular infectious agent, the antibiotic regimen should be tailored accordingly (e.g., antistaphylococcal agents should be included when abscesses occur in the setting of recent head trauma or brain surgery).

2. Endocarditis

Infections in the heart are ideally situated for sending colonies in all directions. Between 10% and 30% of all patients with endocarditis develop embolic occlusion of major cerebral arteries. Emboli from patients with endocarditis can be either sterile or infectious. Sterile emboli result in strokes that are indistinguishable from any other cardioembolic strokes. Infectious emboli can produce strokes by occluding arteries, or they may be deposited in the meninges or parenchyma, serving as foci for the development of meningitis or abscesses. Septic emboli can also infect the walls of the cerebral arteries themselves, leading to aneurysmal dilatation (*mycotic aneurysms*). These aneurysms can themselves embolize, resulting in strokes, or they can rupture, resulting in subarachnoid, intraparenchymal, or intraventricular hemorrhage. The consequences of rupture are often devastating.

Strokes that occur in patients with infectious endocarditis can result from embolization either directly from the heart or from a mycotic aneurysm. The distinction is important because of the risk that a mycotic aneurysm could rupture. Clinical features do not distinguish these two possibilities; cerebral angiography is required. If mycotic aneurysms are found, they are usually treated with antibiotics initially. In at least one-half of patients, this treatment results in reduction in size and eventual resolution of the aneurysms. Thus, the role of angiography is to determine if mycotic aneurysms are present and to document their size so that response to treatment can be monitored. Surgical resection should be considered if aneurysms do not respond to antibiotics.

Although anticoagulation is the standard treatment for most cardioembolic causes of stroke (see Chapter 4), it is generally avoided in patients with infectious endocarditis because it does not prevent the growth of vegetations and may increase the risk of hemorrhagic transformation of a stroke or rupture of a mycotic aneurysm. The one exception is endocarditis on an artificial valve, in which the risk of recurrent embolization is so high that the benefits of anticoagulation probably outweigh the risks.

3. Specific infectious agents

Certain infectious agents are particularly likely to produce multifocal nervous system disease. Most of these infections are relatively indolent, perhaps because more aggressive infections become symptomatic and are treated (or result in death) before they have a chance to form colonies throughout the body.

a. Human immunodeficiency virus

Patients infected with HIV can develop dysfunction at any level of the CNS. At least three factors predispose to CNS involvement. First, these patients are at risk for many opportunistic infections and neoplasms that affect the CNS. Second, HIV itself appears to have a predilection for the CNS and may produce symptoms directly. Third, antigenic cross-reactivity between HIV and CNS elements may occur, so that the inflammatory reaction provoked by HIV infection results in CNS damage.

Peripheral nervous system syndromes reported in HIV patients include polymyositis and other forms of myositis. There also appears to be a myopathy associated with the use of zidovudine, which may lead to diagnostic confusion. Four principal neuropathic syndromes are associated with HIV infection. The most common is a distal, symmetric peripheral polyneuropathy that tends to increase in incidence and severity with disease duration. This polyneuropathy is thought to be a direct effect of HIV infection, although other potential causes are often present (notably nutritional deficiencies and drug toxicity). Didanosine (ddI), zalcitabine (ddC), and stavudine (d4T) have been associated with neuropathy; so have some of the drugs typically used to treat AIDS manifestations. Inflammatory demyelinating polyradiculoneuropathies are much less common than axonal polyneuropathies. Acute inflammatory demyelinating polyradioneuropathy (AIDP) and chronic inflammatory demyelinating polyradioneuropathy (CIDP) may occur in HIV-positive patients who do not have AIDS. These conditions sometimes develop at the time of seroconversion, suggesting that they are caused by the inflammatory response to HIV and not by immunosuppression or some other direct effect of HIV infection. Another less common neuropathic syndrome is mononeuropathy multiplex, which can also occur early in the course of HIV infection. The fourth major variety of HIV-related neuropathic syndrome is progressive polyradiculopathy, typically beginning with leg weakness and bladder or bowel problems, with progression to the arms over several weeks. This generally occurs with advanced immunodeficiency. Cytomegalovirus (CMV) appears to be the cause in many cases. Herpes zoster reactivation is also common in HIV-infected patients, leading to a more localized radiculopathy. Cranial nerves may also be involved in patients with herpes zoster, mononeuropathy multiplex, AIDP, or CIDP.

In the CNS, the most common manifestation of HIV infection is an encephalopathy that is sometimes mistaken for depression because it usually presents with nonspecific mood changes, psychomotor slowing, and concentration problems. It rapidly progresses to generalized cognitive deterioration, often associated with pronounced apathy and social withdrawal. These patients frequently develop tremor or myoclonus. At least one-half of patients with encephalopathy also develop a myelopathy, with characteristic vacuolar changes noted in the spinal cord at autopsy. Incontinence, gait disturbance, and bilateral Babinski signs are frequent late in the course of the encephalopathy, either as a direct result of cerebral involvement or as a consequence of myelopathy. Encephalopathy typically occurs in the setting of advanced immunosuppression, and it improves in response to high doses of zidovudine, suggesting that it is a direct result of HIV infection. Histopathologic evidence of CMV is found in a high proportion of patients with neurologic manifestations of HIV infection, but it is not clear what role CMV plays in AIDS encephalopathy or in producing other clinical manifestations.

Focal lesions in the brain and spinal cord are common manifestations of HIV-associated secondary processes, especially toxoplasmosis, cryptococcus, lymphoma, and progressive multifocal leukoencephalopathy (PML), a disease of white matter caused by the JC virus, an opportunistic papovavirus. All of these can produce progressive, focal symptoms (that is, they can present as mass lesions, usually with a subacute time course), but they can also be asymptomatic or produce diffuse symptoms. Cryptococcus, in particular, usually manifests with a meningitis that typically produces headaches (in 85% of patients), but fever and neck stiffness each occur in only 35% of patients. Approximately 40% of patients with cryptococcal meningitis have altered mental status. Except for cranial neuropathies, focal findings are uncommon in cryptococcal meningitis.

Because of the high incidence of mass lesions in the brain, an imaging study of the brain is usually the first test obtained in HIV-infected patients with headaches or mental status changes, even if there are no focal abnormalities on neurologic examination. When this study is normal, a lumbar puncture is usually performed to look for evidence of cryptococcal meningitis; cryptococcal antigen is present in the spinal fluid of 95% of patients with this infection, and India ink staining is positive in 70–80% of patients.

The conditions that produce abnormalities on brain imaging studies often have similar radiologic characteristics, making diagnosis difficult. Polymerase chain reaction (PCR) testing of CSF shows promise for the diagnosis of PML, which also has a fairly distinctive appearance on MRI scans, but the lesions caused by toxoplasmosis and lymphoma are often indistinguishable on CT and MRI scans. The diagnosis is most often established by treating empirically with sulfadiazine and pyrimethamine, antibiotics that usually produce a dramatic response in patients with toxoplasmosis. When lesions fail to improve despite these antibiotics, or when only a single lesion is evident on an initial MRI scan (unusual for toxoplasmosis, which typically produces multiple lesions), a biopsy may be necessary for diagnosis. CNS lymphoma responds transiently to corticosteroids, and radiation therapy can prolong expected survival by 4 or 5 months, but the life span of AIDS patients with CNS lymphoma is usually less than 1 year even with optimal treatment. No treatment has proved effective for PML. For both toxoplasmosis and cryptococcal meningitis (which usually responds readily to treatment with amphotericin or fluconazole) lifelong maintenance therapy is necessary to prevent relapses.

Patients with AIDS have an increased incidence of syphilis, which may be hard to diagnose because some of the traditional serologic tests are less reliable in this setting. Patients who have AIDS may require more aggressive and sustained treatment for neurosyphilis than is necessary in immunocompetent individuals. Other conditions that may affect the nervous system in patients with AIDS include Kaposi's sarcoma, atypical mycobacterial infections, nocardiosis, and fungal infections (e.g., candidiasis, aspergillosis, histoplasmosis, mucormycosis, and others). Patients with AIDS also have an increased incidence of strokes. It is common for a single patient to have several different processes affecting the nervous system simultaneously.

b. Spirochetal infections

The initial clinical manifestation of syphilis (*primary syphilis*) is a skin lesion, or chancre, at the site of inoculation. In untreated patients, this heals spontaneously over 3–6 weeks, at which point the features of secondary syphilis (flulike symptoms, rash, lymphadenopathy, and mucosal lesions) usually appear. Some patients with secondary syphilis never develop symptoms. Nervous system dissemination of the organism occurs even in the primary and secondary stages of infection, but most patients have no neurologic symptoms. No more than 5% of patients with secondary syphilis develop symptoms of aseptic meningitis. The symptoms (if any) of secondary syphilis resolve without treatment over a period of weeks to months, and patients enter a latent stage in which there are no clinical manifestations of infection for months to years. In 10–30% of untreated patients, the latent stage is followed by tertiary syphilis, which is characterized by skin, osseous, cardiovascular, or neurologic manifestations. Neurosyphilis refers to nervous system involvement at any stage of syphilis. At all stages, most patients with neurosyphilis are asymptomatic. Those who do develop neurologic symptoms typically manifest one of several distinctive clinical syndromes. The earliest is the aseptic meningitis that can occur within the first 1–2 years after the initial infection, often associated with cranial nerve involvement. Meningovascular syphilis can occur 1–10 years (but typically 5–7 years) after the initial infection. It is characterized by diffuse meningeal infiltrates and inflammation and fibrosis of arteries, causing brain and spinal cord lesions that may be focal, multifocal, or diffuse. The most delayed neurologic manifestations of syphilis are general paresis and tabes dorsalis, which generally occur 10–30 years after the initial infection. General paresis is a condition of diffuse cortical dysfunction, producing dementia, upper motor neuron findings, myoclonus, seizures, dysarthria, and pupillary abnormalities. Tabes dorsalis results from involvement of the posterior nerve roots as they enter the spinal cord. Typical symptoms are loss of proprioception, ataxia, and lightning-like pains. Deep tendon reflexes are usually absent in the lower extremities, though Babinski signs may be present. Bladder dysfunction often exists due to sensory involvement, and the pupils are abnormal in more than 90% of patients.

Diagnosis of neurosyphilis is based on serologic studies and spinal fluid analysis. Two types of serologic tests are currently available (tests using PCR or monoclonal antibody reagents hold great promise but are still experimental). Nonspecific antibodies, such as the VDRL or rapid plasma reagent (RPR), are present in the blood of almost all patients with secondary syphilis but revert to normal in approximately one-third of patients with late syphilis. Their presence in the CSF is strong evidence for neurosyphilis, but their absence does not exclude the diagnosis. Specific treponemal antibodies, such as fluorescent treponemal antibody (FTA) or microhemagglutination–*Treponema pallidum* (MHA-TP), are also present in the blood of nearly all patients with secondary syphilis, and persist throughout life even when the infection itself is eradicated. They are therefore a reliable indicator of previous syphilitic infection, but they do not indicate whether the infection is still active. In a patient with clinical features suggestive of neurosyphilis, the first diagnostic test should be to check the serum FTA or MHA-TP. If the result is negative, this excludes the possibility of secondary or late syphilis, so the patient's symptoms are not due to neurosyphilis. If the FTA or MHA-TP result is positive, this simply means that the patient had an active syphilis infection at some point in the past. To determine if the infection is currently active in the CNS, a lumbar puncture should be performed, and the presence of any of the typical abnormalities (i.e., elevated white blood cell count, increased protein concentration, or positive VDRL) warrants treatment for neurosyphilis with IV penicillin.

Lyme disease, like syphilis, can result in neurologic complications months or years after the initial infection. The most common neurologic manifestation is a subacute or chronic meningitis that typically begins a few weeks to a few months after inoculation. The usual symptoms are headache and stiff neck, often with associated mood changes and difficulty concentrating. These symptoms are frequently mild and usually resolve even without treatment, so this stage of the disease is probably unrecognized in many cases. Cranial nerve palsies (almost always including one or both facial nerves) and radicular pain sometimes accompany the meningitis. As with neurosyphilis, some patients in whom Lyme disease is not eradicated in the early stages subsequently develop late neurologic complications, including chronic or subacute encephalitis, hemiparesis, paraparesis, and peripheral neuropathy.

Borrelia burgdorferi, the agent that causes Lyme disease, can almost never be cultured from the blood or spinal fluid, so diagnosis is based on clinical characteristics and serologic studies. Antibodies to the organism can be detected using either enzyme-linked immunosorbent assay (ELISA) techniques or indirect fluorescent antibody testing. These tests (like the specific treponemal antibody assays for syphilis) indicate a history of exposure and not necessarily active infection. Moreover, they are neither 100% specific nor 100% sensitive. Western blot assay can provide specificity by identifying the specific antigens to which the patient's antibodies react, but this is a more laborious and intensive procedure, and criteria for positivity have not been standardized. PCR techniques applied to the spinal fluid offer the advantage of testing directly for bacterial DNA rather than the host response, but there remains a 40–50% false-negative rate that is attributed to the organism's relative scarcity in body fluids.

Neuroborreliosis requires treatment with IV ceftriaxone, cefotaxime, or penicillin for at least 2 weeks, and many experts recommend a 4-week course. IV doxycycline or chloramphenicol may be used as a second-line drug.

c. Tuberculosis

Mycobacterium tuberculosis can spread to the nervous system via the bloodstream either during the initial infection or with subsequent caseation at the primary site or other sites. The resulting tuberculous foci (*tubercles*) can then remain dormant in the CNS for months or years before producing clinical symptoms. The most common neurologic manifestation is tuberculous meningitis, which occurs when a suitably located subpial tubercle grows or ruptures into the subarachnoid or intraventricular space. This meningitis is most marked at the base of the brain, ultimately forming a thick, gelatinous mass that engulfs the cranial nerves and blood vessels passing through it. Less often, tubercles located deep in the parenchyma may grow large enough to present as a mass lesion (a *tuberculoma*).

Tuberculous meningitis usually begins with a several-week pro-drome of headache, malaise, personality change, and low-grade fever. The headache eventually becomes more severe and continuous, and patients develop nausea, vomiting, neck stiffness, confusion, papille-dema, and cranial nerve abnormalities. Because blood vessels passing through the region of basilar meningitis become inflamed and throm-bosed, focal deficits (including hemiparesis, paraparesis, ataxia, and involuntary movements) may occur. Approximately 10% of adults and a higher proportion of children develop seizures. Patients subse-quently progress to stupor and coma, with death typically occurring within 2 months of the onset of illness when no therapy is given.

The diagnosis of tuberculous meningitis can be extremely difficult to establish, and antituberculous treatment often must be initiated even when the diagnosis is only presumptive. A positive tuberculin skin test is helpful, but a negative test is not, because false-negatives are com-mon in all forms of tuberculosis. Similarly, evidence of active tubercu-lous infection elsewhere in the body is helpful when present, but not when absent, because the nervous system can be the only site of active infection. CSF is usually the most important guide to diagnosis. Typi-cal findings are elevated opening pressure, increased protein (usually 100–500 mg/dl), reduced glucose (< 45 mg/dl in 80% of patients), and moderate pleocytosis (100–300 white blood cells/mm^3 in most patients). The cellular reaction is predominantly mononuclear, but polymorphonuclear cells may predominate in a significant minority of patients, especially early in the course. Mycobacterial cultures from the CSF require weeks to months for detectable growth, and even then the false-negative rate is at least 25%. The yield is increased by send-ing samples from several lumbar punctures (usually repeated on a daily basis); there is no need to delay treatment for this, because the yield from cultures remains good even after several days of therapy.

The long delay and high false-negative rate for cultures has prompted a search for alternate means of diagnosis. Some tests involve assaying the spinal fluid for substances that are believed to be unique to *M. tuberculosis*, including tuberculostearic acid and adeno-sine deaminase. Other tests involve the use of ELISA and other immu-nologic techniques to detect specific *M. tuberculosis* antigens or anti-bodies directed against the organism. PCR techniques provide nearly 100% specificity but a sensitivity of only approximately 70%. Promis-ing results have been reported with an assay for mycobacterial riboso-mal RNA.

The optimal treatment regimen for tuberculous meningitis has not been established. Most patients are initially treated with a combination of three first-line drugs. These first-line agents include isoniazid, rifampin, pyrazinamide, ethambutol, and streptomycin. After 2 months, one of the agents is discontinued, and the remaining two agents (usually isoniazid and rifampin) are continued for 4–7 more months. The specific agents used and the duration of therapy may be modified depending on the likelihood of drug resistance. Adjunctive corticosteroids appear to help limit or even prevent the neurologic consequences of tuberculous meningitis, though this has never been convincingly demonstrated. They are typically administered to patients with increased intracranial pressure, spinal block, focal neurologic signs, or depressed level of consciousness. Tuberculomas can usually be adequately treated with medications, although the lesions are sometimes resected when the diagnosis is uncertain. Surgical procedures are sometimes required to treat increased intracranial pressure or hydrocephalus.

d. Herpesviruses

Herpesviruses have a tendency to lie dormant in the nervous system for years at a time, periodically reactivating and causing clinical symptoms. Several distinctive syndromes can result. The most serious is **herpes simplex encephalitis** (HSE). This is mainly due to **herpes simplex virus type 1** which causes HSE in adults, whereas **herpes simplex virus type 2** is the principal cause of neonatal HSE and adult aseptic meningitis. HSE is the most frequent cause of fatal encephalitis, and it is the most common cause of specifically diagnosed acute, sporadic encephalitis. Approximately two-thirds of cases are due to reactivation, and approximately one-third are due to primary infection resulting from exposure to contaminated saliva or respiratory secretions. The clinical presentation is similar to that of any other form of encephalitis, with a prodromal phase characterized by malaise, fever, headache, and sometimes behavioral changes. The distinctive feature of HSE is a tendency to involve the frontotemporal lobes predominantly, resulting in focal signs and symptoms in at least 75% of patients. These include hemiparesis, aphasia, visual field abnormalities, and cranial nerve deficits. Florid behavioral changes, amnesia, seizures, stupor, and coma are also common. The clinical course is extremely variable, with some patients progressing to coma within a few days but other patients stabilizing and demonstrating only a mild to moderate encephalopathy for several weeks.

Spinal fluid examination typically reveals a lymphocytic pleocytosis (50–500 cells/mm^3) with mild protein elevation and normal or moderately reduced glucose. In 25–40% of patients, red blood cells are present in the CSF. Regions of abnormal signal and microhemorrhage, especially in the temporal lobes, may be evident on MRI scans, and unilateral or bilateral periodic lateralized epileptiform discharges in the frontotemporal regions are the characteristic EEG findings. None of these tests is 100% sensitive or specific, however. PCR testing for viral DNA in the spinal fluid is rapidly replacing brain biopsy as the "gold standard" for diagnosis. Viral DNA is detected in 98% of patients with biopsy-proven HSE and only 6% of patients with negative biopsies; brain biopsy has a false-negative rate of 2% when compared with autopsy results. Whenever HSE is suspected, it is best to initiate empiric treatment with acyclovir (30 mg/kg per day in three divided doses for at least 10 days) while awaiting CSF PCR results. Brain MRI scan and EEG can also be helpful. Brain biopsy is of value in confusing clinical presentations, when rapid and reliable PCR testing is not available, or when the PCR results are negative. The mortality rate in patients treated with acyclovir and supportive care is 20–30%, compared with approximately 80% mortality in untreated patients. These data are derived from patients with classic clinical presentations, however; there are suggestions that milder, unrecognized cases may exist.

Herpes varicella-zoster virus remains latent in neurons of sensory ganglia after resolution of the primary infection (varicella, commonly called chickenpox). Zoster, or "shingles," occurs when the virus is reactivated years later. The risk of zoster increases with increasing age and decreasing immune function, but it may occur even in immunocompetent young people. The most common manifestation is sharp, burning pain in a dermatomal distribution, followed 2–5 days later by a characteristic rash in the same distribution (though some patients never develop the rash). The most commonly involved dermatomes are at the thoracic and lumbar levels. Another typical area of involvement is the territory of the ophthalmic division of the trigeminal nerve (*zoster ophthalmicus*). The most common neurologic complication is postherpetic neuralgia, which occurs in roughly 10% of all patients with zoster but in more than one-half of patients older than 60 years. Postherpetic neuralgia is characterized by steady, burning pain with superimposed lightning-like pains in the distribution of the preceding skin involvement, persisting for more than 4 weeks after the rash disappears. The area is often extremely sensitive to touch. Acyclovir, famciclovir, and valacyclovir have all been shown to reduce the duration of the rash and the duration of postherpetic neuralgia. Famciclovir and valacyclovir are generally preferred over acyclovir because they are more convenient to administer. Options for symptomatic pain relief include tricyclic antidepressants, antiepileptic drugs (especially gabapentin and carbamazepine), opioids, and local anesthetics (including capsaicin cream).

Other neurologic complications of zoster can occur when the virus spreads from the sensory nerve to involve other components of the nervous system. For example, spread to the anterior root can cause segmental motor paresis, usually involving the myotome that corresponds to the affected dermatome. Spread of the virus to the spinal cord may result in myelitis, and more diffuse spread may result in encephalitis or aseptic meningitis. Approximately one-third of patients with zoster ophthalmicus develop abnormalities of other cranial nerves, especially the third nerve. Other potential complications of zoster ophthalmicus include ocular involvement (in approximately 20% of patients) and, rarely, a thrombotic cerebral vasculopathy that results in delayed contralateral hemiparesis. Ramsay Hunt syndrome (*zoster oticus*, *zoster auricularis*, or *zoster cephalicus*) is thought to represent spread of the virus from the geniculate ganglion of the facial nerve. It is characterized by vesicular eruption in the external auditory meatus accompanied by ipsilateral facial weakness, and often by hearing loss, tinnitus, or vertigo. Cranial nerves V, IX, and X are frequently involved, and there may be severe pain in the territories of these nerves. Patients with these syndromes of more extensive nervous system involvement are usually treated with acyclovir, although its efficacy remains unknown.

e. Parasitic infections

Parasites are ideally adapted to colonize multiple sites in the nervous system and other organ systems without provoking overwhelming host responses. Many of these organisms are uncommon in the United States, but they account for significant worldwide morbidity and mortality. Parasitic infections that are particularly likely to involve the nervous system include malaria, toxoplasmosis, trypanosomiasis, amebic infections, strongyloidiasis, trichinosis, onchocerciasis (the fourth leading cause of blindness in the world), schistosomiasis, paragonimiasis, echinococcosis, and cysticercosis (the most common cause of adult-onset epilepsy in developing countries and increasingly common in the United States). Detailed descriptions of these parasites, their life cycles, and the diseases they cause are available in textbooks of infectious diseases.

IV. Inherently Multifocal Diseases

A. Multiple Sclerosis

MS is the prototype of multifocal CNS diseases. The cornerstone of diagnosis is still the traditional clinical description of "multiple CNS lesions separated in space and time." These lesions correspond to pathologic findings of perivascular inflammation and destruction of myelin in the CNS white matter. Aggressive investigation has failed to identify a consistent infectious agent or other common factor responsible for inciting the inflammation, so the disease is generally thought to be due to an autoimmune reaction. Genetic and environmental factors also play a role.

Several diagnostic tests can be helpful in supporting or challenging the diagnosis, but no test is completely reliable. The most sensitive test is the MRI scan of the brain, which demonstrates white matter abnormalities in most patients with MS, but identical findings can result from other inflammatory conditions, ischemia, metabolic abnormalities, or even neoplasms. An elevated immunoglobulin G (IgG) index (the ratio of IgG to albumin in the CSF, divided by the corresponding ratio in the serum) or the presence of oligoclonal bands in the CSF can provide evidence of ongoing inflammation, but they do not distinguish between MS and any other condition that provokes CNS inflammation. Evoked potential testing may be useful for demonstrating physiologic abnormalities that may be clinically asymptomatic and radiographically invisible. These tests involve EEG recording after exposing the subject to a sensory stimulus, either visual, auditory, or somatosensory. Because of the large amount of random activity in a routine EEG, the specific response to the stimulus cannot be distinguished from the background noise after a single stimulus. For this reason, the same stimulus is presented repetitively, and time-locked EEG activity is recorded. When these repetitive records are averaged, the random noise activity cancels out, whereas the specific activity triggered by the stimulus summates across records, resulting in a clear signal. Abnormal function of the sensory pathway results in a prolonged latency of the signal (or, less reliably, reduced amplitude or complete absence of the signal). "Multiple lesions separated in space" can therefore be identified using evoked potential studies, but the results provide no information about the time course or underlying cause. Moreover, all of the ancillary tests (MRI, CSF analysis, and evoked potentials) can produce false-negative results in patients with definite MS.

The clinical course of MS is extremely variable. Onset is typically between the ages of 20 and 50 years, with the peak at age 25–30 years.

Most patients have a **relapsing/remitting** course, with discrete episodes of neurologic dysfunction separated by periods in which their clinical condition is stable or improving. They may have episodes as frequently as several times a year, or as rarely as once every few years. Approximately 10–20% of young patients (and a higher proportion of older-onset patients) have a **primary progressive** course, with gradual clinical deterioration from the time symptoms first develop. Particular caution is required before making the diagnosis in these patients, so that a focal or multifocal structural process is not overlooked. Approximately 50% of patients with relapsing/remitting disease evolve within 10 years to a gradually progressive course; this is known as **secondary progressive** MS. **Relapsing/progressive** MS is a fourth clinical pattern, in which patients have discrete relapses and remissions superimposed on a steady overall clinical deterioration.

The particular neurologic manifestations that occur in MS are nearly as diverse as the nervous system itself. The most common initial manifestations are weakness in one or more limbs, optic neuritis, sensory symptoms, diplopia, vertigo, and disturbance of micturition. Other common manifestations include spasticity and other features of upper motor neuron involvement, ataxia, tremor, fatigue, cognitive impairment, and Lhermitte's sign (an electric sensation passing down the back and into the limbs provoked by neck flexion, typically seen in any condition affecting the posterior columns of the cervical spinal cord). Patients may also experience paroxysmal symptoms, including seizures, trigeminal neuralgia (see Chapter 12), other intermittent pains, episodic dysarthria or ataxia (usually lasting less than 20 seconds), and dystonic episodes (often called *tonic seizures*).

Three medications that reduce the frequency of relapses are currently approved for use in patients with relapsing/remitting MS: interferon beta-1b (Betaseron), interferon beta-1a (Avonex), and glatiramer acetate (Copaxone, formerly known as copolymer-1). The first two agents have multiple immunomodulatory actions, and the third was initially developed as a synthetic analogue of myelin basic protein for use in experimental animal models of inflammatory demyelinating disease. All three of these medications are administered by injection— every other day subcutaneous injections for interferon beta-1b, weekly intramuscular injections for interferon beta-1a, and daily subcutaneous injections for glatiramer. All three are extremely expensive. The two forms of interferon frequently produce flu-like symptoms. Thus, patients who take these drugs are making a substantial commitment, and they must have realistic expectations or they are likely to get frustrated by what they perceive as a lack of effect. They must be advised that although the medications reduce the number of relapses by approximately one-third, they do not prevent relapses completely. Although the medications slow disease progression, they do not halt it, and they certainly do not reverse it. Because there is no way for an individual patient to know how many relapses would have occurred or how quickly the disease would have progressed if left untreated, there is no way to gauge the benefit of treatment on an individual basis.

There have been no studies directly comparing any one of the three available agents with another. The choice of agent is usually based on side-effect profiles and ease of administration. Similarly, there have been no studies comparing any of these medications to IV immunoglobulin, which also reduces the frequency of relapses.

No medication is currently approved for patients with primary progressive or secondary progressive MS. Interferon beta-1b reduced the rate of progression in one European study, but the results of additional studies are still pending. Analogous studies of interferon beta-1a and glatiramer are in progress. A variety of forms of immunosuppression or immunomodulation have been studied in MS, including cyclophosphamide, azathioprine, cyclosporine, methotrexate, cladribine, linomide, total lymphoid irradiation, phosphodiesterase inhibitors, monoclonal antibodies, and bone marrow transplant, but the results have been mixed. The most promising results to date have been with mitoxantrone, which was reported to slow the development of disability in patients with progressive MS.

Corticosteroids have traditionally been used to treat patients having acute relapses; the most convincing evidence of benefit has been for IV methylprednisolone, which has been shown to shorten relapses but not alter the ultimate outcome. Some investigators have found the results with methylprednisolone and adrenocorticotropic hormone to be equivalent, but others have found methylprednisolone to be superior. Oral prednisone has probably been used more often than either of these two agents to treat exacerbations, but there are no controlled studies to support this practice. Plasma exchange may improve the outcome in patients with a severe relapse.

Symptomatic treatment is at least as important as disease-modifying therapy. Physical therapy, strict bladder and bowel regimens, drugs to reduce spasticity, and psychologic support are essential components of patient management. Certain symptoms respond to specific medications. Controlled trials have established that amantadine is effective in alleviating fatigue, but only some patients note a benefit, and the response is often incomplete. Selective serotonin reuptake inhibitors may also be helpful. Patients with trigeminal neuralgia are treated with carbamazepine or the other agents used for this disorder in patients without MS. Lhermitte's sign often responds to carbamazepine also. The paroxysmal dystonic episodes of MS usually respond dramatically to carbamazepine, phenytoin, or gabapentin. Tremors are treated in the same way as tremors in non-MS patients.

B. Connective Tissue Diseases

Connective tissue diseases characteristically involve widespread organ systems throughout the body, including the nervous system. Organ damage can be caused by immune complex deposition, vasculopathy, granuloma formation, or secondary damage due to musculoskeletal abnormalities. All levels of the nervous system can be affected. In some patients, nervous system dysfunction is the initial or the predominant symptom of the disease. Because these patients typically have multifocal neurologic deficits, they often resemble patients with MS. The main clues to the correct diagnosis are serologic tests and the eventual development of systemic symptoms.

Systemic lupus erythematosus (SLE) is the connective tissue disease most commonly associated with neurologic dysfunction, which occurs at some stage of the disease in 50–75% of patients. The initial manifestations of the disease are neurologic in as many as 3% of patients. Neuropsychiatric abnormalities—including cognitive impairment, psychosis, and alteration of consciousness—are the most common neurologic manifestations of SLE. Seizures are also common, usually in an active phase of the disease. Focal neurologic deficits in patients with SLE sometime result from focal inflammation, but they are usually due to stroke (which, in turn, is most often related to a hypercoagulable state; see Section D below). Peripheral nerve involvement occurs in 5–27% of patients with SLE. The most common peripheral manifestation is a distal, symmetric polyneuropathy, but mononeuropathy multiplex also occurs.

The main CNS manifestations of **rheumatoid arthritis** result from compression of the spinal cord or brainstem due to arthritic changes in the spinal column. Rheumatoid nodules frequently form in the meninges, but they are usually asymptomatic. Symptomatic CNS vasculitis is rare in patients with rheumatoid arthritis. In contrast, peripheral nerve involvement is common. It may take the form of mononeuropathy multiplex (due to either vasculitis or multiple sites of nerve entrapment) or a distal sensorimotor polyneuropathy.

CNS manifestations occur in fewer than 10% of patients with **Sjögren's syndrome,** although some have suggested that these complications may be underreported. Psychiatric symptoms, cognitive problems, meningoencephalitis, seizures, and focal cerebral and spinal cord deficits have all been described. The most common peripheral nervous system manifestation of Sjögren's syndrome is a distal, symmetric, sensorimotor polyneuropathy. A less common but more distinctive manifestation is pure sensory neuropathy. Mononeuropathy multiplex, cranial neuropathies (especially trigeminal sensory neuropathy), and entrapment neuropathies (especially carpal tunnel syndrome) also occur. Patients may develop focal myositis. Polymyositis and dermatomyositis may also accompany Sjögren's syndrome, but such cases are usually considered secondary Sjögren's (i.e., Sjögren's that is associated with another connective tissue disease).

Progressive systemic sclerosis (scleroderma) only rarely affects the CNS, but focal lesions have been reported on occasion. Trigeminal neuropathy is more common, and peripheral entrapment neuropathies, particularly carpal tunnel syndrome, may occur. There have been occasional reports of a sensorimotor polyneuropathy, with pathology suggesting a microangiopathy. Approximately 20% of patients have diffuse muscle weakness and elevated creatine kinase levels.

The neurologic features of **mixed connective tissue disease** (like the systemic features) overlap with those of SLE, rheumatoid arthritis, progressive systemic sclerosis, and polymyositis. The most common neurologic feature is aseptic meningitis. Trigeminal neuralgia and trigeminal sensory neuropathy are also common. Psychiatric manifestations, movement disorders, and seizures also occur.

Between 10% and 40% of patients with **Behçet's disease** have neurologic signs or symptoms. The most common neurologic manifestation is aseptic meningitis. There may be focal lesions at any level of the nervous system, with the brainstem and basal ganglia being the most commonly affected sites. Lesions often occur simultaneously at multiple locations, and clinical fluctuations are common, sometimes leading to an incorrect diagnosis of MS. Misdiagnosis is particularly likely in the 5% of patients who present with neurologic symptoms. Peripheral nervous system manifestations are rare in Behçet's disease.

Polyarteritis nodosa (PAN) is the prototypical vasculitic condition. It is a necrotizing vasculitis of small- and medium-sized muscular arteries with preferential involvement of vessel branch points. It may produce an acute stroke syndrome with focal manifestations or a global syndrome characterized by headache and encephalopathy. The encephalopathy may present either acutely or chronically. Most patients also have peripheral nervous system involvement. Mononeuropathy multiplex is the classic manifestation, but distal, symmetric polyneuropathies, radiculopathies, and plexopathies also occur. Other systemic necrotizing vasculitides, including **allergic angiitis and granulomatosis (Churg-Strauss syndrome)**, **overlap syndrome**, and **Wegener's granulomatosis**, can all produce similar neurologic manifestations. In addition, the respiratory tract granulomas of Wegener's granulomatosis can extend to involve neighboring nervous system structures, especially the optic nerve in the orbit.

Primary angiitis of the CNS is a rare vasculitis restricted to small- and medium-sized arteries of the CNS. The clinical manifestations resemble the CNS manifestations of PN without the systemic symptoms. **Primary peripheral nervous system angiitis** is an analogous condition in the peripheral nervous system.

Patients with neurologic manifestations of connective tissue diseases are treated in the same way as patients with manifestations in other organ systems, typically with immunosuppressive agents, including corticosteroids and cytotoxic agents. Wegener's granulomatosis is particularly responsive to cyclophosphamide.

C. Sarcoidosis

Sarcoidosis is a chronic, multisystem disorder of unknown cause characterized by noncaseating granulomas in several organs. It affects the nervous system in approximately 5% of patients, and the neurologic involvement is similar in many ways to what occurs in tuberculosis. As with tuberculosis, there may be either parenchymal granulomas or meningeal involvement, particularly involving the meninges at the base of the brain and producing multiple cranial neuropathies. The most common neurologic manifestation of sarcoidosis is transient unilateral or bilateral facial nerve palsy. Cranial nerves II, V, VIII, IX, and X are also commonly involved, but any cranial nerve can be affected. The most common site of parenchymal involvement is the hypothalamus, leading to diabetes insipidus or other endocrine abnormalities. Other intracranial sites may also be involved, resulting in focal signs or obstructive hydrocephalus. Spinal cord involvement can produce a transverse myelopathy. Noncranial peripheral neuropathy occurs in only 9–20% of patients with neurosarcoidosis. The most common pattern of involvement is a chronic sensorimotor polyneuropathy, but mononeuropathy multiplex, pure sensory neuropathy, and plexopathy have also been described. Sarcoidosis commonly affects muscles. Typical granulomas are found on muscle biopsy in up to 50% of patients with sarcoidosis, but these are usually asymptomatic.

When clinical and radiologic findings suggest neurosarcoidosis, the most reliable way to establish the diagnosis is to demonstrate the typical pathologic findings on a tissue specimen. Radiologic evidence alone is not specific enough to permit a definitive diagnosis, and even the pathologic findings are not entirely specific, as non-caseating granulomas can occur in a number of other diseases, including infections and malignancies. Serum levels of angiotensin-converting enzyme (ACE) are typically elevated in patients with sarcoidosis, but this test is neither specific nor sensitive. In patients with neurologic manifestations of sarcoidosis, CSF ACE levels are more likely to be abnormal than serum ACE levels, but they are still normal in approximately 40% of patients with neurosarcoidosis, and they are sometimes abnormal in patients without neurologic involvement.

Patients with neurosarcoidosis usually improve when treated with corticosteroids, but untreated patients can also experience spontaneous remissions, and no controlled trial of corticosteroids in neurosarcoidosis has ever been conducted. Because prednisone at a dose of 0.5–1.0 mg/kg per day has been shown to be effective for most pulmonary cases, this dose usually is initiated for neurologic manifestations also. Even though cyclosporine is ineffective for pulmonary manifestations of sarcoidosis, uncontrolled reports indicate that it may be useful in patients with neurologic manifestations who fail to respond to steroids or who do not tolerate a steroid taper. Occasional reports have indicated success with methotrexate, azathioprine, or radiation therapy.

D. Coagulation Disorders

The physiologic pathways involved in maintaining hemostasis are complicated and can be compromised in many ways. Patients with hemophilia or other diseases predisposing to hemorrhage are usually diagnosed early in life because of uncontrolled bleeding after trivial injuries. Nervous system hemorrhages in these patients are treated as they would be in other patients. Hypercoagulability may occur because of a well-defined abnormality in the coagulation or fibrinolytic systems (primary hypercoagulable states) or in association with some other clinical condition in which the exact pathophysiology of thrombosis is unknown (secondary hypercoagulable states). The most common causes of primary hypercoagulability are antithrombin III deficiency, protein C and protein S deficiency, and abnormalities of plasminogen or plasminogen activator. Most of these conditions are treated with anticoagulant medications. Causes of secondary hypercoagulable states include malignancy, pregnancy, congestive heart failure, extensive trauma, diabetes, nephrotic syndrome, vasculitis, and medications (including oral contraceptives and L-asparaginase). Many of these same conditions, but especially malignancies, can lead to nonbacterial thrombotic endocarditis, which results in an even higher incidence of nervous system involvement due to embolization. An increased risk of thrombosis and stroke is also associated with a heterogeneous family of antibodies known as antiphospholipid antibodies. Lupus anticoagulant and anticardiolipin antibody are two overlapping but not identical groups of antibodies included in this family. These antibodies occur not only in patients with SLE but also in association with other connective tissue diseases, infections, neoplasms, and drugs, and they may be found in otherwise normal individuals. The optimal treatment for patients with secondary hypercoagulable states remains unknown.

V. Discussion of Case Histories

Case 1. In a right-handed patient, aphasia is almost always due to a lesion in the left hemisphere. In this case, the patient is nonfluent with relative sparing of comprehension, suggesting a left frontal lesion. This could not possibly account for the left-sided weakness, which is most likely due to a lesion in the right frontoparietal cortex, given the involvement of face, arm, and leg and the associated sensory loss. A single lesion large enough to produce both the aphasia and the left hemiparesis would involve such an extensive region of cortex bilaterally that impaired consciousness would be expected. Thus, the patient appears to have two separate lesions. The time course is acute, suggesting multifocal vascular disease. This has developed in the setting of an acute or subacute systemic illness. In an IV drug abuser, this clinical picture is suggestive of acute bacterial endocarditis. This patient is also in a risk group for AIDS, which is also associated with an increased risk of stroke, but it would be an unusual coincidence to develop fever, malaise, and cerebrovascular complications simultaneously as a result of HIV infection.

Cerebral emboli suggest left-sided valvular involvement, which is common in endocarditis whether or not the patient abuses IV drugs (in contrast to right-sided involvement, which is much more common in drug abusers than in any other group). Almost all patients with left-sided involvement have a heart murmur at some stage of the disease, but this may be absent on initial presentation.

The most important step in diagnosis is isolation of an organism from the blood. At least three separate venous blood cultures should be drawn. Echocardiography provides useful additional information, but a negative test does not rule out endocarditis. The sedimentation rate is almost always elevated in this condition, but it is nonspecific. An imaging study of the brain should also be performed, because even though the cerebral lesions are most likely ischemic, hemorrhages and even abscesses remain possible. If the lesions appear to be ischemic, the possibility of mycotic aneurysms should be investigated with cerebral angiography. Finally, HIV testing should be offered to the patient, as the results will have an obvious impact on her future medical condition even if unrelated to her current problem.

Even before culture results are available, empiric broad-spectrum antibiotic treatment should be initiated. This should cover *Staphylococcus aureus*, as well as many species of streptococci and gram-negative rods. One such regimen consists of nafcillin, ampicillin, and gentamicin. In areas where nafcillin-resistant *Staphylococcus aureus* species are common, vancomycin should be substituted for nafcillin. Anticoagulation is generally not used in this setting.

Case 2. The examination corroborates this man's complaint of left lower extremity weakness. The hyperreflexia there indicates an upper motor neuron lesion (i.e., a left-sided lesion in the spinal cord or low medulla, or a right-sided lesion above the medulla). The left afferent pupillary defect indicates a lesion anterior to the optic chiasm on the left. A single lesion could not produce both deficits without impairing consciousness. Thus, this patient has a multifocal condition. Based on his history, the two lesions appeared 8 months apart, and the left eye symptoms actually resolved in the interim. Accordingly, there is evidence of multiple CNS lesions separated in space and time, and this patient meets criteria for the diagnosis of MS. Although some connective tissue diseases can mimic MS, these would be unlikely in a patient who has had no other systemic symptoms, even after 2 years of neurologic symptoms.

Given the convincing examination findings, no additional diagnostic tests are necessary. Most practitioners would obtain an MRI scan of the brain in this setting, as it is the single test most likely to lend support to the diagnosis, but a normal scan would not rule out MS.

Because the current exacerbation began 3 weeks ago, has not progressed, and is still producing only mild dysfunction, many clinicians would elect not to treat it. Others would recommend a brief course of steroids, generally IV methylprednisolone followed by a rapid prednisone taper. With three exacerbations in a 2-year period, this patient is in the group most likely to benefit from interferon beta-1a, interferon beta-1b, or glatiramer.

Probably the most important aspect of management at this stage of the disease is patient education. Misconceptions about MS are widespread, and many patients assume that the disease is rapidly disabling or even fatal. Although patients need to be aware that they could eventually become severely disabled, it is equally important that they realize that there is also potential for a relatively benign course. Approximately 15% of patients with MS are able to continue working at full capacity on a long-term basis. Estimates of the percentage of patients able to walk without assistance 15 years after symptom onset vary between 30% and 70%. Unfortunately, there are no reliable prognostic indicators, and patients must understand that the course is unpredictable.

Case 3. In this woman, multiple cranial nerves are impaired. This could conceivably be caused by a mass lesion in the pons and medulla, but with such extensive bilateral impairment in the brainstem, long-tract signs (such as limb weakness, spasticity, hyperreflexia, ataxia, and sensory loss) would be expected, and alteration of consciousness would also be likely. Involvement of the cranial nerves as they exit the brainstem is therefore more plausible. In addition, she has signs and symptoms consistent with a right S1 radiculopathy. This suggests a meningeal process producing multifocal involvement of nerve roots and cranial nerves as they leave the neuraxis. The chronic time course suggests a neoplastic process, such as leptomeningeal metastasis or lymphomatous meningitis, but chronic inflammatory conditions such as tuberculous meningitis, connective tissue diseases, and neurosarcoidosis should also be considered. Diagnosis depends on CSF examination and a search for other systemic manifestations of these conditions.

In this case, CSF cytopathology revealed lymphomatous cells, and there was no evidence for any other systemic involvement. The diagnosis of primary leptomeningeal lymphoma was made. This is an extremely rare condition. The patient was treated with craniospinal radiation and intrathecal methotrexate, but symptoms continued to progress and she died 6 months after diagnosis.

III

Common Symptoms

Acute Mental Status Changes

I. Case Histories

Case 1. You are called by a nurse at 3 PM to evaluate a 72-year-old diabetic woman for an acute alteration in mental status. She had been admitted to the hospital the day before for evaluation of exertional chest pain and had undergone cardiac catheterization earlier today. When you arrive, you find the nurse struggling to restrain the patient, who is awake but agitated and unable to follow commands. The patient makes occasional attempts at speech, but it is unintelligible. She seems to be able to move her limbs symmetrically and withdraws to noxious stimulation in the arms and legs. With difficulty, you examine her further but find no "focal" abnormality.

Case 2. A 19-year-old college student has been brought to the emergency room (ER) by friends after they found him unconscious in his dorm room. He had been to a fraternity party the night before and apparently looked well at 1 AM, just before retiring. His friends report that he is "not a party animal"; he rarely, if ever, drinks alcohol and "never" uses drugs. On examination, his pulse is 110 per minute and his blood pressure is 120/70. Temperature is slightly elevated at 38.3°C. Respirations are 24 per minute. Neurologic examination reveals no response to voice and only brief eye opening to noxious stimulation. Pupils are equal and reactive, and the doll's eyes response is absent. Reflexes are depressed but present, and the plantar responses are mute.

Questions:

1. What initial approach should be taken with both of these patients?

2. How does each clinical setting affect your diagnostic considerations and the workup?

3. How will you manage each of these cases?

Case 3. A 38-year-old weekend softball player was brought to the ER after being hit on the left side of the head with a bat. When first hit he had severe pain and stumbled but did not lose consciousness. He was able to speak to his teammates and initially refused to go to the hospital. On arrival in the ER he was able to speak to the triage nurse without difficulty and signed all of his admission papers. When you first examine him 20 minutes later, he requires constant stimulation to stay alert. The left pupil is slightly larger than the right, but both react to light. The rest of his examination is normal.

Case 4. You are asked to evaluate a 20-year-old woman who was thrown from a horse and hit her head on the ground. There was no loss of consciousness at the time of the fall. She has a severe headache but otherwise feels all right. On examination, she is alert and conversant. Her mental status is normal and there are no focal abnormalities on neurologic examination. She has a large occipital laceration.

Questions:

1. What is the proper approach to these two patients?

2. What determines whether a head injury is complicated or uncomplicated? When do you need the assistance of a neurosurgeon?

3. What advice do you give to a patient who has had an uncomplicated head injury?

4. What problems can follow head injury?

II. Background Information

A. Definitions

coma: a state in which subjects lie with eyes closed and demonstrate no conscious responses to external stimuli, even after vigorous attempts to rouse them.

delirium: a floridly abnormal mental state characterized by clouded, reduced, or shifting attention; often associated with agitation, disorientation, fear, irritability, illusions (misperceptions of sensory stimuli), or hallucinations (imagined perceptions with no basis in the external world).

encephalopathy: any state of altered level of consciousness or clouded sensorium.

stupor: a state of unresponsiveness resembling deep sleep, from which subjects can be roused only by vigorous and repeated stimulation.

B. Mechanisms of Mental Status Changes

Focal brain lesions can produce discrete cognitive deficits such as aphasia or anosognosia. Generalized confusion or behavioral changes can also be caused by focal brain lesions (especially in the right parietal lobe or either frontal lobe), but diffuse cerebral dysfunction is more often the cause. An altered level of consciousness occurs only when there has been damage to both cerebral hemispheres or to the reticular activating system in the brainstem.

III. Approach to Acute Mental Status Changes

There are many potential reasons for an acute change in mental status, and they should be addressed in order from most urgent to least urgent. For the less urgent causes, time is available to be analytical and individualize the management plan, but for the most urgent conditions diagnosis and therapy should proceed rapidly and systematically. The initial management of these patients should be almost automatic. Conceptually, the evaluation should proceed in the following order:

A.   ABCs (airway, breathing, circulation)

B.   Oxygen, glucose, naloxone

C.   Pupils, doll's eyes, motor asymmetry

D.   Other electrolytes, renal, hepatic, temperature

E.   Everything else

In practice, it is often convenient to take some steps out of order. For example, the blood necessary for the tests in step D can be drawn and sent to the laboratory along with the glucose in step B. In fact, as with any other medical emergency, there are bound to be many things happening at once, producing a sense of controlled anarchy. The evaluation may simultaneously reveal several potential causes of altered mental status, which makes it even more important to have a clear idea of which problems must be addressed most urgently.

A. ABCs

As in most other clinical emergencies, the most important initial management goal is to ensure the adequacy of cardiopulmonary function by evaluating the patient's ABCs (Airway, Breathing, Circulation). All other evaluations should be deferred until it is clear that blood pressure and ventilation are adequate. Even if ventilation is adequate, it should be monitored closely, as patients with a depressed level of consciousness are at risk for both hypoventilation and aspiration. If there is any hint that ventilation is failing, elective intubation should be considered.

B. Oxygen, Glucose, Naloxone

Once it is clear that cardiopulmonary function is adequate, hypoxia and hypoglycemia must be addressed most urgently. Both conditions can be treated rapidly and can be fatal or result in irreversible damage if left untreated for even a short period. In fact, **patients should be treated empirically for hypoxia and hypoglycemia unless rapid and**

reliable testing is available. Empiric treatment for possible narcotic overdose should be administered at the same time.

The only reliable way to assess oxygenation is to measure it directly. A clear airway and normal breathing pattern are no guarantee that oxygenation is adequate. A pulmonary embolus, interstitial pneumonitis, or anything else that produces a significant ventilation-perfusion mismatch may cause hypoxia without significantly altering breathing. Arterial oxygen saturation must be determined either with a pulse oximeter or with an arterial blood gas measurement. The blood gas has the advantage of providing additional useful information about pCO_2 and pH, but a pulse oximeter, when it is available, is faster. As a general rule, it should be assumed that there will be a brief but significant delay in obtaining the necessary information about oxygenation status, and during that delay the patient should empirically be given 100% oxygen by face mask. A theoretical risk exists that this concentration of oxygen will lead to respiratory arrest in patients with chronic CO_2 retention who are dependent on hypoxia for respiratory drive. This situation is rare, however, and represents a far less significant risk than the danger of giving insufficient concentrations of oxygen to correct hypoxia.

The issues involved in treating hypoglycemia are analogous to those involved in treating hypoxia. Again, the most rapid tests (e.g., finger stick methods) may not be immediately available, and the most reliable test (analysis of a venous blood sample) is too slow. The best method is to treat empirically by giving a 50-ml IV bolus of a 50% dextrose solution ("one amp of D50") immediately after sending a venous sample to the laboratory. This treatment might seem dangerous, because it could exacerbate hyperglycemia (another potential cause of mental status changes). Even if the patient is hyperglycemic, however, the increased glucose concentration resulting from this dose is unlikely to have a significant impact on the patient's outcome or management. If there is any possibility that the patient might have thiamine deficiency (because of alcoholism or malnutrition), 100 mg of IV thiamine should be given with the dextrose to avoid precipitating or inducing Wernicke's encephalopathy.

The final empiric treatment that should be administered at this stage is naloxone (Narcan), 0.4–0.8 mg IV, unless the cause of coma is obvious. This measure is not as urgent as oxygen or glucose administration because patients often recover fully from narcotic overdose even when it is prolonged. Like oxygen and glucose, however, naloxone is a generally benign treatment that can produce dramatic reversal of mental status changes in the appropriate situations. This rapid improvement may be sufficient to establish the diagnosis and save the patient from more invasive and expensive diagnostic testing.

While treating for drug *overdose*, the possibility of drug *withdrawal* should also be considered. In particular, alcohol withdrawal can produce a delirious state (*delirium tremens*) characterized by agitation, confusion, hallucinations, and autonomic overactivity, including fever, tachycardia, and profuse sweating. This condition typically occurs 3 or 4 days after the last drink; common settings are alcohol detoxification programs or several days after a patient is incarcerated or admitted to a hospital. The diagnosis should always be considered in a delirious patient, even if no history of alcohol abuse is evident. The main goals of treatment are to address the autonomic overactivity, maintain hydration and electrolyte balance, and prevent self-injury. To this end, large doses of benzodiazepines may be required to control agitation. Less severe alcohol withdrawal produces tremulousness and agitation; a similar picture can occur with benzodiazepine or barbiturate withdrawal.

C. Pupils, Doll's Eyes, Motor Asymmetry

After addressing the most urgent conditions that can affect mental status—systemic derangements like hypotension and hypoglycemia—the possibility of structural brain damage must be considered. Not until this stage does the neurologic examination become critical. The most urgent structural problem is cerebral herniation, in which a mass lesion in one cerebral hemisphere expands downward and puts pressure on the brainstem, resulting in a depressed level of consciousness. Assessment of cranial nerve function is the most important way to identify this situation. The examination is restricted to reflex functions in patients with altered consciousness, and the most useful localizing information is provided by the pupillary light reflex and the doll's eyes response.

For the doll's eyes response to be affected by downward expansion of a lesion originating in a cerebral hemisphere, the expansion must progress to the level of the pons and upper medulla, because the afferent limb of the reflex is in the vestibular nerve (cranial nerve VIII), which enters the brainstem at the pontomedullary junction, and the efferent limb depends on the pontine gaze center adjacent to the abducens (cranial nerve VI) nucleus. By the time the lesion has expanded down to this level, it must already have passed through the level of the brainstem involved in the pupillary reflex (the midbrain, at the level of the superior colliculus and the third nerve nucleus). Thus, when the doll's eyes response is abnormal in these patients, the pupillary reflex is almost always abnormal also. This leads to a useful rule: **If the pupils are normal but the doll's eyes response is not, herniation** is not the cause of coma. A systemic metabolic abnormality is more likely than a structural lesion.

Conversely, the presence of abnormal pupillary responses suggests the possibility of an underlying structural lesion. Whereas the doll's eyes response is generated by complicated reflex patterns that can be disrupted by even mild metabolic disturbances, the pupillary reflex is resistant to such disturbances and is often preserved when altered mental status is due to metabolic causes. Exceptions to this rule include certain drug ingestions and metabolic disturbances that can affect pupillary function:

1. Opiates—pinpoint but sometimes fixed and dilated

2. Cholinergics (e.g., eyedrops)—pinpoint

3. Anticholinergics—dilated, fixed

4. Glutethimide—irregular, unreactive, bizarre

5. Barbiturates, lidocaine (Xylocaine)—dilated, fixed

6. Adrenergics (e.g., bronchodilator splashed in eye)—dilated

7. Hypoxia—dilated, fixed

8. Hypothermia—often dilated, fixed

The right and left pupils are affected equally by all of these metabolic factors (except when drugs are applied directly to one eye only). When the pupillary responses are asymmetric, a structural lesion should be strongly suspected.

Even a mass lesion that is not actively herniating has the potential to expand, so patients with altered mental status must also be assessed for asymmetric sensorimotor findings. Even though many components of the standard neurologic examination must be modified or eliminated when impaired cognitive function prevents full patient cooperation (see Chapter 2), deep tendon reflexes and resistance to passive manipulation can still be assessed, and the response to painful stimulation of the limbs often provides important information. An asymmetric withdrawal response to pain can signify hemiparesis or hemisensory loss. When evaluating responses to painful stimuli, one should distinguish purposeful withdrawal from both local reflex responses and central reflexes (decorticate or decerebrate posturing). A useful technique to avoid this problem with interpretation is to pinch the inner aspect of the arm or leg. Abduction of the stimulated limb is purposeful withdrawal; adduction or extension may indicate a local reflex or decerebrate posturing, and flexion of the arm may indicate decorticate posturing.

When the examination suggests an expanding structural lesion, a brain imaging study should be performed immediately. CT scanning is usually the most readily available modality. Even before the CT scan, neurosurgical consultants should be informed that their assistance may soon be necessary. The treatment measures described in Part IV, Section B, may be required when the physical examination provides compelling evidence that intracranial pressure (ICP) is significantly increased. When a metabolic cause of altered mental status is more likely, a brain imaging study may still be necessary eventually, but only if the diagnosis remains obscure after proceeding with the next steps in the evaluation.

D. Other Electrolytes, Renal, Hepatic, Temperature

At this point in the diagnostic process, all of the true emergencies have already been considered, and a little time can be spared for deliberation. Many of the remaining causes of altered mental status are serious conditions requiring prompt treatment, but they can only be corrected gradually. Rapid treatment is impossible for some of these conditions and potentially dangerous for others.

Hyponatremia, hypernatremia, hypocalcemia, hypomagnesemia, hepatic disease, and uremia all commonly result in acute alterations in mental status. These disturbances can produce a wide spectrum of mental status changes, from irritability to coma, and there is nothing specific about the clinical picture associated with any one of them (except that the presence of tetany suggests hypocalcemia or hypomagnesemia). Laboratory testing is required for diagnosis. As noted earlier, the necessary laboratory tests should generally be requested at the same time that blood samples are sent for glucose and blood gas determinations, so the results will be available by the time this step in the evaluation process is reached. Treatment for each of these conditions is discussed in textbooks of internal medicine.

Body temperatures below approximately 34°C or above 39–40°C can produce mental status changes ranging from lethargy or agitation to stupor or coma. They can also produce many systemic abnormalities, including many of the metabolic derangements listed in the previous paragraph. These metabolic problems are often resistant to treatment until the underlying thermal disorder has been corrected. Treatment of hyperthermia and hypothermia is discussed in textbooks of intensive care medicine and emergency medicine.

E. Everything Else

The first four steps in the evaluation process address problems that are common, and patients often have more than one of these problems. For example, a hyperglycemic patient will often be dehydrated, resulting in both hypotension and hyponatremia. Narcotic overdose may be associated with hypothermia and hypotension. Thus, it is usually appropriate to proceed through all of the first four steps even if one of the initial steps has already revealed an abnormality. For the majority of patients with acutely altered mental status, those four steps will uncover the likely cause (or causes). It is only necessary to search further when the first four steps have been unrevealing or when something specific in the patient's history or examination suggests another potential cause (e.g., a febrile patient should be evaluated for infection, even if hypotension and hypoglycemia have already been discovered).

Narcotics are not the only drugs that can produce altered mental status. Drugs with anticholinergic activity (including atropine, scopolamine, and tricyclic antidepressants), amphetamines, cocaine, LSD, and phencyclidine are other potential culprits. Friends and relatives of the patient should be asked explicitly about drug use. A brief search may reveal an empty pill bottle or an unfilled prescription. A urine toxin screen should be sent whenever a possibility of a drug overdose exists.

Patients may be agitated or stuporous in the postictal period after a seizure (see Chapter 5). The diagnosis is straightforward when the seizure was witnessed or when the patient is known to have epilepsy but may not be suspected when this information is unavailable. Witnesses should be questioned about abnormal movements or behavior preceding the alteration in mental status and about any history of similar events. Again, a search for medications or prescriptions may be helpful.

Bacterial, viral, and fungal meningitis and encephalitis can all cause alterations in mental status. Fever, stiff neck, and headache are all clues to the diagnosis. Subarachnoid hemorrhage can mimic meningitis. The approach to these disorders is discussed in Chapter 12. Mental status changes also occur with sepsis and even with apparently localized infections such as pneumonia or urinary tract infections (especially in elderly or demented patients), presumably because of clinically undetectable spread of the organism to the nervous system or because of metabolic effects of the infection. If the first four steps of the evaluation are unrevealing, patients should probably be evaluated with chest x-ray and cultures of blood, sputum, urine, and spinal fluid, even if they are afebrile and have normal white blood cell counts.

Other inflammatory conditions, such as lupus and isolated central nervous system vasculitis, may also produce acute mental status changes. Hyperthyroidism, hypothyroidism, addisonian crisis, and Cushing's syndrome (either iatrogenic or endogenous) are other potential causes. Unless there are specific features pointing to these diagnoses, they should only be considered when more common conditions have been excluded.

IV. Special Circumstances

A. Head Trauma

When a patient has sustained trauma to the head, there is no mystery about the cause of altered mental status. Even so, the initial evaluation should proceed through the same steps as for any other cause of altered mental status in order to assess the patient's overall condition and to exclude additional causes of encephalopathy. Indeed, these other factors may even have precipitated the head trauma (e.g., a motor vehicle accident could have resulted from depressed consciousness caused by hypoglycemia).

Management should be aimed at determining whether the head trauma caused any structural damage to the nervous system and whether that damage will require neurosurgical intervention. Neurosurgical consultation should be obtained whenever an operative procedure may be necessary, such as with an intracranial hematoma (especially epidural or subdural); cerebrospinal fluid leak; compound, comminuted, or depressed skull fracture; or cervical spine injury.

Clues to the nature and severity of the injury can be gleaned from the history and general physical examination. For example, a patient who hit his head on a rafter while installing insulation is less likely to have sustained a serious injury than a patient who was violently struck in the head with a club. The head and scalp should be carefully inspected and palpated for evidence of laceration, fracture, or hematoma. Any scalp laceration detected should be probed with a sterilely gloved finger to exclude the presence of a fracture or foreign body. The periorbital and temporal regions should be inspected for evidence of ecchymoses that suggest basilar skull fracture, and the nares and external auditory canals should be examined for evidence of a cerebrospinal fluid leak or hemotympanum.

Progressive focal abnormalities on neurologic examination increase the likelihood of intracranial hemorrhage (see Chapter 3). It is also crucial to monitor changes in the patient's level of alertness that could indicate progressive brain damage. Every effort should be made to speak to someone who observed the patient's behavior at the scene of the injury and since. The level of alertness should be assessed at regular intervals. One quick, reproducible method for assessing level of alertness is provided by the Glasgow Coma Scale (Table 11-1).

Table 11-1. Glasgow Coma Scale*

I.	Best motor response	
	Obeys	6
	Localizes	5
	Withdraws	4
	Abnormal flexion	3
	Extensor response	2
	Nil	1
II.	Verbal response	
	Oriented	5
	Confused speech	4
	Inappropriate words	3
	Incomprehensible sounds	2
	Nil	1
III.	Eye opening	
	Spontaneous	4
	To speech	3
	To pain	2
	Nil	1

*Coma score = score I + II + III.

When a neurosurgical intervention is contemplated, a CT scan of the head should be obtained. Specifically, a CT scan should be performed when the patient is unconscious, lethargic or confused; the level of alertness is declining or fluctuating; there are focal neurologic findings; a cerebrospinal fluid leak is present; or a basilar skull fracture is suspected.

Head injuries are often accompanied by injury to the cervical spine. *Never* remove a cervical collar or manipulate the neck of a head-injured patient without first excluding the possibility of an unstable cervical fracture by x-ray. Traumatic events that result in head injury can cause intra-abdominal or intrathoracic injury as well; these possibilities should not be ignored.

When no evidence exists for a process that might require surgical intervention, many patients with uncomplicated head injuries can be allowed to return home under close supervision by friends or family members. Patients' families should be instructed to awaken the patient every 2 hours during the first 12 hours after the injury and to return to the ER if the patient has severe headache, nausea and vomiting, or reduced responsiveness. Many ERs publish a "head sheet" with instructions that a patient can take home; be sure that these instructions are clearly understood before allowing the patient to leave the ER.

In the days and weeks after a head injury, patients can develop a condition known as *postconcussion syndrome* or *post-traumatic syndrome*, characterized by any combination of a diverse set of symptoms that include headaches, diffuse pain, vertigo, difficulty with thinking and memory, depression, behavioral changes, and seizures. The mechanism underlying this syndrome is not understood, and there is an ongoing debate about the role played by secondary gain and compensation issues. Treatment is symptomatic. Fortunately, the symptoms usually resolve spontaneously over a period of months, although they may last several years in some patients.

B. Increased Intracranial Pressure

The only definitive treatment for increased ICP is eliminating the underlying cause. In many cases, this requires a neurosurgical procedure. Several measures can reduce ICP transiently, limiting neurologic deterioration while awaiting definitive treatment.

Hyperventilation results in decreased arterial pCO_2, which induces cerebral vasoconstriction and hence a reduction in intracranial blood volume. This treatment requires intubation and mechanical ventilation. Levels of pCO_2 below 25 mm Hg should be avoided because of the risk of ischemia from excessive vasoconstriction. This technique lowers ICP within 2–30 minutes, but the effect is transient.

Hyperosmolar agents that do not readily cross the blood-brain barrier produce an osmotic gradient that pulls fluid out of the brain parenchyma and into the blood vessels. The increased intravascular water content results in decreased viscosity and hence improved perfusion. An osmotic diuresis also occurs because these agents are not reabsorbed from the renal tubule. It is not clear which of these effects is most significant in lowering ICP. In any event, the effect is transient, presumably because the agents eventually do permeate tissue barriers, eliminating (and eventually reversing) the osmotic gradient. The most commonly used osmotic agent is mannitol, 1.0–1.5 g/kg over 10–20 minutes, administered in a 20% solution (100 g of mannitol in 500 ml of D_5W). The same dose can be repeated every 4–6 hours. Serum osmolality is sometimes used as a treatment end point.

For tumors and abscesses, increased ICP is usually a result of edema formation around the lesion. In these cases, glucocorticoids often produce dramatic improvement. In fact, improvement may be so dramatic that the underlying lesion is no longer evident on imaging studies, complicating subsequent attempts to establish a specific diagnosis and management plan. Thus, when a brain biopsy of a mass lesion may be necessary, glucocorticoids should generally be deferred until immediately before the procedure as long as the patient's medical condition and neurologic status are stable. A typical glucocorticoid regimen is 10 mg of IV dexamethasone (Decadron) followed by 4 mg every 6 hours, but the optimal dosing regimen is unknown. There is no evidence that steroids are effective in treating edema related to ischemic or hemorrhagic stroke or in treating edema related to metabolic or hypoxic injury.

These measures do not in any way constitute definitive treatment of increased ICP. They are at best temporizing maneuvers to minimize deterioration while awaiting definitive treatment. Neurosurgical consultation should be requested as soon as possible whenever operative intervention is a consideration. The neurosurgeon may also elect to monitor ICP directly by means of an epidural, subdural, or intraventricular catheter, using these measurements to guide therapy.

C. Brain Death

With the development of mechanical ventilators and other means of artificial support, it has become possible to maintain some bodily functions indefinitely. As a result, philosophical questions regarding the definition of death have immediate practical relevance, especially with the advent of organ transplantation. Is it ethical to remove a kidney from a donor whose heart is still beating?

The concept of brain death was formulated primarily because of the issues raised by these new technologies. The United States and almost every industrialized nation in the world formally recognize the principle that conscious and unconscious brain functions are fundamental to human life, so a person who has permanent loss of all brain function is dead. Explicit rules governing the determination of brain death have been developed. In essence, they require that there be no evidence of cortical or brainstem function. Other than reflexes mediated at the level of the spinal cord, there should be no response to noxious stimuli. There must be no response to visual or auditory stimuli. All brainstem reflexes must be absent, including the pupillary reflex, oculocephalic (doll's eyes) reflex, vestibulo-ocular (ice water caloric) reflex, corneal reflex, and the respiratory reflex in response to hypercarbia. Finally, the cause of coma must be known and it must be irreversible.

Determination of brain death is necessary only in specific circumstances, usually to decide if a patient is eligible to be an organ donor. In some circumstances, disagreements among family and caregivers require formal determination that the patient is actually dead, so further medical treatment is pointless. Most decisions about withdrawal of medical support do not involve brain death, however. Many comatose patients who still have some brainstem function have a poor prognosis. *In such cases,* **even though the patient is clearly not brain dead,** *it is appropriate to withdraw support if family members agree that this is what the patient would have wanted.* Published guidelines are available to help determine the prognosis in patients with coma due to a hypoxic-ischemic event.

V. Discussion of Case Histories

Case 1. The initial approach to this patient should be the evaluation discussed in the text: (1) ABCs; (2) oxygen, glucose, naloxone; (3) pupils, doll's eyes, motor asymmetry; and (4) other electrolytes, renal, hepatic, temperature. Particular concerns in this setting would be the possibilities of hypoglycemia (if she was given her usual doses of insulin or oral hypoglycemic agents despite being NPO for the procedure), drug toxicity (from opiates or sedatives given for the catheterization), or multiple cerebral emboli dislodged from the heart or aorta because of the catheterization (less likely given the nonfocal examination).

Comment: In this case, none of the initial steps provided an explanation for the patient's altered mental status. Careful review of her medication chart revealed that she had received several sedative-hypnotic drugs before and after the catheterization. After she was successfully controlled with soft restraints, her physicians ordered a sitter to stay by her bedside and she gradually returned to normal. She had little recall of her agitated state. Follow-up examinations were normal.

Case 2. The initial management of this patient is the same as that in Case 1. Starting to get the picture? This is the initial approach that should be followed in *all* cases of altered mental status. The normal pupillary response in a patient with no doll's eyes response is strong evidence that the cause of this patient's coma is toxic/metabolic.

Comment: Despite the history given by his friends, this patient had opiates and benzodiazepines on his toxicology screen, and drug ingestion was the ultimate diagnosis. A lumbar puncture was performed because of the patient's fever, and the results were normal. His remaining blood tests, including complete blood cell count and electrolytes, were normal. He awoke quickly after naloxone was administered and went home 1 day later.

Case 3. This patient has progressively worsening mental status, and his asymmetric pupils suggest a structural lesion of the brain. A neurosurgeon must be consulted urgently because of these findings.

Comment: He had suffered a fractured skull with laceration of the middle meningeal artery and epidural hemorrhage. Prompt evacuation of the hematoma saved his life, and he went home after a 2-week hospital stay.

Case 4. Because the patient has a normal mental status and normal neurologic examination, the patient can be allowed to go home (after the laceration is stitched) if friends and family members agree to observe her closely.

Comment: Aside from mild residual headache, she felt well at a follow-up visit 4 weeks later.

12

Headache

I. Case Histories

Case 1. A 28-year-old man came to the ER complaining of the worst headache of his life, starting 12 hours ago. He first started having headaches when he was 16 years old, but they used to occur only two or three times a year. In the last 2 years they have been more frequent, up to twice a week. They always start on one side of the head, usually the right, but sometimes the left, and progress to involve the entire head. They are associated with photophobia and nausea. They usually go away if he takes two aspirin and lies down in a dark room. His current headache is qualitatively similar to his previous headaches, but more severe. The pain is continuing to get worse, even though he has taken eight aspirin.

Questions:

1. What diagnoses should be considered?

2. What tests are necessary?

3. What treatment would you give?

Case 2. A 54-year-old man with a history of chronic obstructive pulmonary disease and hypertension has come to your office for his routine quarterly check-up. He mentions in passing that he has been having daily headaches for the past 3 or 4 months. They are always on the right side of his head. The pain is not severe, just a nagging ache that usually gets better when he takes two aspirin and goes away completely when he takes two more aspirin 4 hours later. He can live with the pain at this level, but he thought he should mention it because he never used to have headaches at all. On examination, he has his baseline level of wheezing, and a chronic cough. You note a mild left hemiparesis, and when you point it out he says he never noticed it before, but it's probably just because he is strongly right-handed and hardly uses his left side. You also find mild but definite hyperreflexia on the left, and he tends to extinguish left-sided stimuli on double simultaneous stimulation.

Questions:

1. What diagnoses should be considered?

2. What tests are necessary?

3. What treatment would you give?

II. Background Information

Headaches can occur independently of any other disease processes (*primary headache disorders*) or they can be associated with a wide variety of underlying neurologic and systemic conditions (*secondary headache disorders*). The pathophysiologic mechanisms are incompletely understood. Most research has focused on migraine headaches, in which activation of the trigeminovascular system appears to play a major role. Nociceptive fibers convey information about painful stimuli from the head and neck to the trigeminal ganglion, which transmits the information centrally and at the same time sends retrograde impulses down fibers that innervate meningeal and parenchymal blood vessels. This results in perivascular release of neuropeptides and produces an inflammatory response. The neurologic symptoms that often accompany migraine are generally attributed to cortical spreading depression. This phenomenon can be induced by a variety of stimuli in experimental animals and is characterized by dramatic ionic shifts and changes in electrical excitability and blood flow that march across large regions of the cortex. The factors that trigger the trigeminovascular activation and the cortical spreading depression are not known, and the sequence and interrelationships of these processes remain unclear. Several different neurotransmitter systems are involved, but serotonergic pathways appear to play a prominent role. It is not clear to what extent migraine and other primary and secondary headache conditions share the same pathophysiologic mechanisms.

III. Approach to Headache

Three questions must be addressed in managing a patient with headaches:

A.   Is the situation an emergency?

B.   Are the headaches primary or secondary?

C.   If the headaches are primary, which of the established headache syndromes do they most resemble?

A. Is It an Emergency?

When a patient has a severe headache that is qualitatively different from all previous ones, or when a headache is accompanied by fever, stiff neck, or a focal neurologic abnormality not documented with previous headaches, **this is an emergency!** The patient must be assumed to have either a subarachnoid hemorrhage (SAH) or bacterial meningitis until proven otherwise.

A similar approach is to assume that any patient complaining of the "worst headache of my life" has a life-threatening illness until proven otherwise. However, any patient with chronic headaches who happens to develop a particularly severe headache can legitimately complain of "the worst headache of my life." In fact, any patient who goes to the trouble of coming to an ER will probably use this or a similar phrase to impress the ER staff that the pain is severe. The important thing to determine is whether this headache is *qualitatively* different from other headaches the patient has experienced in the past. If the difference is only quantitative—that is, if the patient has a long history (>2 years) of similar headaches, and the current one is simply lasting longer or hurting more than usual—no diagnostic studies are required, and the patient can be treated with medications appropriate for his or her chronic condition.

On the other hand, if the current headache is different in character from anything the patient has ever experienced before, **this is an emergency!** Patients with SAH must be evaluated for an aneurysm so that it can be repaired before it bleeds again and causes further damage. Bacterial meningitis is an extremely aggressive condition and has a high mortality rate; antibiotics must be started as early as possible in the course. No completely reliable method exists to distinguish SAH from meningitis based on clinical characteristics. The onset of pain is typically more abrupt in SAH, and fever is more common (and usually more pronounced) in meningitis, but there are exceptions to these generalizations. Patients should be evaluated for both conditions simultaneously, and they should immediately receive a single IV antibiotic dose (either 2 million units of penicillin or 2 g of either cefotaxime or ceftriaxone). Antibiotics should only be deferred if the clinical suspicion of meningitis is low and the patient is afebrile with completely normal cardiovascular, respiratory, and mental status. Conversely, if bacterial meningitis seems likely, glucocorticoids may be beneficial, but the only conclusive evidence for this is in children with *Haemophilus influenzae* meningitis.

The diagnostic test for meningitis is a lumbar puncture (spinal tap). Once antibiotics have been given, CSF must be obtained within 4 hours, or cultures may be falsely negative. Because SAH can also be diagnosed by examining the CSF, one reasonable approach would be to perform a lumbar puncture immediately. This is an invasive test, however, with the potential to provoke herniation in patients who have a cerebral mass lesion. It is usually possible to detect SAH on a noncontrast CT scan, so if a CT scan can be obtained immediately, it should be done first. If the CT scan clearly establishes the cause of the headache (either SAH or a mass lesion), a lumbar puncture is not necessary. If there is any possibility of delay, however, the CT scan should be omitted and a lumbar puncture performed immediately, unless the examination strongly suggests that the patient has a mass lesion.

Even when a CT scan can be obtained immediately, it will fail to detect at least 10% of cases of SAH, so a normal CT scan necessitates a lumbar puncture both to evaluate further for subarachnoid hemorrhage and to diagnose meningitis. If there are no white blood cells in the CSF, no further antibiotics are necessary. If there are more than five white blood cells per mm^3, however, the patient should be treated for presumed bacterial meningitis. A CSF white blood cell count less than 100 per mm^3, a lymphocytic predominance, and a normal glucose increase the likelihood that the meningitis is viral rather than bacterial, but there are exceptions to all of these rules, so IV antibiotics should be continued until cultures have been negative for 48 hours.

The hallmark of SAH is the presence of red blood cells in the CSF. This must be distinguished from a traumatic tap, in which local blood vessels are punctured during the procedure and blood enters the CSF at the puncture site. For this reason, whenever SAH is a consideration, it is imperative to spin down the CSF immediately. Blood cells that have been present for 12 hours or more will already have started to break down, producing xanthochromia (a yellow tinge to the supernatant). If all the blood present in the CSF was introduced at the time of the lumbar puncture, the cells will aggregate at the bottom of the tube and the supernatant will be completely colorless.

If the CT or lumbar puncture suggests SAH, neurosurgical consultation should be obtained immediately. The patient will need an angiogram to search for the source of hemorrhage. If an aneurysm is present, the patient should be admitted to a closely monitored bed in a dark, quiet room. Several emergency treatment measures should be initiated, but those are beyond the scope of this discussion.

B. Are the Headaches Primary or Secondary?

Once an emergency situation has been ruled out, the next step is to decide whether the patient needs to be evaluated for generalized systemic or neurologic conditions that can occasionally cause headaches. Such conditions are usually apparent from a thorough review of the patient's medical history, with particular attention to any recent medication changes or new symptoms that developed at about the time the headaches began. If the history and examination are unrevealing, further testing is generally not necessary. In particular, patients whose headaches are due to structural abnormalities in the brain, such as tumor, abscess, stroke, parenchymal hemorrhage, subdural or epidural hematoma, or hydrocephalus, typically have papilledema or focal neurologic abnormalities. If the lesion is of recent onset, however, it might not have produced these findings yet. Thus, there are two features that necessitate a brain CT scan or MRI: a focal abnormality on the neurologic examination or recent onset (or major change in character) of the headaches.

The one other diagnosis to consider, even in patients whose history and physical examination are unremarkable, is **temporal arteritis**, which produces head pain that is usually dull and superficial, with superimposed lancinating pains. It may be unilateral or bilateral, and although it is often temporal, it may occur in any location. Patients frequently report temporal artery tenderness and jaw claudication. Approximately 40–50% of patients also have polymyalgia rheumatica, manifested by pain and stiffness of the limbs.

Temporal arteritis is a generalized disorder of medium and large arteries. It can result in a variety of focal neurologic deficits, or it may present with generalized mental status changes. The most common complication is permanent bilateral blindness, which occurs in up to 50% of untreated patients. Thus, while the clinical course is self-limited and lasts only 1–3 years, prompt treatment is essential. A sedimentation rate should be checked in all patients older than age 50 with headaches of recent onset (temporal arteritis is rare in patients younger than age 50). The sedimentation rate is a useful screening test because it is elevated in 95% of patients (and >100 mm per hour in 60%), but it is not specific. The diagnosis should be confirmed with a temporal artery biopsy. When the clinical suspicion is high enough, a temporal artery biopsy should be performed even if the sedimentation rate is normal. As it happens, false-negative biopsies are fairly common, because the arteries are typically involved only in patches, so if the biopsy result is negative and the clinical suspicion is high, the biopsy should be repeated on the contralateral temporal artery. Patients should be treated with high-dose (60–80 mg per day) prednisone during the 1 or 2 days they may have to wait before the biopsy can be arranged. If the diagnosis is confirmed, they should remain on these doses for at least 6–8 weeks, with a subsequent slow taper guided by clinical symptoms and sedimentation rate.

C. Which Syndrome Fits Best?

In the majority of patients with headache, emergency measures and diagnostic testing are not necessary. Generally, there is a long history of similar episodes, the neurologic examination is nonfocal, and there is no fever or neck stiffness. These patients (and the patients who merit diagnostic testing that proves to be normal) have "benign" headache conditions. The next step is to classify the patient's headache as carefully as possible so that the appropriate treatment can be given. This classification is based purely on the history. The character of pain, accompanying symptoms, and time course should be delineated. Provoking, exacerbating, and alleviating factors should be identified. A history of motion sickness and a family history of headaches are also relevant.

Character: Is the pain throbbing, pulsing, burning, squeezing, "lightning-like," "bursting," or a sensation of pressure? Is it a combination of these? Is it unilateral or bilateral? Is it frontal, temporal, parietal, occipital, facial, nuchal, a combination, or generalized? Does the patient have more than one type of headache?

Accompanying symptoms: Are the headaches associated with nausea, vomiting, photophobia, phonophobia, visual disturbance, numbness, weakness, dizziness, language difficulty, or confusion? Is there nasal congestion, rhinorrhea, unilateral tearing, conjunctival redness, ptosis, or pupillary asymmetry?

Time course: In an individual attack, what symptom occurs first, and what is the progression? Is the pain maximal at onset or does it build gradually? If it builds, over how many minutes or hours? How long does each symptom last? Do the symptoms resolve suddenly or gradually?

How frequently do the headaches occur? Can they occur at any time of day? Do they occur in clusters? How long have they been happening? Has there been any change in character, severity, or frequency over time?

Provoking/exacerbating/alleviating factors: Do any specific foods (especially chocolate, caffeine, cheese, monosodium glutamate, processed meats, pickled items) tend to bring on a headache? Does alcohol (especially red wine) cause a headache? Does the position of the patient's head or body affect the pain? Is there a relationship to emotional stress? Was there any change in living situation when the headaches began (or got worse)? Was any new medication (including birth control pills) introduced at the time? Is there any relationship to the menstrual cycle? Did headaches get better or worse during pregnancies? What medications has the patient taken for headaches in the past? What other measures has the patient tried? Which have worked and which have not?

The rationale for asking each of these questions is explained in Part IV.

IV. Primary Headache Conditions

A. Migraine and Tension Headaches

The vast majority of patients with headaches have symptoms that fall somewhere on a spectrum that includes the symptoms of migraine and tension headaches. These have traditionally been viewed as two completely separate conditions with distinct etiologies, but some investigators believe that they may simply be varying manifestations of a single underlying pathophysiologic process. Certainly, many patients report that they have some headaches that are typical of migraine and other headaches that have features characteristic of tension headaches. It is also common for individual headaches to have some attributes of migraine and other characteristics that suggest tension headache. The same medications are effective for treating both classes of headache. Despite this overlap, it is useful to characterize patients' headaches as precisely as possible in order to monitor them over time and assess their response to therapy. This information could also be useful if the distinction between migraine and tension headache is ultimately shown to have therapeutic implications. At present, management is the same whether patients have migraines, tension headaches, or some combination.

Migraine headaches are typically unilateral (although the side of the headache may vary from one episode to the next). The pain is usually throbbing or pulsing. Nausea, vomiting, photophobia, and phonophobia are common accompaniments. In some cases, there are focal neurologic abnormalities. The most common are visual (scintillations and scotomata), but focal numbness, weakness, aphasia, dysarthria, dizziness, and even syncope may occur. Patients who experience focal neurologic symptoms during, after, or immediately before a migraine are said to have **migraine with aura**, and patients with no neurologic symptoms are classified as having **migraine without aura**.

Migraines may last from hours to days. Many patients note that specific triggers can precipitate their headaches. These can include alcohol (especially red wine), chocolate, cheese, pickled items, processed meats, monosodium glutamate, menstrual periods, weather conditions, irregular eating or sleep habits, and stress. Many patients also have a history of motion sickness, and 50–60% have other family members with headaches (compared to 10–20% of the headache-free population).

Tension headaches are typically bilateral, often involving either the forehead or the back of the head and neck, and sometimes the entire head. The pain is described as a pressure or squeezing sensation. Nausea may occur, but most of the other features that can accompany migraine are absent. The only common precipitating factor is stress.

Some patients with migraine or tension headaches can achieve adequate control simply by identifying and eliminating triggers. In particular, many women only develop severe headaches after starting oral contraceptives, and they may want to consider alternative forms of birth control. Even when there does not seem to be a clear correlation between the headaches and initiation of contraceptive pill use, an empiric trial off the pills sometimes produces significant improvement in headaches. A separate concern for patients on birth control pills is the risk of thromboembolic events, including stroke. Migraines, birth control pills, and smoking are all independent risk factors. The incidence of such events in young women is so low that the increased risk with one of these three factors is still negligible. Even with two factors present, the risk is usually acceptable (although the patient should be informed of the issue). With all three factors present, however, the risk becomes more of a concern: in general, a patient with headaches should either stop smoking or stop taking birth control pills.

For most patients, elimination of trigger factors does not produce adequate headache control, and medications are necessary. Nonpharmacologic treatments such as neck stretching exercises, relaxation techniques, and biofeedback may be helpful, but they are usually not adequate to control headaches by themselves. Pharmacologic treatment is centered around two kinds of medications: **abortive agents** and **prophylactic agents**. An abortive agent is one taken as soon as possible when a headache begins, in an attempt to shorten the headache. A prophylactic agent is one taken on a regular basis, even when the patient does not have a headache, in an attempt to prevent headaches or reduce their frequency. The most commonly used abortive and prophylactic agents are listed in Tables 12-1 and 12-2, respectively.

Patients with infrequent migraine or tension headaches do not require prophylactic medications if they can find an abortive agent that consistently and rapidly relieves their symptoms. The key factor in deciding whether to start a prophylactic agent is the degree to which patients' headaches disrupt their lives. Even patients who have found an effective abortive regimen often experience a substantial period of discomfort before the drug takes effect, and this can be severe enough to interfere with normal activities. If this happens frequently, work productivity and quality of life can be affected. Furthermore, most abortive agents seem to be less effective if used too frequently. For these reasons, patients with frequent headaches often need a prophylactic medication. No absolute criterion exists to determine when such treatment is necessary, but as a general guideline, a patient with more than one headache a week should probably be on a prophylactic medication. Some patients with only one headache a month may require a prophylactic agent if the headaches last several days and are disabling. Other patients may have more tolerable headaches or may get prompt relief from an abortive agent, so that they will choose to experience several headaches a week rather than take a medication regularly.

Table 12-1. Abortive Agents

Generic (Trade) Name	Dosing Regimen
Oral and sublingual agents	
Aspirin	325–650 mg q4h p.r.n. (some patients respond best to 1950 mg all at onset)
Acetaminophen (Tylenol)	325–650 mg q4h p.r.n.
Naproxen (Naprosyn, Anaprox, Aleve)	500–750 mg at onset, 250–375 q4h p.r.n.
Ibuprofen (Motrin, Advil, Nuprin)	400–800 mg at onset, 300–800 q4h p.r.n.
Indomethacin (Indocin)	25–50 mg at onset, 25–50 q4h p.r.n.
Ketorolac (Toradol)	10 mg at onset, 10 q6h p.r.n.
Ergotamine tartrate/caffeine (Wigraine, Ercaf, Cafergot)	1–3 pills at onset, 1 pill q1/2h p.r.n.; maximum 5 pills/day, 12 pills/wk
Ergotamine tartrate sublingual (Ergomar)	2 mg at onset, 2 mg ql/2h p.r.n.; maximum 3 pills/day, 5 pills/wk
Isometheptene/acetaminophen/ dichloralphenazone (Midrin, Duradrin)	1–3 pills at onset, 1 pill q1/2h p.r.n.; maximum 5 pills/day, 12 pills/wk
Sumatriptan (Imitrex)	25–100 mg at onset, 25–100 q2h p.r.n.; maximum 300 mg/day, 4 days/wk
Naratriptan (Amerge)	1.0–2.5 mg at onset, repeat in 4 hrs p.r.n.; maximum 5 mg/day, 4 days/wk
Rizatriptan (Maxalt); pills or orally disintegrating tablets	5–10 mg at onset, 5–10 q2h p.r.n.; maximum 30 mg/day, 4 days/wk
Zolmitriptan (Zomig)	2.5–5.0 mg at onset, 2.5–5.0 q2h p.r.n.; maximum 10 mg/day, 4 days/wk
Aspirin/butalbital/caffeine (Fiorinal)	1–2 pills q4h p.r.n.; maximum 6 pills/day; **avoid if possible—addictive**
Acetaminophen/butalbital/caffeine (Fioricet, Esgic)	1–2 pills q4h p.r.n.; maximum 6 pills/day; **avoid if possible—addictive**
Nasal sprays	
Dihydroergotamine (Migranal)	0.5 mg (one spray) in each nostril, repeat in 15 mins p.r.n.; maximum 2 mg/day, 4 mg/wk
Sumatriptan (Imitrex)	5–20 mg (in one nostril or split between the two nostrils); repeat in 2 hrs p.r.n.; maximum 40 mg/day, 4 days/wk

Table 12-1. *Continued*

Generic (Trade) Name	Dosing Regimen
Butorphanol (Stadol)	1 mg (one spray) in one nostril q1h p.r.n.; maximum 4 mg/day; **avoid if possible—addictive**
Subcutaneous injections	
Sumatriptan (Imitrex)	6 mg sc; maximum 8 doses/mo
Suppositories	
Indomethacin (Indocin)	50–100 mg at onset, q1h p.r.n.; maximum 150 mg/day, 4 days/wk
Ergotamine tartrate/caffeine suppositories (Cafergot, Wigraine); may be unavailable	1/2–1 suppository at onset, 1/2–1 q1h p.r.n.; maximum 2/day, 5/wk
Emergency room options (besides all of the above)	
Dihydroergotamine (DHE-45)	0.5–1.0 mg IV; premedicate with 10 mg Metoclopramide or Prochlorperazine, repeat q8h p.r.n.
Chlorpromazine (Thorazine)	25–50 mg IM or 25 mg IV (slowly)
Prochlorperazine (Compazine)	10 mg IV
Metoclopramide (Reglan)	10 mg IV
Hydroxyzine (Vistaril)	25–100 mg IM
Ketorolac (Toradol)	30–60 mg IM, repeat q6h p.r.n.
Oxygen	100% by mask at 8–10 liters/min × 30 mins
Hydrocortisone	100–250 mg IV over 10 mins; may repeat in 8–12 hrs
Dexamethasone (Decadron)	12–20 mg IM or IV; may repeat in 8–12 hrs
Narcotics	Use cautiously

The choice of which abortive or prophylactic agent to use is generally based on the side effect profiles and dosing characteristics. For example, a patient with asthma should generally not be given a beta blocker, but this might be the first choice in a patient with borderline hypertension. A patient with an ulcer should not be given a nonsteroidal anti-inflammatory drug, but most other patients tolerate these agents quite well. A patient who can't manage to take medications regularly throughout the day should be given a medication with a long half-life.

Side effect profiles are a particular concern in pregnant patients. No medication is considered absolutely safe during pregnancy (and similar

Table 12-2. Prophylactic Agents

Generic (Trade) Name	Dosing Regimen
Nonsteroidal anti-inflammatory drugs	
Naproxen (Naprosyn, Anaprox, Aleve)	250 mg b.i.d. up to 375 mg t.i.d.
Indomethacin (Indocin)	25 mg t.i.d. up to 50 mg t.i.d.
Beta-blockers	
Propanolol (Inderal)	20 mg t.i.d. up to 80 mg q.i.d.*
Nadolol (Corgard)	40 mg b.i.d. up to 80 mg q.i.d.
Metoprolol (Lopressor, Toprol-XL)	50 mg b.i.d. up to 100 mg q.i.d.*
Calcium channel blockers	
Verapamil (Calan, Isoptin, Verelan)	80 mg t.i.d. up to 160 mg t.i.d.*
Tricyclic antidepressants	
Amitriptyline (Elavil)	50 mg q.h. (but start lower, build slowly!) up to 200 mg q.h.
Nortriptyline (Pamelor)	50 mg q.h. (but start lower, build slowly!) up to 150 mg q.h.
Serotonin reuptake inhibitors	
Fluoxetine (Prozac)	20 mg/day up to 40 mg b.i.d. (last dose in early afternoon)
Sertraline (Zoloft)	50 mg/day up to 200 mg/day
Paroxetine (Paxil)	20 mg/day up to 50 mg/day
Other antidepressant medications	
Venlafaxine (Effexor)	25 mg b.i.d. up to 75 mg t.i.d.
Nefazodone (Serzone)	100 mg b.i.d. up to 300 mg b.i.d.
Ergots	
Methylergonovine maleate (Methergine)	0.2 mg t.i.d. up to 0.4 mg t.i.d.
Methysergide (Sansert)	2 mg t.i.d. (but start at 2 mg/day) up to 4 mg t.i.d.; need abdominal CT every 9–12 months to watch for retroperitoneal fibrosis
Monoamine oxidase inhibitors	
Phenelzine (Nardil)	15 mg t.i.d. up to 30 mg t.i.d.
Miscellaneous	
Cyproheptadine (Periactin)	4 mg t.i.d. up to 8 mg t.i.d.
Valproic acid (Depakote)	250 mg t.i.d. up to 500 mg q.i.d.
Gabapentin (Neurontin)	100 mg t.i.d. up to 900 mg q.i.d.

*Long-acting preparations can be given less frequently.

considerations apply to women who are breast-feeding). Fortunately, headaches often subside during pregnancy. If a patient requires medication, it is best to try to control the headaches with abortive agents alone. Ergots and triptans are absolutely contraindicated. Acetaminophen is generally thought to be the safest abortive agent. Codeine may be added if necessary, but indiscriminate use has been associated with various congenital malformations. Meperidine (Demerol) is considered relatively safe, and isometheptene (Midrin) probably is also. If a prophylactic agent is necessary, cyproheptadine may be the safest choice, but it is not always effective. Nonsteroidals can cause premature ductus closure and consequent pulmonary hypertension; they may also increase bilirubin and impair renal function. They are generally considered relatively safe in the first two trimesters. Fluoxetine (Prozac) and metoprolol (Lopressor) are also considered fairly safe. Propanolol (Inderal) has an oxytocic effect and may cause growth retardation, respiratory depression, and hypoglycemia. It carries more risk than metoprolol but may be more effective for some patients. Calcium channel blockers may be relatively safe in pregnancy, but there is a theoretical risk of reduced uterine blood flow due to hypotension. Limb reduction abnormalities, other bone deformities, and hand swelling have been reported with amitriptyline (Elavil) and nortriptyline (Pamelor).

B. Cluster Headaches

The most distinctive feature of cluster headache is the time course: the patient may go for months or years without headaches but then experiences a cluster of daily headaches. Clusters usually last 4–8 weeks and occur once or twice a year, but this is quite variable. The headaches themselves typically last 30 minutes to 2 hours (an average of 45 minutes), and the onset is explosive. Patients often cannot sit or stand still and prefer to be upright; many will even hit their head against a wall. Within a cluster there may be one or more headaches a day, but at least one of the headaches typically occurs at the same hour every day (patients say they "could set the clock" by them). Most of the headaches occur at night, frequently awakening the patient from REM sleep.

Like typical migraine, cluster headaches are unilateral, but unlike migraine, they are almost always on the same side. Cluster headaches are frequently associated with ipsilateral lacrimation, redness of the eye, nasal congestion, and rhinorrhea. An ipsilateral partial Horner's syndrome is sometimes present. While migraine headaches are twice as common in women as in men, cluster headaches are six times more common in men than women.

Any abortive agent used for migraine can also be used to abort a cluster headache, but certain agents are particularly effective:

1. Oxygen, 100% at 8–10 liters per minute for 10–15 minutes

2. Intranasal (aerosol) ergotamine, 0.36–1.08 mg (1–3 puffs)

3. Intranasal lidocaine, 4% (1 ml) in the ipsilateral nostril

4. IV dihydroergotamine (DHE); see Table 12-1 for dose recommendations

5. Subcutaneous sumatriptan, 6 mg

In some cases, the cluster can be managed purely with abortive treatments (e.g., by providing a home oxygen tank). In many cases, this is not practical, however, and medication must be given to try to stop the cluster. One commonly used medication is prednisone, 80 mg per day for 1–2 weeks, followed by a rapid taper. Alternatives include verapamil (360–480 mg per day in divided doses), ergotamine tartrate (1 mg twice a day), valproic acid (500–2,000 mg per day in divided doses, lithium carbonate (600–900 mg per day in divided doses, adjusted to keep the serum level in the therapeutic range), or methysergide (4–10 mg per day in divided doses). Whichever medication is used, the dose should be gradually tapered after the patient has been free of headaches for 2 weeks. For patients who have very frequent clusters (or who have entered a chronic phase, which may last 4–5 years), prophylactic medication may be necessary even between clusters. All of the same prophylactic agents may be useful, but lithium and verapamil are the ones prescribed most commonly. Surgical intervention is an option for the 10% or less of patients who are refractory to medications.

C. *Trigeminal Neuralgia*

Trigeminal neuralgia (*tic douloureux*) is characterized by a paroxysmal, "electric shock-like" pain, usually beginning at the maxilla or mandible and lasting approximately 1 second. It tends to occur in trains lasting 5–30 seconds. The pain can sometimes be triggered by lightly touching a particular spot on the face, called a *trigger zone*. The location of the trigger zone differs among patients. The pain may also be triggered by cold wind, brushing the teeth, or chewing. It usually does not wake patients from sleep. There is often a superimposed dull, continuous ache, especially when the condition has been present a long time.

Trigeminal neuralgia is usually a benign condition, either idiopathic or associated with compression of the trigeminal sensory root by blood vessels, but it can also be associated with other structural lesions of the fifth nerve, and it occurs fairly frequently in patients with multiple sclerosis. Symptoms usually begin after age 50 but may occur from the second decade on. The younger the patient, the greater the likelihood that the trigeminal neuralgia is secondary to some other condition, especially multiple sclerosis. An MRI scan of the brain, with special attention to the posterior fossa, should be done if symptoms began or changed in character within the past 2 years, if the patient is younger than age 50, or if there are focal abnormalities on examination. A substantial number of patients develop trigeminal neuralgia as a result of dental problems, including microabscesses, so all patients should be carefully evaluated for dental disease.

Initial treatment is usually with carbamazepine (Tegretol), starting at a dose of 100 mg b.i.d. or t.i.d., but increasing if necessary to doses as high as 1,500 mg per day. If this is ineffective (or if its effect is only temporary), the following drugs are often effective also:

1. Baclofen (Lioresal), 10 mg b.i.d.; up to 20 mg q.i.d., if necessary

2. Gabapentin (Neurontin), 300 mg t.i.d.; up to 900 mg q.i.d., if necessary

3. Lamotrigine (Lamictal), 25 mg b.i.d.; up to 200 mg b.i.d., if necessary

4. Phenytoin (Dilantin), 100 mg b.i.d.; up to 100 mg q.i.d., if necessary

5. Amitriptyline (Elavil), 25 mg q.h.s.; up to 150 mg q.h.s., if necessary

6. Valproic acid (Depakote), 250 mg b.i.d.; up to 500 mg q.i.d., if necessary

7. Clonazepam (Klonopin), 0.5 mg b.i.d.; up to 2.0 mg q.i.d., if necessary

At least several of these agents should be tried before considering surgical treatment. There are two principal surgical options. The most reliable method, but also the most invasive, is microvascular decompression of the trigeminal sensory root. The less invasive method is a percutaneous lesion of the trigeminal ganglion or root, either with radiofrequency pulses or with glycerol injection. Unfortunately, a few patients develop "anesthesia dolorosa" after the percutaneous procedures. This is a condition of numbness and extremely painful paresthesias over part of the face, notoriously refractory to treatment. As a general rule, microvascular decompression is probably preferable to percutaneous ganglion lesions, except in older patients or others who might be poor surgical candidates. A third option is to destroy a branch of the trigeminal nerve, but results are often inadequate.

D. Glossopharyngeal Neuralgia

The pain characteristics and clinical features of glossopharyngeal neuralgia are similar to those of trigeminal neuralgia, except that the pain typically starts in the oropharynx and extends upward and backward toward the ear (sometimes in the reverse direction). Swallowing (especially sour or spicy foods), yawning, sneezing, coughing, cold liquids in the mouth, or touching the ear can be triggers. Unlike trigeminal neuralgia, the pain frequently awakens patients from sleep. The pain sometimes is associated with syncope. Medical treatment is the same as for trigeminal neuralgia, and surgical treatment is analogous. Glossopharyngeal neuralgia is rare (trigeminal neuralgia is 75 times more common).

E. Chronic Paroxysmal Hemicrania

Chronic paroxysmal hemicrania is also a rare condition. The clinical features of the pain and accompanying symptoms are the same as for cluster headache, but the temporal profile is different: The headaches are short (3–46 minutes, an average of 13 minutes) and recur frequently throughout the day (4–38 attacks a day, an average of 14). No nocturnal predominance is apparent, and the headaches usually occur daily throughout the year, rather than in clusters. Chronic paroxysmal hemicrania is five times more common in women than in men and is responsive to indomethacin (Indocin), though dose requirements may vary.

F. Atypical Facial Pain

Patients who do not fit cleanly into any well-defined category are classified as having atypical facial pain. They often have some features of migraine, but others of neuralgia, and other features that are not typical of either. This diagnosis obviously has no consistent pathophysiologic correlate, and treatment is usually a matter of trial and error with medications used for one of the more well-defined conditions. As with other headache syndromes, diagnostic testing is only necessary if the neurologic examination shows focal abnormalities or if there has been recent onset or change in the character of the patient's symptoms.

V. Secondary Headaches

Although most patients with isolated headaches have a primary headache syndrome, occasional patients have an underlying neurologic or systemic disease. This is most likely when patients have additional symptoms or signs that suggest a generalized disease process, when there are focal neurologic abnormalities on examination, or when the headaches are of recent onset (see Part III, Section B, of this chapter). Several conditions merit special consideration, because some physicians think that these conditions are responsible for headaches in large segments of the population, whereas others question their significance.

A. Sinus Disease

Patients with acute sinusitis often experience headaches that are typically exacerbated by changes in head position. The diagnosis is usually apparent because these patients also have nasal discharge, congestion, conjunctival injection, cough, and sinus tenderness. Sphenoid sinusitis may be difficult to detect because the sphenoid sinus does not communicate directly with the nasal passages, so patients may experience headaches without any of the other associated symptoms that are typical of sinusitis. Patients with sphenoid sinusitis are at substantial risk for developing meningitis and require a prolonged course of antibiotic therapy, often IV.

The role of *chronic* sinusitis in producing headaches is less clear. Many patients with chronic headaches have some opacification in one or more sinuses on imaging studies, but many patients without headaches have similar findings. There is no compelling evidence that these patients respond to antihistamines, antibiotics, or sinus surgery, so they should be treated with the same medications used for tension and migraine headaches.

B. Temporomandibular Joint Disease

Structural malalignment of the temporomandibular joint can produce both local and referred pain. There is wide variation in the way this diagnosis is made, and the condition is probably overdiagnosed. Still, if a patient reports a correlation between chewing and headaches, and if the temporomandibular joint is easily dislocated on examination, the diagnosis should be considered. Initial treatment is usually a soft diet; jaw bracing and surgery are used for more severe cases.

C. Postconcussion (or Post-traumatic) Syndrome

It is common for patients who have had head trauma to develop headaches that generally have features typical of the migraine/tension spectrum. The pain is often continuous, waxing and waning in severity. These patients often report memory difficulties, sleep disturbance, mood swings, depression, neck and back pain, and diffuse sensory symptoms. Imaging studies are usually normal (but should be obtained once, to exclude chronic subdural hematomas and to exclude structural problems in the spine if the patient has symptoms there). This syndrome is often complicated by superimposed legal and disability issues, and because all features are subjective, there is no way to rate the severity of this condition or even to be sure it is present. In most cases, the symptoms resolve spontaneously—usually within a year—but they sometimes last as long as 3 years. In approximately 10% of patients, symptoms persist beyond that point. While waiting for resolution, only symptomatic treatment is available. The headaches should be treated in the same way as migraine and tension headaches; antidepressants are often used because the patients also have symptoms of depression.

VI. Discussion of Case Histories

Case 1. Even though this patient complains of the worst headache of his life, it is not qualitatively different from headaches he has been having for 12 years. If his examination (particularly temperature, assessment of neck stiffness, and thorough neurologic examination) is normal, no imaging study is necessary. The patient is too young to have temporal arteritis, so a sedimentation rate is not necessary. The features are in the migraine/tension spectrum (mostly migraine, although the progression to the entire head is not classic). He should be given an abortive agent. Nonsteroidal medications should be avoided because he has already taken eight aspirin; subcutaneous sumatriptan (Imitrex) or IV DHE would provide the most rapid relief. Since he is now having up to two headaches per week, he should be sent out of the ER with a prescription for a prophylactic agent; either naproxen (Naprosyn) or propanolol (Inderal) would be a reasonable first choice.

Case 2. Although this patient's headache is not severe, it has two features that increase the likelihood of an underlying systemic or neurologic process: It has only been present 3 months, and there are focal abnormalities on examination (localizing to the right frontal and parietal lobes). The patient seems to have some anosognosia (unawareness of his own deficits), a common accompaniment of nondominant parietal lobe lesions. Given a focal lesion and a chronic time course, a neoplasm is a prime concern (see Chapter 3). This patient needs an imaging study of the brain as soon as possible, and treatment will depend on what it shows. At the same time, he could be given symptomatic treatment for his headaches, using the same approach that would be followed in a patient with migraine or tension headaches.

Comment: A CT scan revealed a ring-enhancing lesion in the right frontal and parietal lobes, with substantial edema surrounding it. A chest x-ray showed an apical lesion in the right lung that had not been present on previous studies, the most recent of which had been obtained 9 months earlier. A non–small cell lung cancer was found at bronchoscopy. The cerebral mass was presumed to be a metastasis, and the patient was started on dexamethasone to treat the cerebral edema. This eliminated the headaches also. He was referred to an oncologist for management of his primary cancer. The patient refused resection and radiation of the cerebral metastasis.

13

Visual Symptoms

I. Case Histories

Case 1. A 22-year-old woman has been experiencing discomfort and blurring of vision in her left eye for several days. She has never had similar symptoms and has otherwise been healthy. She has 20/20 vision in her right eye, measured with a near vision card while her left eye is covered. With the right eye covered, she is unable to read newsprint and her acuity is 20/300. Her pupils are equal, but she has a left afferent pupillary defect. The left optic disk appears slightly pale; the right appears normal. She complains of discomfort in the left eye during testing of visual pursuit. The remainder of her examination is normal.

Case 2. A 75-year-old man complains of "blurred vision" in his left eye. The symptoms began several days ago and have progressed slowly. There is no eye pain. He also complains that he has been unable to chew meat because of pain in his jaw. With glasses he is barely able to count fingers with the left eye, but right eye visual acuity is normal. He has a left afferent pupillary defect and a swollen left optic disk. The remainder of his examination is normal.

Case 3. A 60-year-old woman reports episodes of loss of vision in the left eye. Each spell begins suddenly and gradually worsens over 15–30 seconds, "like a shade being drawn over the eye." The vision loss lasts for several minutes before resolving completely. She has no pain or other symptoms with these spells. The first episode occurred 2 months ago, and she has had four more episodes since. Her examination is normal.

Questions:

1. How is the approach to these patients the same?

2. How does their evaluation differ?

3. What steps must be taken urgently?

II. Background Information

A. *Definitions*

diplopia: double vision.
homonymous: affecting the same side of the visual field in both eyes.
heteronymous: affecting different sides of the visual field in each eye.

B. *Overview of the Visual System*

Information from each eye travels separately to the optic chiasm, where fiber pathways cross and sort themselves so that fibers carrying information from analogous portions of the visual fields of the two eyes travel together to the primary visual cortex in the occipital lobe. The visual information is subsequently forwarded to many other specialized regions of cortex where such features as form, color, depth, and motion are analyzed. Most of the individual cells in these different regions of visual cortex receive input from both eyes. For these cells to function properly, the two eyes must be exquisitely aligned. This is the function of the ocular motor system, which directs the output of cranial nerves III, IV, and VI in such a way that both eyes are always fixated on the same point.

When the ocular motor system malfunctions so that the two eyes fixate on slightly different points, the brain receives two visual images of the world that are a little displaced from each other. The result is diplopia. In contrast, lesions of the visual pathways produce a degraded image in the affected visual field regions, but the visual fields of the two eyes remain aligned, so vision loss occurs, rather than diplopia.

III. Approach to Visual Symptoms

An accurate description of visual symptoms is the key to diagnosis. Does the patient have diplopia or vision loss? If the problem is vision loss, does it involve one eye or both, and does it involve the entire visual field of the affected eyes or only a portion of the field? Are the symptoms transient, static, or progressive? If the symptoms are transient, are there any precipitating factors? Are the episodes stereotyped, and, if so, what is the temporal progression of the symptoms?

Patients with static or progressive deficits can be examined while symptoms are present. When the symptoms are transient, however, the patient is often completely free of symptoms when examined and may have trouble providing a detailed description of the episodes. In these cases, it is helpful to instruct patients to cover each eye in turn during subsequent episodes and pay careful attention to how this affects their symptoms.

IV. Monocular Vision Loss

Symptoms confined to a single eye imply a lesion anterior to the optic chiasm because this is the only portion of the visual pathway that does not include input from both eyes. The cause of monocular vision loss can usually be deduced from the age of the patient and the time course of symptoms.

Examination findings are helpful in distinguishing diseases of the optic nerve from other ocular causes of vision loss. Unless the vision loss is mild, the "swinging flashlight test" (see Chapter 2) almost always reveals an afferent pupillary defect when the problem is in the optic nerve. A careful ocular examination (including measurement of intraocular pressure) will usually reveal disease situated in the nonneural tissue of the eye. Regardless of the cause of monocular vision loss, the most straightforward way to determine severity and follow the clinical course is to measure visual acuity in each eye separately. In a few conditions, especially glaucoma and increased intracranial pressure, visual acuity is relatively spared, so disease progression must be assessed in other ways.

A. Acute Monocular Vision Loss in Young Patients

In young patients, the acute onset of monocular vision loss usually signifies **optic neuritis** (much less common causes include sinus mucocele, vasculitis, and optic nerve infiltration by carcinomatous or granulomatous processes). The vision loss may progress over 7–10 days. Eye pain may precede or accompany the vision loss; it is usually exacerbated by eye movement. Optic neuritis may occur in isolation or as a manifestation of multiple sclerosis (MS). Patients should be asked explicitly about any previous neurologic symptoms that might suggest the latter diagnosis. Those with no prior history of neurologic symptoms have a 30% risk of developing MS within 5 years. Patients with white matter lesions on MRI scan of the brain have a higher (up to 50%) likelihood of developing MS than patients with normal MRI scans.

Patients with optic neuritis who receive a 3-day course of high-dose IV methylprednisolone (followed by oral prednisone for 11 days) recover slightly more quickly than those who receive placebo, but the difference in visual function between the two groups 6 months later is minimal. Patients who receive oral prednisone alone for 14 days recover at the same rate as those receiving placebo. In one large, randomized study, patients who received IV methylprednisolone had a lower incidence of MS in the subsequent 2 years than did patients who received placebo, whereas patients who received oral prednisone without a preceding dose of IV methylprednisolone had a *higher* incidence of recurrent optic neuritis within 2 years than patients who received placebo and the same incidence of MS as the placebo group. These differences between groups were not evident at a 5-year follow-up. Although these results are difficult to interpret, many clinicians use IV methylprednisolone followed by prednisone to treat patients with optic neuritis, especially if an MRI scan of the brain reveals white matter lesions.

Acute vision loss can also result from traumatic injury to the eye, but this is usually obvious from the history and examination. In young diabetic patients, vitreous hemorrhage should be considered. Acute iritis typically presents with blurred vision, pain, and redness, sometimes in one eye only. Iritis can be a symptom of systemic autoimmune disease, so these patients should be asked about problems of the skin, joints, or visceral organs.

B. *Acute Monocular Vision Loss in Older Patients*

In older patients, monocular vision loss may be due to acute glaucoma, retinal detachment, macular degeneration, cataracts, and acute ischemic optic neuropathy. Glaucoma (increased intraocular pressure) is usually a chronic condition causing gradually progressive field loss, but acute obstruction of aqueous outflow results in sudden vision loss accompanied by severe eye and face pain, nausea, vomiting, and dilation of the pupil. Retinal detachment is usually associated with a history of trauma, though it may be surprisingly minor (e.g., jogging). Cataracts and macular degeneration (and most cases of glaucoma) produce gradual vision loss progressing over years and are usually evident on examination.

Acute ischemic optic neuropathy is particularly important because it is sometimes caused by **temporal arteritis,** which can usually be successfully treated but may progress to complete blindness in both eyes if left untreated. Historical clues to the presence of temporal arteritis include headache, jaw or tongue claudication, and aches or discomfort in the shoulder and pelvic girdles (polymyalgia rheumatica). On examination, temporal pulses may be absent or there may be evidence of temporal artery tenderness and tortuosity. Biopsy of the temporal artery is the "gold standard" for diagnosis and should be obtained whenever the clinical setting suggests temporal arteritis, even if the sedimentation rate is not elevated (see Chapter 12). Whenever the diagnosis of temporal arteritis is seriously considered, treatment with high-dose corticosteroids (prednisone, 1 mg/kg per day) should begin immediately even if temporal artery biopsy must be delayed. Histopathologic changes will still be seen if the biopsy can be performed within several days.

V. Transient Vision Loss (Monocular or Binocular)

Transient visual obscuration in one or both eyes may be caused by ischemia, migraine, or increased intracranial pressure. The visual phenomena associated with migraine are typically distinctive: Patients describe flashing lights or jagged lines on the edge of a scotoma in which vision is obscured or totally absent. The abnormal region often expands gradually or moves off toward one side of the visual field. When patients have a typical headache before, during, or after experiencing characteristic visual symptoms, the diagnosis is usually straightforward. Diagnosis can be more difficult when patients have the visual symptoms without any headache, or symptoms that are atypical in some way; some of these patients may need to be evaluated for vascular disease or structural abnormalities before concluding that their symptoms are due to migraine.

Transient vision loss in one eye can represent a transient ischemic attack (TIA) due to atherosclerotic disease in the ipsilateral carotid artery (or, less likely, due to cardioembolism). The vision loss typically progresses over a matter of minutes and is described as being "like a shade being pulled down from the top or up from the bottom" of the visual field. After some minutes, the same process occurs in reverse. The entire episode usually resolves completely in less than 60 minutes. Not all patients describe such stereotypical episodes, however, and the possibility of TIAs should always be considered when patients at risk for atherosclerotic disease experience transient monocular vision loss.

Patients can also experience transient vision loss as a result of cortical TIAs, but in this case the symptoms involve only one-half of the visual field, and both eyes are affected. Patients sometimes mistakenly report that they were unable to see out of one eye during the episode, so they should be questioned carefully about whether they checked their vision in each eye separately. In addition to the homonymous nature of the visual symptoms, the time course and the presence of risk factors are clues to the diagnosis.

Patients with increased intracranial pressure sometimes experience transient episodes of altered vision triggered by even minor increases in the pressure. For example, they may note visual disturbance in one or both eyes whenever they bend over. The characteristic physical finding is bilateral papilledema in the presence of normal optic nerve function. Increased pressure results from obstruction of cerebrospinal fluid outflow. This can be caused by an appropriately placed mass lesion (see Chapter 11), or it may occur without any obvious structural cause; this is called **pseudotumor cerebri**. Pseudotumor cerebri is most common in obese women of childbearing age. It is generally a self-limited condition but may lead to permanent vision loss. Pseudotumor is generally treated with acetazolamide (Diamox); other treatments include periodic removal of cerebrospinal fluid or fenestration of the optic nerve sheath.

VI. Binocular Vision Loss

Soon after the visual pathways leave the optic chiasm, the input from the two eyes is aligned so closely that any lesion produces a homonymous visual field defect. Lesions anterior to the chiasm cause exclusively monocular symptoms. With lesions in the chiasm itself, a variety of patterns of visual field defect may occur, depending on the exact placement of the lesion. The most central lesions affect only those fibers in the process of crossing from right to left or vice versa; these are the fibers from the nasal half of each retina, corresponding to the temporal half of each eye's visual field. The result is a **heteronymous hemianopia.** As noted in Chapter 2, this lesion may go undetected by the patient, because the "bad" field in each eye corresponds to the "good" field in the other eye. They are only evident when each eye is tested separately.

Lesions affecting the visual pathway posterior to the optic chiasm are conceptually equivalent to any other focal cortical lesions. The differential diagnosis is based on demographic considerations and the time course of symptoms, as described in Chapter 3, and management is predicated on the underlying disease process.

VII. Diplopia

A. *Localization in Diplopia*

Diplopia can result from lesions anywhere in the ocular motor system starting in the brainstem nuclei of cranial nerves III, IV, and VI and proceeding along the pathways of those nerves to the individual extraocular muscles. Generalized diseases of muscle or the neuromuscular junction can also interfere with the ability to keep the eyes aligned, and so can anything affecting the mechanical properties of the eyeballs themselves (e.g., a soft tissue mass in the orbit restricting movement of the eyeball).

The first issue to address in a patient with diplopia is whether all of the patient's findings could be caused by dysfunction of a single cranial nerve. There are three specific patterns to recognize:

1. Sixth nerve lesion: limitation of abduction (lateral gaze) of *one eye only*; all other movements intact.

2. Fourth nerve lesion: impaired ability of *one eye* to look down and in (i.e., toward the nostril); patients often compensate by tilting the entire head in the direction the affected eye cannot move (i.e., away from the affected side).

3. Third nerve lesion: limitation of adduction (medial gaze), elevation, and depression of *one eye only*, associated with ipsilateral ptosis and dilated pupil.

If one of these patterns is found, then the correct localization is almost always at the level of the cranial nerve or its nucleus. The same is true even if some components of the pattern are missing (e.g., a patient with a third nerve lesion may have all the eye movement abnormalities without a dilated pupil or ptosis). A disease of muscle or neuromuscular junction (or even a structural abnormality in the orbit) can sometimes produce one of these patterns also, but this is rare because there is no particular reason for these conditions to affect only the muscles innervated by a single cranial nerve (just as it is theoretically possible for motor neuron disease or myasthenia gravis to produce the same pattern of weakness as an L5 root lesion, but it is not likely).

If the patient's eye movement problems do not all fit into the syndrome expected with a lesion of a single cranial nerve, the next question is whether the findings could all be explained by combined lesions of two cranial nerves, especially two that are neighbors at some point in their course (such as both sixth nerves, or the left third and left fourth nerves). If so, this is the likely localization.

Whenever the cause of the eye movement abnormality appears to be malfunction of one or more cranial nerves, the next issue to address is whether the lesion is intra-axial (within the substance of the brainstem itself) or extra-axial (affecting cranial nerves after they have exited the brainstem). This requires a search for involvement of fiber tracts passing through the brainstem but not entering or exiting at that level, so that a purely extra-axial process could not possibly affect them. Thus, patients should be examined closely for limb weakness, ataxia, hyperreflexia, and sensory changes.

When the pattern of eye muscle abnormality cannot be explained by a lesion of one or two cranial nerves, and there is no suggestion of an intra-axial brainstem lesion, a primary muscle or neuromuscular junction problem should be considered, especially when muscles of both eyes are involved. Meningeal inflammation or cancer can also affect multiple cranial nerves (see Chapter 10), and mechanical limitation of eye movement from structural problems in the orbit (including soft tissue swelling) should not be ignored.

B. Differential Diagnosis and Management

Diseases primarily affecting the neuromuscular junction or muscle are discussed in Chapter 6. Initial symptoms may be restricted to extraocular muscles, and sometimes these are the only muscles involved throughout the entire course of the illness. The principles of diagnosis and management are the same as for patients with more widespread muscle involvement.

When the localization of disease appears to be at the level of the cranial nerve, the differential diagnosis depends on whether the process is intra-axial or extra-axial and on how many cranial nerves are affected. An intra-axial lesion can be analyzed according to the approach presented in Chapter 3, using the time course and epidemiologic factors to guide diagnosis and management. An extra-axial process affecting multiple cranial nerves is almost always due to meningeal infiltration, from either inflammatory disease (including infection) or neoplastic disease. The diagnosis is usually established by examining cerebrospinal fluid and searching for systemic evidence of a neoplasm or inflammatory disease. On rare occasions, meningeal biopsy may be diagnostic when less invasive studies are not.

Extra-axial involvement of a single cranial nerve is usually caused by either compression or focal ischemia. Diabetic patients are particularly likely to develop isolated third, fourth, or sixth nerve palsies, and these are generally attributed to small-vessel ischemia. As with small vessel disease elsewhere in the nervous system, no specific treatment is available; fortunately, spontaneous recovery gradually occurs in approximately 50% of cases. Compressive lesions, in contrast, often signal the need for urgent treatment, because an expanding mass at this level may go on to produce brainstem compression and death. Because treatment of a compressive lesion can potentially prevent devastating consequences, patients with extra-axial involvement of a single cranial nerve should be considered to have a compressive lesion until proved otherwise. An MRI of the brain with attention to the brainstem should be obtained as soon as possible.

The best-known example of a life-threatening situation presenting with a lesion of a single cranial nerve is the "blown pupil" seen when transtentorial herniation of a cortical lesion compresses the third nerve. Third nerve compression may also result from an expanding arterial aneurysm, which is almost as urgent a problem as herniation, because of the high morbidity and mortality associated with aneurysmal rupture. Aneurysm repair before rupture may prevent permanent neurologic consequences altogether. Thus, it is important to distinguish a compressive third nerve lesion from an ischemic lesion. Pupillary involvement is the key to this distinction. Ischemic lesions usually affect the extraocular muscles innervated by the third nerve but "spare" the pupil. Occasionally, however, the pupil may also be spared with compressive lesions, especially early in the course, so patients with weakness but not complete paralysis of the extraocular muscles innervated by the third nerve should be observed closely for evidence of pupillary involvement if the weakness progresses. If the pupil remains normal even when all muscles innervated by the third nerve are completely paralyzed, an ischemic lesion is likely.

Treatment of a compressive lesion usually requires surgical intervention and the techniques of treating increased intracranial pressure discussed in Chapter 11.

VIII. Discussion of Case Histories

Case 1. The monocular visual symptoms indicate a lesion in the visual pathway anterior to the optic chiasm, and the left afferent pupillary defect implies that the lesion is in the left optic nerve. The relatively acute onset suggests optic neuritis in this age group, and her examination is typical of that condition.

Comment: Although she had not volunteered the information, when asked explicitly about previous sensory symptoms, she recalled an episode of numbness from the neck down 3 years earlier. She had attributed this to stress, and the symptoms had resolved after 2 weeks. An MRI scan of the brain showed several 2- to 3-cm white matter lesions. MS was diagnosed, and she was given a brief course of IV methylprednisolone. The variable and unpredictable prognosis of MS was discussed with her at length. After learning about the available treatment options, she decided to begin treatment with glatiramer.

Case 2. This patient also has monocular visual symptoms and a left afferent pupillary defect, again suggesting a lesion in the left optic nerve. Of the various potential causes of monocular vision loss in this age group, the time course is most consistent with acute ischemic optic neuropathy. The jaw pain when chewing (jaw claudication) suggests that this patient's acute ischemic optic neuropathy is due to temporal arteritis.

Comment: His sedimentation rate was greater than 100 mm per hour, and temporal artery biopsy showed arteritis. He was treated with prednisone for just over 6 months, and all of his symptoms resolved.

Case 3. This patient had amaurosis fugax, a TIA involving the retinal artery. Evaluation and management of TIAs are discussed in Chapter 4.

Both Case 2 and Case 3 represent urgent problems because the symptoms described by each of the two patients may be associated with underlying conditions (temporal arteritis and TIAs) for which prompt treatment can prevent serious and irreversible consequences (blindness in Case 2 and permanent ischemic deficits in Case 3).

14

Dizziness and Disequilibrium

I. Case Histories

Case 1. A 40-year-old school bus driver is terrified that she is going to lose her job. For the past 6 weeks, she has been experiencing severe nausea and a spinning sensation every time she turns her head to the far right. She has stopped driving, because even though the symptoms always resolve within 30 seconds, she reasons that this is plenty of time for an accident to happen. A routine physical examination is entirely normal.

Questions:

1. Does this patient have vertigo? If so, is it central or peripheral?

2. What additional examination techniques would be useful in this case?

3. What is the likely diagnosis?

4. What additional diagnostic and treatment measures should be taken?

5. What is the prognosis?

Case 2. A 45-year-old right-handed man is "having problems walking straight." For the past 6 months, he has needed to hold on to walls or furniture for support when he walks, because it feels as if the ground slants to the left. He thinks the problem is getting worse, because 3 days ago he actually fell down for the first time. He has also noticed that the right side of his face "feels funny," but thinks he may be imagining it. His handwriting is getting sloppier, but it has always been poor. He also mentions that he has had tinnitus and hearing loss in the right ear for the past 2 or 3 years, but attributes it to "all those rock concerts in college."

His examination is notable for reduced sensation on the entire right side of his face, with an absent corneal reflex on the right. He has left-beating nystagmus with a slight rotatory component, most prominent when looking to the left. His hearing is reduced in the right ear, and his right arm and leg movements are ataxic.

Questions:

1. Does this patient have vertigo? If so, is it central or peripheral?

2. What is the likely diagnosis?

3. What additional diagnostic and treatment measures should be taken?

4. What is the prognosis?

Case 3. A 60-year-old man has an unsteady gait that has been getting progressively worse over the past 6 months. He stumbles so much at times that others worry for his safety. He has had increasing trouble climbing ladders because of "stiffness" in his legs. He has a long history of mild neck discomfort. He has had several episodes of urinary incontinence that have embarrassed him significantly. On examination, his mental status and cranial nerves are normal. His gait is stiff and unsteady, and he tends to fall if not supported. There is mild wasting of the intrinsic muscles of the hands, along with spasticity and weakness in the lower extremities, brisk knee and ankle jerks, normal arm reflexes, and bilateral extensor plantar responses.

Questions:

1. Does this patient have vertigo? If so, is it central or peripheral?

2. Where's the lesion?

3. What is the likely diagnosis?

4. What additional diagnostic and treatment measures should be taken?

Case 4. A 65-year-old man has finally been persuaded by his family to see a doctor for his trouble walking. He has difficulty relating a coherent history, especially regarding the time course of his symptoms, but his family is certain that his walking is getting worse. He seems afraid to walk and will only do so when he can hold on to somebody's hand. He denies incontinence but smells like urine. His examination is notable for global cognitive deficits, but they are mild. His gait is wide-based. He is very hesitant when he walks and needs significant support. His lower extremity strength and coordination are normal, however, and in fact, the remainder of his examination is notable only for diffuse hyperreflexia.

Questions:

1. Does this patient have vertigo? If so, is it central or peripheral?

2. Where's the lesion?

3. What is the likely diagnosis?

4. What additional diagnostic and treatment measures should be taken?

II. Approach to Dizziness

Patients use the word *dizzy* in many different ways. It can refer to light-headedness, a sense of spinning or other movement, balance difficulty, clumsiness, confusion, or a vague sense of malaise. Thus, the first step in evaluating a dizzy patient is to clarify exactly what symptoms the patient is experiencing. The subsequent steps will differ depending on the precise nature of the patient's symptoms.

III. Light-Headedness (Presyncope)

Light-headedness is probably the most commonly experienced kind of dizziness. Patients often say they feel as if they are about to faint, and at times they do lose consciousness. This symptom usually results from global cerebral hypoperfusion. The potential causes are discussed in Chapter 5.

IV. Vertigo

Many people (including many physicians) think that vertigo refers specifically to a sense of spinning, and this is probably the most common manifestation, but in fact, it means any false sensation of movement. Vertigo results from dysfunction of the vestibular system, either in the periphery (the labyrinth and the vestibular nerve) or centrally (the vestibular nuclei and the cerebellum).

A. Localization

The processes that affect the peripheral vestibular system are distinct from those that affect it centrally. Several features help to distinguish central from peripheral lesions. Because the vestibular end-organ (the labyrinth) is adjacent to the auditory end-organ (the cochlea), and the vestibular and cochlear nerves remain next to each other all the way to the brainstem, **hearing loss and tinnitus frequently accompany peripheral vertigo.** In contrast, because the auditory pathways proceed bilaterally as soon as they enter the brainstem, a unilateral central lesion generally does not produce significant hearing loss, so it is unusual for central vertigo to be associated with prominent auditory symptoms. Instead, the **typical abnormalities accompanying central vertigo include dysarthria, dysphagia, diplopia, and numbness or weakness in the limbs,** reflecting the fact that this portion of the vestibular pathway is located in the brainstem and cerebellum.

Both central and peripheral vertigo are commonly associated with ataxia and nystagmus because of the strong connections between the cerebellum and the vestibular system. The specific characteristics of the nystagmus help to distinguish between central and peripheral lesions, but there are no absolutely reliable rules. The most dependable rule is that **nystagmus that changes direction depending on the direction of gaze ("multidirectional nystagmus") is almost always due to a central lesion.** Peripheral lesions always cause unidirectional nystagmus; the direction can be remembered by recalling that in testing caloric responses, cold water in one ear (which mimics a destructive lesion) results in slow deviation of the eyes toward that ear, and (in a conscious patient) the fast beat of nystagmus is away from that ear (see Chapter 2).

In general, peripheral nystagmus usually has both a horizontal and a rotational component; pure horizontal, pure rotatory, or pure vertical nystagmus usually indicates a central lesion. Also, nystagmus is usually more intense and more persistent with a central lesion than with a peripheral one. In contrast, the intensity of the subjective sensation of vertigo is often greater with peripheral lesions. There are exceptions to all of these rules, however.

In summary, peripheral vertigo is typically associated with hearing loss and tinnitus; the accompanying nystagmus is always unidirectional and usually has both horizontal and rotatory components. Central vertigo is typically associated with symptoms or signs of brainstem function; the accompanying nystagmus may be either unidirectional or multidirectional, and it may be purely horizontal, purely vertical, purely rotatory, or any combination. Nystagmus is usually more prominent with central lesions, and vertigo is often more severe with peripheral lesions.

When these clinical features are not sufficient to determine whether the lesion is central or peripheral, additional information can be obtained by specialized testing in a vestibular laboratory. Brainstem auditory evoked potentials (see Chapter 10) can help in localizing blocks in the auditory pathway, which parallels the vestibular pathway in the periphery. An audiogram can also be useful in documenting unilateral eighth nerve dysfunction. When localization remains uncertain, imaging studies of the brain (especially the posterior fossa) and skull (especially the auditory canal) may be necessary.

B. Differential Diagnosis

The differential diagnosis of vertigo depends primarily on two factors: whether the lesion is central or peripheral and the time course of symptoms.

1. Central vertigo

Central vertigo that is getting progressively worse is usually due to a neoplasm or abscess (see Chapter 3). Central vertigo of acute onset usually signifies a vascular process (or trauma, in the appropriate setting). Recurrent, transient spells can represent transient ischemic attacks, migraines, or seizures; the time course and associated symptoms usually distinguish these possibilities (see Chapters 4, 5, and 12). Episodic vertigo may also occur in multiple sclerosis.

2. Peripheral vertigo

Peripheral vertigo that is getting progressively worse also suggests inflammatory or neoplastic disease. The most common tumors in the cerebellopontine angle are meningiomas and vestibular nerve schwannomas; the latter have traditionally been referred to as *acoustic neuromas*, but this term is misleading, because these tumors usually arise from the vestibular division of the eighth nerve. Even so, the initial symptoms are usually auditory. Disequilibrium, ipsilateral facial numbness and weakness, and ipsilateral ataxia often develop later in the course. A few specific toxins also cause progressive eighth nerve dysfunction, notably aminoglycosides and cisplatin.

Most often, peripheral vertigo begins acutely and does not progress (though it may persist for days, weeks, or even months). The major differential point in this circumstance is whether similar episodes of vertigo have occurred in the past. There are several conditions that produce recurrent episodes of vertigo.

a. Recurrent episodes

The distinction between peripheral and central vertigo may be especially difficult when the symptoms are episodic, and the patient is only available for examination during asymptomatic periods. Thus, even when the symptoms sound peripheral, central disorders such as migraines, vertebrobasilar TIAs, seizures, and multiple sclerosis must be considered in a patient with recurrent episodes of vertigo. Most often, though, a peripheral condition is the cause.

Benign paroxysmal positional vertigo (BPPV) is the most common cause of recurrent vertigo. Patients with BPPV experience brief episodes of vertigo whenever the head assumes certain positions. The vertigo usually begins about 5–10 seconds after the head assumes the symptomatic position. It typically lasts less than 30 seconds and almost always less than a minute. The vertigo usually becomes less severe if the head is placed in the symptomatic position several times in a row. These features can often be demonstrated by performing the Hallpike maneuver: The patient starts by sitting on the examination table, close to one end, and then reclines to a supine position with the head hanging over the edge of the table and extended 30–45 degrees. The patient remains in this position for 60 seconds and is asked to report any symptoms of vertigo; at the same time, the patient's eyes are observed for nystagmus. The patient is then returned to the seated position, and the maneuver is repeated with the head rotated 45 degrees to one side. The patient is again returned to an upright, seated position, the head is rotated 45 degrees to the other side, and the maneuver is repeated.

BPPV is thought to be due to degenerative debris in the posterior semicircular canal, either adherent to the cupula or floating free in the endolymph. The condition may follow head trauma or "labyrinthitis," but usually no obvious precipitant is apparent. BPPV is typically treated by performing particle repositioning maneuvers designed to dislodge debris from its postulated location and expel it from the posterior canal or by teaching the patient positional exercises. Most exercise programs require the patient to assume the head position of greatest discomfort many times a day for several weeks. This treatment is presumed to dislodge the degenerative debris. Alternatively, it may produce central habituation.

Ménière's disease is characterized by episodic vertigo and tinnitus superimposed on a condition of hearing loss. The hearing loss is fluctuating and completely reversible early in the disease, but it eventually becomes progressive. The episodes of vertigo typically begin with a sensation of fullness and pressure in one ear, accompanied by tinnitus and reduced hearing in that ear. The vertigo reaches maximum intensity within minutes and slowly subsides over the next few hours, but the patient usually continues to feel vaguely unsteady and dizzy for the next few days. Nausea, vomiting, and ataxia may accompany the episodes. These attacks occur irregularly, at intervals of weeks, months, or years.

Ménière's disease is associated with increased endolymph volume throughout the labyrinth. It can occur after labyrinthitis but is usually idiopathic. It is typically treated with salt restriction and diuretics, although the only evidence that these treatments are effective is anecdotal. Endolymphatic shunts have been attempted, without consistent benefit. When all else fails, ablative therapy may be attempted, because the brain can eventually habituate to the complete loss of vestibular function on one side better than it can adjust to fluctuating vestibular function. The least complicated ablative procedure is labyrinthectomy, but this is only feasible when the patient has already lost all functional hearing on that side. Otherwise, a vestibular nerve section is performed.

Perilymph fistula is characterized by episodes of vertigo that are often precipitated by sneezing, coughing, loud noises (*Tullio's phenomenon*, which may also occur in Ménière's disease), exertion, or airplane flights. The fistula consists of a small tear in the oval window or the round window, but the mechanism by which this produces symptoms is unclear. Most patients recover spontaneously, so conservative treatment is recommended: bed rest, head elevation, and measures to reduce straining. Surgical correction is possible when conservative measures are ineffective.

b. Single episode

Acute labyrinthitis is characterized by the sudden or subacute onset of severe vertigo, nausea, vomiting, and ataxia, sometimes associated with hearing loss and tinnitus. Symptoms are usually severe for hours to days, with residual symptoms gradually resolving over days to months. This condition may occur with a documented bacterial infection of the middle ear or in association with a systemic viral illness. Much more commonly, however, the vestibular symptoms occur in isolation. These isolated attacks are widely presumed to be viral or postviral based on some epidemiologic and pathologic evidence, but the etiology has not been convincingly demonstrated. Such attacks are most appropriately termed acute vestibulopathy, but the terms acute labyrinthitis, vestibular neuronitis, or even viral labyrinthitis are often used synonymously.

When a clear infectious cause can be found, appropriate antibiotics should be given. Otherwise, treatment is symptomatic and may include bed rest, antiemetics, and antihistamines.

All of the conditions in the differential diagnosis of recurrent peripheral vertigo must also be considered in a patient with a single episode; after all, there must be a first episode even for recurrent symptoms. The specific characteristics of the patient's symptoms will determine which (if any) of these recurrent conditions are realistic possibilities.

V. Disequilibrium

To maintain balance, the brain must receive detailed, accurate information about the position of the body relative to the environment and generate an appropriate, coordinated motor response. Any condition that disturbs either the sensory input or the motor output can produce disequilibrium. The visual, proprioceptive, and vestibular pathways are the most important sensory systems for determining body position. The auditory pathway also contributes, but to a lesser degree. The history and examination should be directed at detecting dysfunction in any of these pathways. The Romberg test is a useful screen. Normal individuals can maintain balance with their eyes closed, because the remaining sensory modalities are sufficient to provide a sense of body position even when visual information has been removed. In contrast, patients with dysfunction of the proprioceptive or vestibular systems rely heavily on visual input, and while they may be able to maintain equilibrium with their eyes open, they lose their balance when they close their eyes.

Patients with disequilibrium because of an inadequate motor response usually have difficulty maintaining their balance even with their eyes open, so the Romberg test does not apply. An inadequate motor response can result from a purely mechanical problem (such as a fracture), weakness, stiffness (either because of spasticity or due to extrapyramidal disease), ataxia, or cognitive deficits. All of these possibilities should be evaluated in the course of the history and the physical examination.

If any sensory or motor abnormalities that could contribute to disequilibrium are found, they should be evaluated and treated according to principles presented elsewhere in this book. For example, vestibular diseases are discussed in Part IV of this chapter, neuromuscular causes of proprioceptive disturbance are discussed in Chapter 6, normal pressure hydrocephalus is discussed in Chapter 7, and so forth. Disequilibrium is often multifactorial; patients may have several minor abnormalities combining to produce significant impairment of balance even though each of the abnormalities in isolation would be unlikely to cause serious problems.

Treatment of gait difficulty should include an assessment of the patient's home environment. Patients with gait disturbances who have difficulty climbing stairs can be helped by a stair-lift or by moving to a ground-floor apartment or bedroom. Loose rugs are a hazard and should be removed whenever possible. Strategically placed handrails can help to make the home safer. Wall-to-wall carpeting is more easily negotiated in smooth-soled shoes than sneakers, whereas sneakers are better for walking on the sidewalk or street.

VI. Discussion of Case Histories

Case 1. This patient clearly has recurrent episodes of vertigo based on her description. The consistent relationship to a specific head position, the brevity of the symptoms, and the intensity of the vertigo all suggest a peripheral lesion, and specifically, BPPV. Positional vertigo can occasionally occur with central lesions, however, so Hallpike maneuvers or specialized vestibular testing should be performed. If such testing confirms the diagnosis of BPPV, the patient can be reassured and treated with a particle repositioning procedure.

Case 2. This patient also has vertigo, because he feels as if he is falling in one direction. The association with tinnitus and hearing loss makes a peripheral lesion almost certain. The unidirectional nystagmus with both horizontal and rotatory components also suggests a peripheral lesion (a right-sided lesion, in particular). All of the examination findings are consistent with a focal lesion located at the right cerebellopontine angle. In this case, the symptoms were progressive, suggesting inflammatory or neoplastic disease.

Although the history is typical of an *acoustic neuroma*, other inflammatory and neoplastic diseases are certainly possible, so an imaging study is necessary (preferably an MRI scan). If it is consistent with an acoustic neuroma, the treatment of choice is surgical excision using microsurgical techniques, with intraoperative electrophysiologic monitoring of the facial nerve. Radiosurgery is sometimes used for small tumors. The prognosis is good.

Case 3. This patient has disequilibrium, not vertigo. He has upper motor neuron signs in the lower extremities and lower motor neuron signs in the intrinsic hand muscles. Although a combination of upper and lower motor neuron signs can indicate motor neuron disease, this patient's lower motor neuron findings are confined to the distribution of the C8 and T1 nerve roots. A lesion compressing the spinal cord at this level would produce upper motor neuron signs in the lower extremities while sparing structures higher up, explaining the normal arm reflexes (mediated by roots C5–C7), cranial nerves, and mental status. The symptoms have been progressive, with a chronic time course. A chronic, focal lesion is generally a neoplasm. An imaging study of the cervical spine is therefore indicated.

Comment: In this case, an MRI scan of the cervical spine showed degenerative spine changes and compression of the spinal cord. A multilevel decompressive laminectomy was performed with slight benefit.

Case 4. This patient also has disequilibrium rather than vertigo. Like the patient in Case 3, he has a gait disorder and urinary incontinence. The diffuse hyperreflexia suggests upper motor neuron involvement. Cervical spine disease is once again an important consideration, and this could be an urgent problem. In addition, however, this patient has dementia, indicating diffuse involvement of the cerebral hemispheres. It is possible that this is unrelated, as dementia and cervical spine disease are both relatively common in 65-year-old people, and some patients have both conditions just on the basis of chance. On the other hand, the triad of gait disturbance, dementia, and incontinence suggests the diagnosis of normal pressure hydrocephalus (see Chapter 7). One reasonable approach to evaluating this patient would be to obtain an imaging study of the head, and if it did not show prominent hydrocephalus, to proceed with an imaging study of the cervical spine.

Comment: In this case, a head CT scan confirmed markedly enlarged ventricles with only mild sulcal enlargement. The patient's gait and incontinence improved with shunting, and his dementia stopped progressing but did not resolve.

15

Back Pain and Neck Pain

I. Case Histories

Case 1. A 55-year-old woman with a history of heavy tobacco use and right lung resection for cancer 1 year ago has come to your office because yesterday, while lifting a heavy box, she suddenly developed a sharp pain that started in her low back and shot into her right buttock, posterior thigh, and posterior leg. On examination, you note a positive straight leg raising sign on the right, slight weakness of right ankle plantar flexion, and a reduced right ankle jerk.

Case 2. A 50-year-old hypertensive, diabetic man has come to the ER "to get some relief." Over the years, his back would "go out" on him now and then, but he would stay in bed for 1 day, apply heat, and wear a corset for the next 2 weeks and he would be "as good as new." Six weeks ago his back went out on him again, but it did not resolve as it had previously. If anything, it seems to be getting worse. It keeps him awake at night, and he is having trouble concentrating at work. He has no pain in his legs, and no difficulty with bladder or bowel function. His examination is notable only for obesity, tight muscles throughout the lower back, and mild tenderness in that region. He has no tenderness along the spine. His motor examination, reflexes, and sensory examination are all normal.

Questions:

1. What diagnoses should be considered?

2. What tests should be ordered?

3. What treatment should be prescribed?

II. Approach to Back or Neck Pain

There are two principal questions to address in evaluating a patient with back or neck pain:

A.   Does the patient have a condition that might require urgent treatment?

B.   Should the patient be managed surgically?

A. Emergency Situations

Urgent treatment may be required if a patient's back or neck pain is due to a process that threatens to produce rapidly progressive neurologic impairment. In practice, this means a rapidly expanding structural lesion that compresses multiple nerve roots or the spinal cord. The two groups of patients for whom this is a reasonable consideration are those with known cancer and those with progressive symptoms or signs suggestive of damage to the spinal cord or more than one nerve root.

Any patient with known cancer who develops back or neck pain should be assumed to have a spinal metastasis until proven otherwise. If plain x-rays of the symptomatic region of the spine suggest a metastasis or if the neurologic examination suggests damage to the spinal cord or roots, an MRI scan or myelogram of the symptomatic region of the spinal canal must be obtained. Only if both plain films and the neurologic examination are normal is it safe to treat the patient symptomatically without further testing. If a metastatic lesion is found, high-dose dexamethasone (Decadron) should be started immediately and arrangements made for starting radiation therapy. The role of surgery is still being evaluated.

Even if a patient has no *known* cancer, symptoms or signs suggesting rapidly progressive damage to the spinal cord or multiple nerve roots could be due to a metastasis. Acute disk herniation, spinal abscess, and hematoma are other considerations that could require urgent treatment. This situation warrants an immediate MRI scan or myelogram of the involved area of the spinal canal. If a soft tissue mass is compressing the spinal cord or multiple nerve roots in a patient with no known cancer, the patient will generally need a surgical procedure to decompress the lesion and to establish a diagnosis if it is not clear from the imaging characteristics. If imaging studies do not reveal a compressive lesion, the patient's pain should be treated in the same way as patients with musculoskeletal pain (see Part III of this chapter). At the same time, the patient should be evaluated for noncompressive causes of the neurologic abnormalities (e.g., multiple sclerosis or vitamin B_{12} deficiency in a patient with myelopathy).

B. Is Surgery Appropriate?

Even when patients do not require urgent decompression, their back or neck pain could still be caused by a structural lesion that might eventually require surgical intervention. The main indications for surgery are the following:

1. Spinal cord compression

2. Compression of one or more nerve roots causing persistent motor deficits or abnormal control of bladder or bowels

3. Lumbar spinal stenosis

4. A mass lesion of unknown etiology

Surgery is also performed on occasion when patients have pain that is refractory to all nonsurgical treatment, if the pain is in a distribution that clearly corresponds to the structural lesion.

Thus, patients who have symptoms or signs that suggest lumbar spinal stenosis or damage to the spinal cord or to one or more nerve roots should have an MRI scan (or myelogram) of the appropriate region of the spinal canal. The imaging study can be scheduled electively to be done within the next few weeks as long as the patient has no known cancer, no erosive bone lesions on plain films of the spine, and no clinical evidence of rapid progression.

III. Specific Conditions Causing Back or Neck Pain

A. Musculoskeletal Pain

In the vast majority of patients with back or neck pain, the pain is diffuse, with no specific signs or symptoms to suggest damage to any single nerve root. This is a very common problem, but it is not well understood. It is generally thought to be a musculoskeletal problem related to frequent excessive stress on the bones, muscles, and connective tissue elements that support the back. The pain generally improves over time. Treatment approaches include bed rest, physical therapy, heat, ultrasound, and analgesics. The evidence that any of these treatments can change the long-term course of the condition is actually quite weak, although most provide at least temporary relief. A common approach is to prescribe a nonsteroidal anti-inflammatory drug and to instruct the patient to remain at strict bed rest (getting up only for meals and bathroom) for at least 2 days. Some physicians recommend up to 2 or even 4 weeks of bed rest, but there are no data to support this approach. Patients should also be instructed in correct postures and should begin physical therapy if no improvement is observed. They may require trials of several medications or physical therapy regimens.

B. Disk Herniation

A small number of patients with back pain demonstrate a herniation of an intervertebral disk, exerting pressure on a nerve root. The classic history for a lumbosacral disk herniation is a sudden pain in the low back during heavy lifting, later radiating into one lower extremity in a band conforming to the distribution of the L5 or S1 nerve root. Pain in this distribution is often referred to as *sciatica*, but wide variations in the way this term is used can lead to confusion. The pain of a herniated disk is worst when sitting and is exacerbated by coughing, sneezing, or straining at bowel movements, but these classic features are not always present.

Many patients have no precipitating event, some patients have only lower extremity pain with no back pain, and others have the opposite.

A straight leg raising sign is usually present: patients experience extreme pain when the hip is passively flexed while holding the knee extended. This pain is exacerbated by dorsiflexion of the ankle and relieved by flexion of the knee. This sign is sensitive but not specific. Some patients with a herniated disk will have weakness in the distribution of the involved nerve root, and some may have a reduced tendon reflex. When the nerve root irritation is severe, abnormalities may be detected on EMG and nerve conduction studies.

Cervical disk herniation is analogous. When an antecedent injury occurs, it often involves rapid head turning. Pain or numbness extends from the neck into one arm. If the disk herniates centrally, pushing on the spinal cord, it may also affect function of the lower extremities, bladder, or bowels.

Disk herniation, like musculoskeletal pain, is incompletely understood. Although the symptoms suggest nerve root irritation, and imaging studies show impingement on the nerve root by the disk, many patients' symptoms resolve without resolution of the imaging abnormalities. Other patients with no history of any pain or neurologic symptoms have disk herniation as an incidental finding on imaging studies. It may be that the degree of inflammatory reaction around the nerve root is an important factor in determining whether a herniated disk produces symptoms.

The symptoms of disk herniation, like those of musculoskeletal pain, often resolve even without specific therapy. The same treatment modalities are used, with the same lack of clear evidence that they improve the already favorable natural course of the disease. Decompressive surgery is another option. Although the evidence is primarily retrospective, surgery appears to reduce pain in the short term. Little long-term benefit can be found, and therefore surgery is usually reserved for patients who have failed to respond to conservative treatments (especially bed rest, analgesics, and physical therapy), patients with substantial motor deficits (especially when they are progressive), or patients with involvement of bladder or bowels. Patients who do not fall into one of these categories should be treated in the same way as patients with musculoskeletal pain, and imaging studies may not even be necessary.

C. Spinal Stenosis

Over time, there may be growth of bony elements in the spinal canal, resulting in significant narrowing of the canal (especially when superimposed on a congenitally narrow canal). In the cervical spine, this produces the same symptoms as a disk herniation, and the management is analogous. In the lumbar canal, spinal stenosis often produces a syndrome known as *neurogenic claudication*—pain in the low back or legs provoked by standing and relieved by bending over or sitting down. Unlike vascular claudication, the pain is related to position and not to exertion (walking is no worse than standing, and riding a bike may produce no pain at all). This condition is less likely than disk herniation to respond to conservative measures and generally requires surgical decompression.

IV. Discussion of Case Histories

Case 1. This patient has characteristic features of an acute S1 radiculopathy and most likely has a disk herniation at L5-S1. Even so, with the history of recent cancer, you must be sure she does not have a metastatic lesion at this level. You should order an urgent MRI (or CT or myelogram) of the lumbosacral spine. If metastatic disease is present, start dexamethasone (Decadron) and arrange radiation therapy; if it is not, prescribe a nonsteroidal anti-inflammatory drug and 2 days of bed rest, followed by a gentle stretching program.

Case 2. This is an example of musculoskeletal pain. There is no radiation of the pain along a nerve root, and there are no focal findings on examination. The long history of similar problems makes it very unlikely that the patient has a new structural lesion, and there is no need for imaging studies. This kind of pain may be just as severe as the pain from a herniated disk or metastatic cancer. The patient has already discovered for himself several of the conservative measures that are often used to treat this problem. Because his symptoms persist, he should be given a prescription for a nonsteroidal anti-inflammatory drug and possibly a tricyclic antidepressant (which may be synergistic), while undergoing a physical therapy program designed to teach him gentle stretching exercises and educate him about correct posture. Ultimately, weight loss would help to relieve the mechanical stress on his spine and might prevent future exacerbations.

16

Incontinence

I. Case Histories

Case 1. A 55-year-old multiparous woman complains of "accidents" with her bladder whenever she sneezes or coughs. Otherwise, she is able to void normally and has no bowel or sexual dysfunction. She has no other complaints and has a normal neurologic examination.

Case 2. A 40-year-old man with limb-girdle muscular dystrophy has had episodes of bowel and bladder incontinence for the past several months. He has no difficulty sensing when he "needs to go." He has started using a bedside commode, and this has solved his problem with nocturnal incontinence, but he still has difficulty when he is away from his home. He has started scouting out the rest rooms anytime he goes to a new place, because he can avoid accidents as long as he can make it to the rest room quickly enough. He has also noticed progressive difficulty with walking over the past year. He has no sensory complaints. His sexual function has been normal. His examination is notable for profound proximal weakness of the legs and arms and a slow waddling gait. Perianal sensation and anal-wink reflex are normal. Muscle stretch reflexes are normal and plantar responses are flexor.

Case 3. A 60-year-old woman with chronic back pain due to degenerative lumbar spine disease has developed urinary incontinence characterized by frequent dribbling of small amounts of urine without any sensation of a need to void. She has also noted mild lower extremity weakness and an increase in her baseline lower extremity numbness. Examination is notable for weakness of ankle dorsiflexion, absent ankle jerks, and numbness on the lateral borders of the feet and in the perianal region. Rectal tone is decreased.

Questions:

1. Give a plausible explanation for incontinence in each of these cases.

2. Which of these is an urgent problem?

II. Background Information

The normal bladder unconsciously stores a large volume of urine at low pressure. Continence is maintained by contraction of muscle fibers in the bladder neck (*internal sphincter*) and urethra (*external sphincter*). A micturition reflex is triggered when a sufficient volume of urine collects in the bladder. Except at extremely high bladder volumes, a normal individual is able to inhibit this reflex until a socially convenient time. The reflex produces a coordinated event in which the urethra and sphincter open and the detrusor muscle in the bladder wall contracts, while the junctions between the ureters and the bladder are compressed to prevent reflux toward the kidney. The coordination between bladder and sphincter contraction is largely mediated by a micturition center in the pons.

The majority of detrusor motor innervation is cholinergic from the pelvic parasympathetic plexus, which derives from the S2–S4 nerve roots. Sympathetic adrenergic fibers originating at the T10–L2 levels provide the major motor innervation of the distal ureters, trigone, and bladder neck. Voluntary sphincter control is mediated by the pudendal nerve, which is derived from the S2–S4 nerve roots.

III. Evaluation of Incontinence

Incontinence is a particularly distressing symptom for patients and their families, and this would be reason enough to evaluate it promptly.

In addition, although incontinence is not an emergency in and of itself, it can indicate the presence of an underlying neurologic condition that must be addressed urgently. This chapter focuses on urinary incontinence, but the same principles apply when evaluating neurologic causes of fecal incontinence. Neurologic conditions more often produce urinary incontinence than fecal incontinence, and when both occur, urinary incontinence generally appears first.

Two questions must be addressed in evaluating a patient with urinary incontinence:

A. Is the problem related to nervous system control of bladder function?

B. If so, what level of the nervous system is involved?

A. Neurologic vs. Urologic Causes of Incontinence

The most common cause of incontinence is weakness of the mechanical structures supporting the urethral sphincters. This produces **stress incontinence,** characterized by leakage of small amounts of urine during any activity that results in increased intra-abdominal pressure, such as coughing or sneezing. In normal individuals, increased abdominal pressure is transmitted equally to the bladder and proximal urethra, so that the pressure across the sphincter remains constant. Stress incontinence occurs when there is relaxation of pelvic floor musculature and partial herniation of the proximal urethra through the pelvic floor, so that increases in abdominal pressure result in an increased pressure gradient across the sphincter. This problem is common in elderly women, especially those who have had several vaginal deliveries. It is unusual in men unless there has been damage to urinary sphincters during surgery. There are generally no associated abnormalities on neurologic examination. Treatment consists of pelvic floor exercises, pessaries (instruments placed in the vagina to support the uterus), and various surgical procedures designed to augment the mechanics of the external sphincter.

The term **functional incontinence** applies to any condition that results in difficulty reaching a toilet quickly in a patient whose bladder, its associated sphincters, and their nerve supply all function normally. The most trivial example is a patient in mechanical restraints. Limb pain or weakness may be less obvious but no less an obstacle to patient mobility. Confused patients may manifest functional incontinence simply because they can't find the bathroom. Making the diagnosis of functional incontinence can sometimes be tricky, especially when the condition limiting mobility is a neurologic problem that could also be affecting bladder function directly. The main question is whether the problem would persist even if the patient could get to the bathroom quickly. It sometimes suffices to ask this directly. If patients have trouble answering this question, they should be asked whether they can at least tell when the bladder is full and whether they can inhibit urination for a brief time. Functional incontinence is managed by maximizing mobility, providing adult diapers, and placing commodes in strategic locations in the home.

A damaged urinary sphincter may be inadequate to maintain a tight seal, resulting in leakage of urine from the bladder. This can be caused by neurologic injury or may be the result of prior surgery or trauma. The standard surgical procedures for stress incontinence are not helpful in this condition, but use of a pubovaginal sling is effective. In males, an artificial urinary sphincter can be inserted. Other non-neurologic causes of incontinence include medication side effects (e.g., diuretics and alpha-adrenergic antagonists), volume overload, diabetes mellitus, diabetes insipidus, urinary tract infection, and reduced bladder compliance.

B. Central vs. Peripheral Nervous System Causes of Incontinence

Lesions at any level of the nervous system can cause incontinence. The main localizing distinction is between a **spastic bladder** and a **flaccid bladder**. Patients with a spastic bladder experience **urge incontinence**—a sudden, uncontrollable urge to void, with complete emptying of the bladder contents. In patients with a flaccid bladder, the muscle in the bladder wall does not contract either voluntarily or reflexively; these patients tend to retain urine, and the bladder expands passively until its capacity has been surpassed, at which point urine may leak out in small volumes. This is called **overflow incontinence**. Unlike stress incontinence, this can occur even without any elevation of intra-abdominal pressure.

A spastic bladder indicates an upper motor neuron problem and can result from lesions in the brain or spinal cord. Associated symptoms and examination findings may permit a more precise localization. For example, limb hyperreflexia and a sensory level suggest myelopathy. The coexistence of dementia and gait disorder suggests normal pressure hydrocephalus (see Chapter 7). Other dementing illnesses may also result in incontinence because of disinhibition.

A flaccid bladder corresponds to a lower motor neuron lesion. It can result from any condition that disturbs the nerves that supply the bladder after they have exited the spinal cord. For example, overflow incontinence is the typical pattern that occurs in patients with diabetic polyneuropathy. Associated symptoms and signs again provide clues to the site of pathology; a patient with sacral numbness, leg weakness, and hyporeflexia, for example, may have a lesion of the cauda equina. Overflow incontinence can also occur in patients who have an upper motor neuron lesion that is below the level of the pontine micturition center. Such lesions produce not only a spastic bladder but also **detrusor-external sphincter dyssynergia,** in which the timing of bladder and sphincter contraction is poorly coordinated so that the bladder contracts against a closed sphincter. This condition often leads to ureteral reflux.

When historical information and examination findings are insufficient to discriminate between a flaccid bladder and a spastic bladder, useful information may be obtained from urodynamic studies, in which the bladder pressure is measured at different volumes. The point at which the subject feels an urge to void and the point at which the urge to void cannot be overcome are recorded, as is any residual volume in the bladder after voiding. This study is called a *cystometrogram.*

Neurogenic incontinence is treated by addressing the underlying neurologic problem to the extent possible. When there is a structural lesion affecting the spinal cord or the cauda equina, urgent decompressive surgery may be necessary. In addition, symptomatic improvement can often be achieved using anticholinergic medications or other drugs that inhibit bladder contraction or increase sphincter tone. Timed voiding may help prevent the bladder from filling to the point where reflex emptying occurs. In some patients, catheterization is necessary, especially when detrusor-external sphincter dyssynergia is present.

IV. Discussion of Case Histories

Case 1. This patient is describing typical stress incontinence. In the absence of other symptoms or examination abnormalities, no tests are indicated. This is not an urgent problem. Treatment is described in the text.

Case 2. This patient has functional incontinence that is the result of progressive inability to walk because of his progressive muscle disease. The diagnosis is based on the history; no tests are indicated. This is a serious but not urgent problem. Treatment of the incontinence is described in the text. Unfortunately, no treatment is available for his underlying muscular dystrophy.

Case 3. This patient's incontinence is an important clue to an urgent neurologic problem. The lower extremity weakness and decreased reflexes suggest a lower motor neuron problem, and this is consistent with the flaccid character of her urinary symptoms. The distribution of her weakness and sensory abnormalities (including abnormal sacral sensation) suggest involvement of several different nerve roots bilaterally, and the most likely lesion localization would be the cauda equina. The time course is difficult to determine. Her urinary symptoms are subacute, but she has had chronic back pain and lower extremity numbness. This suggests a chronic process that has recently accelerated. A chronic, focal lesion is most likely a tumor. This patient needs an imaging study urgently, and she may need emergency surgery for diagnosis and decompression.

Comment: An MRI scan of the lumbosacral spine showed a prominent disk herniation with compression of multiple sacral nerve roots. This is yet another example of how the rules of Chapter 3 are approximations, lumping many different "new growths" into the category of neoplasm. Even so, cancer was a realistic possibility, and use of the rules resulted in the appropriate diagnostic test with the correct level of urgency. This patient was taken for decompressive surgery immediately, because a delay could have resulted in permanent loss of bladder and bowel function.

IV

Bookends

17

Pediatric Neurology

I. Case Histories

The five questions below apply to all of the case histories that follow:

1. What additional historical information would be most useful?

2. Which parts of the neurologic examination would most likely provide helpful data?

3. What diagnoses should be considered?

4. How should the patient be evaluated?

5. How should the patient be managed?

Cases 1 and 2: Spells

Case 1. A 5-year-old boy was well until about 1 month ago, when he started having spells characterized by speech arrest and subtle, unilateral facial twitching. The episodes last 1–5 minutes. During the spells, he appears to understand what people say to him, and he sometimes says a few words. There have been at least 20 such episodes so far.

Case 2. An 8-year-old boy has been exhibiting unusual repetitive movements for the past 3 months. For the first 2 months, he repeatedly blinked his eyes and jerked his head. These symptoms resolved spontaneously, but they were followed 2 weeks later by intermittent episodes of repetitive hand clapping and throat clearing.

Cases 3 and 4: Ataxia

Case 3. Seven days after a 7-year-old girl developed chickenpox, her parents noted that she was very unsteady. She was able to sit up, but she was unable to walk. She was mentally alert, and when she was lying down she had normal strength in all four limbs.

Case 4. A 4-year-old boy has been experiencing occasional headaches for the past several months. He has also had some vague stomach problems and vomiting over the same period. For the past week, his gait has been increasingly unsteady, and he has fallen a few times.

Cases 5 and 6: Toe Walking

Case 5. A 3-year-old girl has always walked on her toes. Her parents were initially told that this would probably resolve, and they are concerned because it hasn't. The patient and her twin sister were born at gestational age 32 weeks. The patient has made regular developmental gains, but all motor milestones have been delayed relative to her twin.

Case 6. A 3-year-old boy has recently developed a tendency to walk on his toes. He was born at term, and his initial development was considered normal, although he lagged a little behind his twin sister in all aspects of development. He walked at age 18 months. He has always had trouble running or climbing stairs, but recently he has been stumbling and falling more frequently.

Cases 7, 8, and 9: School Problems

Case 7. A 9-year-old girl has been referred for unusual behavior and problems at school for the past 3 months. She had been an A student last year, but lately her school performance has been inconsistent. The girl's teacher has observed that she often appears to be daydreaming, and she sometimes fails to complete assignments. The family had noted similar behavior at home but had not considered it abnormal.

Case 8. A 9-year-old boy has just transferred to a new school, and an initial evaluation indicates that he is 18 months behind in his reading skills. He has previously been diagnosed as dyslexic and hyperactive, and he is being treated with methylphenidate (Ritalin). The boy's parents and pediatrician all think that his attention and behavior have improved markedly with this treatment. The boy's family is also concerned because he has not learned how to ride a bicycle, and he is awkward and uncoordinated.

Case 9. A 10-year-old boy is being evaluated for a decline in school performance over the past 6–9 months. He had always been an A student before but is now failing in all subjects. He is apathetic and insolent to his teacher, who says that he "seems like a different boy." His parents divorced about 1 year ago, and when the boy's difficulties were first noted they were attributed to psychosocial stress. He has had no headaches, seizures, or loss of motor skills.

II. Developmental Issues

Children are immature. This is hardly a revelation, yet it expresses a fundamental principle of human biology. Although the human brain has an enormous capacity for complex processing, most of its potential is unrealized at birth. In other species, a newborn is able to walk, swim, or fly almost immediately, with full adult function acquired within a few years at most. In humans, the process takes more than a decade (and, of course, "some kids never grow up"). This confers great flexibility, allowing children to develop functions that are directly adapted to their particular environment. In essence, the process results in "custom-made" brains, rather than assembly line products. The most obvious example is language. Children learn the languages they hear around them. They do not come with a "factory-installed" default language, and none of us learn foreign languages effortlessly. At first glance, this might appear to be a disadvantage. A single human language spoken and understood across the globe by individuals of all ages would be preferable in many ways. But how would the "standard" vocabulary be determined? Would it include words like *daguerreotype, pneumoencephalogram,* and *slide rule*? What about *cell phone* and *website*? Would every child be born knowing the words *tuatara, mortmain,* and *khamsin*? Or *forsooth, groovy, Pokemon,* and *shagadelic*? Different cultures, different regions, and above all, different eras have vastly different vocabulary needs, and the rate at which evolution proceeds is far too slow to accommodate them. Instead, heredity provides a general program for linguistic processing, but environmental exposure determines the specific language elements that an individual acquires. The same principle of developmental plasticity applies to most aspects of perception, motor function, and cognition.

Developmental plasticity is the main feature distinguishing pediatric neurology from adult neurology. The diagnostic principles presented in the first three chapters of this book still apply, but many of the nervous system functions typically assessed in adults are not fully operational until months or years after birth. Obvious examples are walking, talking, and control of bladder and bowel function. Incontinence in an adult patient is clearly abnormal and suggests a set of specific lesion sites (see Chapter 16). Incontinence in a pediatric patient may be significant or not, depending on the patient's age. The same is true of the inability to walk or talk. Conversely, some reflexes normally present in infancy disappear as children age. In short, a child's developmental stage determines not only how the examination is interpreted but how it is performed.

The effects of disease also vary depending on an individual's developmental stage. The developing nervous system is extremely vulnerable to some injuries that have little effect on the mature nervous system, whereas developmental plasticity permits more complete recovery from some injuries in children than in adults.

This chapter is not meant to be a comprehensive survey of the vast array of diseases that affect the developing nervous system. Rather, the goal is to present a general approach to some of the more common clinical situations that occur primarily in the pediatric population.

III. Hypotonic Infants

Newborn infants have very limited behavioral repertoires. The most common manifestation of neurologic disease at this age is abnormal motor activity. In particular, parents report a "floppy baby," and physicians observe hypotonia. There are several ways to assess an infant's tone. One way is to pull the baby by the hands from a supine to a seated position. A normal, full-term baby will flex the neck to lift the head from the surface along with the body. When a normal infant is suspended so that the baby's abdomen lies on the examiner's outstretched hand, the infant's back straightens, the limbs flex, and the head is held straight or extended. A hypotonic infant held in this way is limp, with head and limbs drooping down over the examiner's hand. A normal infant can be held vertically by supporting the axillae, whereas a hypotonic infant tends to "slip through" the examiner's hands. The assessment of tone requires a fair amount of experience with the expected range of variation among normal infants.

Hypotonia can result from a lesion anywhere in the motor pathway represented in Figures 1-1 and 1-6. The first step in diagnosis is to distinguish between central and peripheral lesions. Infants with peripheral hypotonia (due to lesions at the level of anterior horn cell, nerve root, peripheral nerve, neuromuscular junction, or muscle) typically have severe weakness, with reduced or absent tendon reflexes. When hypotonia is due to lesions at the level of the spinal cord or higher, the hypotonia is usually more profound than the weakness, and tendon reflexes are normal or brisk. When the lesion is in the cerebral hemispheres, there are often additional manifestations of cerebral malfunction (such as seizures or reduced alertness).

Central hypotonia may be idiopathic, or it may result from intrauterine or perinatal hypoxic-ischemic events, chromosomal abnormalities (such as Down syndrome, Prader-Willi syndrome, or Turner's syndrome), congenital malformations, infections, and a variety of metabolic derangements including hypoglycemia, hyperbilirubinemia, hypothyroidism, leukodystrophy, and drug intoxication. Many of these conditions can be evaluated by obtaining an imaging study of the brain, checking serum electrolytes and glucose, and taking a careful history of intrauterine and postnatal drug exposure.

Some of the peripheral causes of hypotonia are hereditary (especially myotonic dystrophy, some metabolic myopathies, and some neuropathies), so the diagnosis can sometimes be made by taking a careful family history or examining family members. Approximately 15% of infants born to mothers with myasthenia gravis have hypotonia and weakness. These symptoms are thought to be caused by passive transfer of maternal antibodies, and they resolve within 3 months. Spinal muscular atrophies (SMAs) are hereditary forms of lower motor neuron disease. Type 1 SMA is an acute, fulminating form that begins at birth or within the first 6 months. Mothers often report marked reduction or disappearance of fetal movements during the final months of pregnancy. Type 2 SMA usually becomes symptomatic between the ages of 6 and 24 months, and the course is milder and more slowly progressive. Type 1 and type 2 SMA are both associated with a defect on chromosome 5. Infantile botulism is caused by ingestion of the bacterium itself, not the toxin. The source may be the environment or food, most often honey. Other historical information may provide clues to other metabolic or toxic conditions, and nerve conduction studies, EMG, and muscle biopsy may help clarify the diagnosis.

IV. Developmental Delay and Developmental Regression

The process of development varies considerably from one child to the next, but it proceeds in the same general sequence and in a similar time frame in all children. When children reach developmental milestones at a slow rate that is clearly outside the normal range, it is called *developmental delay*. This definition requires comparison to expectations for "normal" children. Because the range of normal is so broad, children should not be labeled developmentally delayed until it is clear that they lie outside this range.

When children who develop at a normal rate begin to lose some of the skills they have already acquired, it is called *developmental regression*. This diagnosis can be assigned even without reference to "normal" ranges, because it is based purely on a child's own previous development. Caution must be exercised in diagnosing developmental regression, because even normal children intermittently regress slightly.

An isolated insult to the nervous system, such as an infection or head trauma, can result in developmental delay. Although the event itself may be transient, the damage it produces may severely limit or even abolish the nervous system's capacity to develop further. On the other hand, regression usually implies an ongoing disease process. Although a one-time event may retard or halt forward progress, it does not usually result in backward movement.

The differential diagnosis for developmental delay depends on the pattern of impairment. When the delay primarily affects **motor** skills, the differential diagnosis is essentially the same as for hypotonic infants (see Part III). Hearing impairment is the most common cause of an isolated delay in **language** development. When language delay is accompanied by abnormal social development, autism is a consideration (but hearing should still be tested). Dyslexia is an important consideration in older children who have difficulty with reading and writing despite normal initial language development. Uncontrolled generalized seizures may also result in learning problems, or even in intellectual deterioration (though it is often difficult to determine how much of the deterioration is due to the seizures themselves and how much is a result of the disease process that underlies the seizures). Attention deficit disorder is a potential cause of delayed learning. It has received a great deal of publicity in recent years, to the point where the most common treatment, methylphenidate (Ritalin), has been inappropriately prescribed for many children who do not meet specific diagnostic criteria. Psychological factors can also impede school performance; a useful clue is that the child's problems are often restricted to particular activities, with relative sparing of language skills, self-care ability, and performance in recreational activities. **Global** developmental delay is most often a result of an infectious, toxic, or hypoxic-ischemic injury that occurred in utero or perinatally. Less often, global developmental delay may result from the same kinds of ongoing disease processes that typically produce developmental regression.

A vast array of disease processes can cause intellectual and motor regression. These include infections, tumors, toxic exposure, vascular conditions, congenital malformations, metabolic conditions, and endocrine disorders. Many of these conditions involve components of the nervous system and other organ systems in specific patterns that provide clues to the diagnosis. The family history is helpful in diagnosing the many metabolic conditions and malformations that are genetic. The age of onset is also helpful in narrowing the diagnosis. More detailed algorithms and tables are available in standard textbooks of pediatric neurology.

V. Paroxysmal Symptoms

As noted in Chapter 3, the most common causes of paroxysmal focal neurologic symptoms in adults are transient ischemic attacks, seizures, and migraines. Atherosclerosis is a disease of adults, and although other cerebrovascular diseases may occur in children, they are not usually associated with transient ischemic attacks. Seizures and migraines are therefore the most important causes of sudden and recurrent focal neurologic symptoms in children. Other paroxysmal conditions that can occur in childhood include breath-holding spells, night terrors, narcolepsy/cataplexy, tics, syncope, psychogenic spells, and benign paroxysmal vertigo. Most of these conditions are discussed in previous chapters. Some features of *childhood* headaches, seizures, breath-holding spells, and benign paroxysmal vertigo are discussed below.

A. Headaches

Headaches are common in childhood, causing 10–12% of children to consult a physician. The same principles of evaluation and treatment that apply to adults (see Chapter 12) also hold for children. In children, of course, there is a lower likelihood that the patient will report a long history of similar symptoms over many years, so diagnostic tests are more often necessary to exclude structural disease. The abortive and prophylactic medications that are prescribed to adults are also effective in children, but the specific drugs used may differ because of different concerns about side effects. **Cyclical vomiting** (characterized by recurrent episodes of nausea and vomiting) and **periodic abdominal pain** are two variants of migraine that arise almost exclusively in childhood. These two syndromes frequently overlap. There is often no accompanying headache, but approximately 75% of these children develop typical migraine later in life, and the cyclical vomiting responds to typical migraine medications. Much less commonly, similar symptoms may be associated with EEG changes and represent epileptic spells.

B. Seizures

Seizures in children are classified, evaluated, and managed according to the same principles that apply in adults (see Chapter 5). It is sometimes more difficult to recognize seizures in children than in adults, however. In neonates especially, the immaturity of the nervous system interferes with propagation of epileptic discharges, so classic tonic-clonic convulsions are rare. More common are brief episodes of hypertonia, atonia, or localized clonic movements. Neonatal seizures may also manifest with rhythmic or sustained eye movements, chewing, or unusual limb movements. Another unique feature of pediatric epilepsy is that certain seizure types arise only at particular ages. **Infantile**

spasms are characterized by sudden muscular contractions that produce head flexion, arm extension, and drawing up of the legs. They may occur singly or in series, and they are sometimes associated with giggling or a piercing cry. Onset is usually between the ages of 3 and 8 months; the first episode occurs during the first year of life in 75% of patients and before 2 years of age in 92%. **Absence seizures** were discussed in Chapter 5; they almost always begin in childhood, with 64% of cases arising between the ages of 5 and 9 years. **Rolandic epilepsy** is a partial seizure disorder with a strong genetic predisposition that presents between the ages of 18 months and 13 years, usually between the ages of 5 and 10 years. The seizures often begin with a sensory aura in the region of the mouth, followed by speech arrest, salivation, and tonic or tonic-clonic movements of the face. In some cases there is secondary generalization, and seizures may be prolonged. The attacks are most common during sleep. They can usually be controlled with antiepileptic medications, and they are typically outgrown by puberty.

The same underlying processes that produce seizures in adults can cause seizures in children. Congenital brain defects and antenatal or perinatal injuries (especially hypoxic-ischemic and infectious) are common causes. Febrile seizures represent a separate category. These seizures occur in the setting of fever in patients who do not have any infection of the nervous system or other known cause. They usually present between the ages of 3 months and 3 years. Approximately 30–40% of children who have a febrile seizure will have another one with a subsequent febrile illness, but only 2–4% of children with febrile seizures subsequently develop epilepsy. The risk of developing epilepsy is increased in patients with a pre-existing neurologic or developmental abnormality, a family history of epilepsy, or complex febrile seizures (defined as prolonged, focal, or multiple). Most children with febrile seizures do not require antiepileptic drugs. Children with frequent and prolonged febrile seizures can be provided with diazepam to be administered rectally at the start of a seizure, or they can take diazepam orally every 8 hours during a febrile illness. Medication is sometimes prescribed for febrile seizures in children who have an abnormal neurologic examination or developmental delay. Some clinicians also start antiepileptic drugs when the initial febrile seizure is complex and there is a family history of epilepsy.

C. Breath-Holding Spells

Small children commonly hold their breath when crying, typically when fright, anger, or frustration precipitated the crying. When prolonged, breath-holding spells may result in seizures. The first attacks usually occur between the ages of 6 and 18 months, become less frequent with advancing age, and disappear by the age of 5 or 6 years. The family should be educated and reassured. No other treatment is necessary.

D. Benign Paroxysmal Vertigo

Benign paroxysmal vertigo is characterized by recurrent episodes of vertigo, vomiting, pallor, nystagmus, and diffuse pallor. The attacks usually last a few minutes, but sometimes last several hours. Children may fall during the attack, but they do not lose consciousness. Onset is usually between the ages of 1 and 4 years. The episodes eventually become less frequent and either disappear or are replaced by symptoms that are characteristic of migraine.

VI. Gait Disturbance

In both children and adults, abnormal gait can be a result of either focal lesions or diffuse processes. When the history and examination implicate a focal lesion, evaluation and treatment proceed in the same manner in children as in adults. When the symptoms are symmetric, the three most likely problems in all age groups are spasticity, weakness, and ataxia. The diagnostic considerations for each of these problems differ in children and adults, however.

A. Spasticity

Gait disturbances in children are commonly associated with developmental delay. This, in turn, is often related to intrauterine or perinatal damage, especially from hypoxic-ischemic events and infections. Infants with these problems are usually hypotonic, but as they mature they develop spasticity, especially in the legs. The main evidence for early brain injury comes from historical information about intrauterine or perinatal complications and delayed motor or intellectual milestones, and from the examination finding of lower extremity spasticity. Structural lesions in the spinal cord or metabolic diseases (such as leukodystrophies) can also produce lower extremity spasticity, but the symptoms are usually progressive, resulting in loss of previously acquired function.

B. Weakness

The most important consideration in evaluating a diffusely weak child is whether the weakness is central or peripheral. Associated hyperreflexia and spasticity suggest a central process. As discussed in the previous paragraph, intrauterine or perinatal damage commonly result in spasticity that remains static over time, and spinal cord damage or metabolic disease typically cause progressive spasticity. Hypotonia, hyporeflexia, and muscle atrophy suggest disease at the level of the anterior horn cell, nerve root, peripheral nerve, neuromuscular junction, or muscle. The evaluation of neuromuscular disease is discussed in Chapter 6. The same principles apply in children and adults, but the particular diseases differ in the two groups. Muscular dystrophies and hereditary neuropathies are more likely to be important diagnostic considerations in children than in adults, for example, whereas conditions like inclusion body myositis or diabetic neuropathy are common in adults but not in children.

C. Ataxia

In children, acute ataxia most commonly occurs in the setting of an infection or nonspecific febrile illness. A wide variety of organisms have been implicated, with varicella virus the most common. The condition may occur at any age, but it is most common between the ages of 1 and 5 years. It is characterized by the sudden onset of truncal ataxia resulting in rapid deterioration of gait. Nystagmus is present in approximately one-half of the patients, and there may be prominent tremors of limbs, head, or trunk. The symptoms resolve completely in most children, usually within several months, but some children have permanent residua.

Another cause of acute ataxia is toxic exposure, primarily to antiepileptic drugs, alcohol, antihistamines, heavy metals, and mercury. There is also a paraneoplastic syndrome, consisting of **ataxia, myoclonus**, and **opsoclonus** (irregular, multidirectional involuntary eye movements), associated with occult neuroblastoma. The same syndrome may occur for no apparent reason in some patients. Intermittent episodes of acute ataxia may occur with some metabolic diseases, such as disorders of amino acid metabolism and ion channel diseases. Posterior fossa tumors can also cause acute ataxia, but they are much more likely to produce gradually progressive, chronic symptoms. Other causes of chronically progressive ataxia include Friedreich's ataxia (see Chapter 8) and **ataxia telangiectasia,** a disorder of DNA repair that is caused by a mutation on chromosome 11 and inherited in an autosomal recessive pattern, characterized by progressive ataxia that usually begins during the first few years of life. Patients subsequently develop telangiectasias (dilated, tortuous capillaries and very small arteries), characteristically located in the conjunctiva, ear, bridge of nose, and antecubital fossa, and they experience frequent sinus and pulmonary infections because of various immunologic abnormalities, particularly involving immunoglobulin A and immunoglobulin E. Patients with ataxia telangiectasia are exquisitely sensitive to radiation, and they are very prone to systemic malignancy. A number of other metabolic conditions can also cause progressive ataxia.

VII. Discussion of Case Histories

Case 1. This boy has paroxysmal symptoms. They sound most like seizures; they could conceivably be tics, but tics usually occur more randomly, rather than in discrete episodes lasting up to 5 minutes. Migraine is unlikely, as the symptoms are not typical of migraine and he has no associated headache. None of the symptoms suggest any of the other paroxysmal conditions of childhood. Given the focal nature of the symptoms and the apparent preservation of consciousness, these would be classified as simple partial seizures. In particular, they are suggestive of rolandic seizures.

The history and examination should be directed at confirming this diagnostic impression and excluding any other type of seizures that might signal the need for more extensive evaluation. Thus, questions about family history are important. The patient and family should be asked about any symptoms that might suggest other kinds of seizures and about any progressive neurologic deficits. Any focal abnormality on examination should prompt further evaluation, because children with rolandic epilepsy typically have normal neurologic examinations. In the absence of any historical or examination evidence of progression, focality, or multiple seizure types, the diagnosis of rolandic epilepsy can be confirmed by finding characteristic abnormalities on EEG (epileptiform activity in the region of the Sylvian fissure). This condition ultimately resolves, so lifelong treatment is not necessary. Antiepileptic drugs may be used to reduce the frequency of seizures in the interim.

Case 2. This patient also has paroxysmal symptoms. They could conceivably be seizures, but the change in clinical characteristics after 2 months would be atypical. This would be more suggestive of a tic disorder. None of the other paroxysmal conditions of childhood are considerations in this case.

Further historical information that would be useful could be obtained by asking whether there is any impairment of awareness associated with the spells (which would favor seizures) and whether the boy can voluntarily suppress the movements, at least temporarily (which would favor tics). The boy's parents should be asked whether he has exhibited any other potential vocal tics in addition to his repetitive clearing of the throat. The patient and family should also be questioned about exposure to stimulants such as methylphenidate (Ritalin) and about weight loss, exercise tolerance, and behavioral changes to evaluate the possibility of hyperthyroidism, which can precipitate tics. A family history of similar involuntary movements, attention deficit disorder, or obsessive compulsive disorder would be consistent with Tourette's syndrome. On examination, direct observation of the involuntary movements would be particularly helpful. Unfortunately, since children can often suppress the movements transiently, they may disappear in the doctor's office even when they are reported to be very frequent at home or at school. Even so, close observation sometimes reveals subtle involuntary movements that the family had never even noticed.

If the information gathered from the history and examination confirms that the movements are most likely tics, no further diagnostic testing is necessary. Symptoms often resolve spontaneously, so treatment is usually reserved for symptoms that have persisted beyond 12 months and are significantly disruptive to the child. Pimozide, haloperidol, and clonidine are helpful for treating tic disorders.

Case 3. This history is very suggestive of postinfectious ataxia, especially since varicella is the infectious agent most commonly associated with this disorder. If the history and examination confirm that the patient has ataxia rather than weaknes and if there are no other deficits, no evidence of pre-existing neurologic dysfunction, and no other potential causes of ataxia (especially toxic exposure), then additional tests may be unnecessary. It is sometimes appropriate to obtain an MRI scan of the brain (looking for hydrocephalus or a mass lesion in the posterior fossa) and a lumbar puncture (to exclude ongoing infection). If these tests are normal (or at most show a mild lymphocytic pleocytosis in the cerebrospinal fluid), only supportive therapy is required.

Case 4. This patient is also ataxic, but the several month history of associated symptoms suggests a more chronic condition. If his ataxia were intermittent, migraine would be a consideration, but this boy's gait has been growing progressively worse over the past week. The headaches and vomiting suggest increased intracranial pressure, making a posterior fossa mass lesion or hydrocephalus the two leading considerations. The history and examination should focus on any focal abnormalities that might help localize a mass lesion. In addition, increased intracranial pressure often causes papilledema, and the examiner should look carefully for eye movement abnormalities that can result from pressure on cranial nerves III, IV, or VI. In younger children, it would also be important to measure head circumference, because subacute decompensation of long-standing hydrocephalus may produce increased intracranial pressure.

If the examination confirms elevated intracranial pressure, an imaging study should be obtained urgently, because even children who look healthy may deteriorate rapidly. Either a CT scan or an MRI scan would be adequate to diagnose hydrocephalus, but an MRI scan is the optimal imaging technique in this setting because it provides much better resolution in the posterior fossa. Immediate neurosurgical evaluation is indicated if either hydrocephalus or a mass lesion is found. Temporizing treatment of increased intracranial pressure with dexamethasone, mannitol, or hyperventilation may also be necessary (see Chapter 11).

Case 5. This history suggests developmental delay rather than regression. Additional historical information about intellectual and motor milestones should be elicited to confirm or refute this impression. In a patient with gait disturbance due to developmental delay, the examination usually reveals roughly symmetric lower extremity spasticity and hyperreflexia. If these examination findings are present in this patient, with a clear history of prematurity, consistent delays in motor development, and no regression, no additional diagnostic tests are necessary. Periventricular white matter injury is typically seen when a brain MRI scan is obtained. The cornerstone of management is physical therapy. Additional interventions for spasticity, such as tendon release procedures or botulinum toxin injections, are sometimes necessary.

Case 6. Although this patient also had delayed motor development, the history also indicates motor regression, suggesting an ongoing disease process. The main goal in the history and examination is to determine whether the prominent abnormality is ataxia, weakness, or spasticity. If there were no history of regression, and the patient had a normal neurologic examination and serum creatine kinase (CK) level (making muscular dystrophy unlikely), it would be reasonable simply to observe the child over time, because some children who toe walk have no specific neurologic deficits, but the history of recent deterioration requires prompt evaluation.

Comment: In this case, the examination was notable for prominent calf muscles and proximal weakness in all four limbs. He exhibited Gower's sign: He marched up his legs with his hands in order to stand up from the floor. These findings suggest a primary muscle disorder, and in particular, the prominent calf muscles are typical of muscular dystrophy. Elevated CK and genetic testing confirmed the diagnosis of Duchenne's muscular dystrophy. The patient was referred to a muscular dystrophy clinic, where he was enrolled in an ongoing physical therapy program and started on prednisone.

Case 7. Although the prominent feature of this case is intellectual regression, there is also a suggestion of paroxysmal symptoms. Frequent daydreaming had been observed both in school and at home. This is often the only symptom reported for children with absence seizures, and physicians must be alert to this possibility. Complex partial seizures may also manifest as daydreaming spells. Absence or partial complex seizures may go unrecognized until they lead to problems at school. Further historical information about the daydreaming spells would be helpful: Can the patient respond during the spells? Are there any associated eye or face movements? Does she have any unusual feelings before, during, or after the spells? The examiner should search for focal neurologic abnormalities, which would support the diagnosis of complex partial seizures. The child should be instructed to hyperventilate for at least 2 minutes while the examiner watches her for absence seizures.

Comment: This girl's neurologic examination was normal, and hyperventilation provoked a typical absence attack. Her EEG showed the classic finding of 3-Hz spike-and-wave activity, and ethosuximide was started. Her daydreaming spells and school problems resolved promptly.

Case 8. In contrast to the previous case, nothing suggests that this boy has a paroxysmal condition. There has been no regression noted, and if further questioning reveals no evidence of a seizure disorder or developmental deterioration, the clear response to methylphenidate would suggest that the diagnosis of attention deficit-hyperactivity disorder is correct. A family history of this condition would also support the diagnosis. The main goal of the examination is to exclude a structural lesion. It would not be unusual if this patient's examination revealed some "soft neurologic signs"—subtle abnormalities that do not clearly correlate with discrete, focal lesions, and that might be considered normal in a younger child. These are present in many patients with attention deficit disorder and other learning disorders, and they have uncertain significance.

If the history shows no evidence of a paroxysmal or progressive disorder and the examination reveals no significant focal abnormalities, then no diagnostic studies are indicated. The methylphenidate treatment should continue.

Case 9. Like the girl in Case 7, this boy has experienced intellectual regression, but in this case, nothing suggests paroxysmal symptoms, so the likelihood of progressive neurologic disease is greater. On the other hand, the problems began at a time of significant psychologic stress, and it was reasonable for his teachers and physicians to wonder about a connection. Historical information should be elicited regarding his behavior outside of school. If he continues to perform well at extracurricular activities he enjoys and still gets along with his friends, an underlying neurologic disease is unlikely. Historical evidence for a focal lesion (such as language disturbance or hemiparesis) and focal examination deficits should also be sought. A family history of neurologic disease would help considerably in narrowing the differential diagnosis.

If the above considerations fail to reveal a specific diagnosis, an MRI scan of the brain should be done, looking for either a focal abnormality or a diffuse process such as leukodystrophy or hydrocephalus. Depending on the age of onset, time course, family history, associated physical examination findings, and MRI findings, more specific tests for particular metabolic, chromosomal, infectious, and neoplastic diseases may be indicated.

Comment: This boy's behavior problems extended to the playground, where he had been getting in more and more fights. Even though he had not lost any motor skills, his examination revealed lower extremity spasticity. This prompted an MRI scan of the brain, which showed symmetric abnormalities in the cortical periventricular white matter bilaterally. This suggested the diagnosis of adrenoleukodystrophy. The diagnosis was confirmed by measuring very long chain fatty acids in serum. This boy was treated with an experimental diet.

18

Geriatric Neurology

I. Case Histories

Case 1. An 82-year-old man who was diagnosed with Alzheimer's disease a year ago has had four episodes of urinary incontinence in the past 3 weeks. His family members understand that people with Alzheimer's disease are often incontinent, and they want advice on how they should deal with the problem. The patient is unable to describe the episodes of incontinence in any detail. He cannot remember whether he felt any urge to void before any of the episodes, and he is embarrassed to talk about them at all. Despite his dementia, he still converses normally, has no difficulty showering or dressing, does simple chores like dishwashing and yard work, and plays golf twice a week.

His general physical examination is unremarkable. He is alert, attentive, and jovial. His speech is fluent, but he has some word-finding problems. He can follow one-step and two-step commands but typically makes slight errors when given three-step commands. He has a normal digit span. He can only remember one of three items after 5 minutes, even with prompting. He cannot name the current president and cannot remember the ages or birth order of his children. He has eight grandchildren but cannot name any of them. He is able to perform one-digit addition and subtraction but no calculations more complicated than that.

His cranial nerve examination is normal. He walks stiffly, with no obvious asymmetry. He has marked spasticity in both lower extremities, but his strength is normal throughout all four limbs, and individual limb coordination is intact. He has diminished biceps and brachioradialis reflexes, but triceps reflexes are brisk bilaterally, and he has unsustained clonus at the knees and ankles, with bilateral Babinski signs. His mental status makes a detailed sensory examination difficult, but he seems to react much more strongly to pinprick in the upper extremities, neck, and face than in the trunk and lower extremities.

Questions:

1. Is this patient's incontinence likely to be due to Alzheimer's disease?

2. Are any other investigations necessary?

3. What interventions are indicated?

Case 2. A 78-year-old woman complains to her family physician that she has chronic pain in her elbows, hips, and knees, and it is worse at the end of the day. The woman's history, examination, and x-rays are all consistent with degenerative joint disease, but she is noted to have absent ankle jerks and markedly diminished vibration sense in her toes.

Questions:

1. Is this woman's pain likely to be caused by peripheral polyneuropathy?

2. What additional diagnostic tests are necessary?

Case 3. A 70-year-old man complains of unsteady gait since an open reduction and internal fixation procedure for a hip fracture 2 months ago. He received physical therapy after discharge, and it helped, but he continues to feel like "any puff of air would blow me over." He has fallen on two occasions when he got up in the middle of the night. He is afraid that he may sustain another fracture if he falls again.

His past history is notable for non–insulin-dependent diabetes. His general physical examination is normal. He has normal mental status, although he is clearly anxious. His cranial nerves are notable only for decreased visual acuity and reduced hearing bilaterally. He notes that he was scheduled for cataract surgery, but it was canceled because he fractured his hip 4 days before the operation date. His wife has been urging him to get his hearing checked, but he has been too busy. His gait is tentative, and he limps favoring the side of the surgery, but he needs no support and has no tendency to sway to either side. He has normal coordination and strength throughout all four limbs. His upper extremity reflexes are normal, his knee jerks are brisk, and ankle jerks cannot be elicited. His plantar responses are flexor. Vibration sense is absent at the toes, moderately reduced at the ankles, and mildly reduced at the knees. Position sense is reduced at the toes, but normal elsewhere. He can distinguish sharp from dull throughout his body but says a pin is less sharp in his feet and lower calves than it is elsewhere.

Questions:

1. What might be responsible for this patient's gait disturbance?

2. What diagnostic tests should be done?

3. What interventions are necessary?

II. Geriatric Issues

Three principles distinguish the neurologic assessment of older patients. First, and most important, people accumulate more diseases the longer they live. Second, some diseases occur primarily in the elderly. Third, even in the absence of any apparent disease, some components of the aging nervous system gradually deteriorate.

As a consequence, older patients often have complicated complaints involving numerous symptoms referable to more than one organ system. The standard approach of trying to localize all symptoms to a single lesion is untenable in many cases. Instead, the question is whether the patient has a degenerative disease affecting sites distributed diffusely throughout the nervous system or a combination of unrelated diseases. The neurologic examination provides useful information for answering this question, but accurate interpretation of the examination requires knowledge of the changes that occur during normal aging.

III. The Neurologic Examination in Normal Aging

It is harder than it might seem to characterize the changes that normally occur with aging. Because there is a wide range of variation even among normal subjects, a population study is required. The simplest kind of population study to conduct is a cross-sectional study, in which specific features are systematically observed in a random group of people of a certain age and then compared to the same features in a separate group of people of a different age. Cross-sectional studies can be misleading, however, because it is difficult to ensure that the groups being compared differ only in age and are identical in all other respects. For example, the elderly group might have a higher proportion of subjects with mild hypertension, cervical stenosis, or subclinical strokes than the younger group. An intended comparison of two "normal" groups then becomes a comparison of two groups with different (and often unrecognized) disease profiles.

Longitudinal studies are more reliable in this regard, but they are much more difficult to conduct: a single group of randomly selected normal people of a certain age is observed serially over many years. Even with this kind of study it is impossible to control for the fact that a given individual might develop a disease during the period of observation, converting from "normal" to "abnormal." This would result in overestimation of the changes that occur with normal aging. Alternatively, the changes could be underestimated if individuals with changes proved to be more difficult to follow over time. For example, suppose that even in the absence of any disease, 50% of normal individuals become so absentminded as they age that they are unable to keep their appointments, whereas memory function remains completely normal in the other one-half of the population. A study based only on the people who were able to return for regularly scheduled memory testing would conclude that no memory problems occur in normal aging.

Additional complications arise in trying to interpret any abnormalities that are observed in the elderly. It is often difficult to unravel the role played by intrinsic processes in the nervous system and the contribution of other, non-neurologic factors. For example, changes in gait can be related to fractures, sprains, and vascular disease as well as neurologic problems. Moreover, even within the nervous system there is interaction between different components. Gait changes may relate to abnormalities of sensation, strength, or coordination. Apparent changes in mental status may simply be due to primary sensory problems, especially hearing loss. Elderly people may seem to forget things just because they never heard them in the first place, and this can also cause them to ask the same question repeatedly. Speed of response is often important in interpreting the mental status examination, and this can be influenced by motor system problems. An extreme example is parkinsonism, which sometimes causes patients to respond so slowly that examiners assume they don't know the answer and move on to another item.

Despite these limitations, some age-related changes in the "normal" neurologic examination have been consistently identified. All of these changes are of relatively low magnitude—that is, the variability *between* individuals of a given age is much greater than the change that occurs in any individual with aging. Even so, an awareness of these age-related changes is important when interpreting the neurologic examination in elderly patients.

A. *Mental Status*

The interpretation of age-related changes in the mental status examination is confounded by the deterioration that occurs in other processes (such as hearing loss and motor slowing), as discussed in the preceding paragraphs. Nonetheless, careful testing strategies that minimize these confounding factors permit the following general observations. First, older patients have difficulty thinking of words but relative sparing of vocabulary (i.e., they are still able to recognize and define words). Second, a generalized slowing of central processing occurs with aging. Third, impairment of recent memory and learning is evident with relative sparing of remote memory. Note that the boundary between normal aging and isolated memory impairment (see Chapter 7) is not sharply defined.

B. *Cranial Nerves*

The most common age-related changes noted in the cranial nerve examination relate to changes in sensory end-organs rather than intrinsic nervous system deterioration. The lens grows less clear and less elastic, the pupil becomes smaller and less elastic, rods and cones decrease in number, and the receptive fields of retinal ganglion cells change. As a result, older subjects have decreased light perception, reduced light/dark adaptation, impaired near vision (*presbyopia*), and changes in contrast sensitivity and color vision. Similarly, pure tone hearing declines with aging (*presbyacusis*), especially for high-frequency tones, and speech discrimination is diminished. Taste and smell discrimination often deteriorates slightly with aging also.

The only other clinically important change in the cranial nerve examination with aging is impairment of upward gaze. This is a supranuclear problem, so reflex maneuvers elicit full upward excursion even though the subject cannot achieve this voluntarily.

C. Motor System

The single greatest change in station and gait that occurs with aging is a reduced ability to stand on one leg with the eyes closed. Older subjects have increased postural sway and reduced postural reflexes. They walk with a widened base, a stooped posture, shortened steps, and reduced arm swing. In short, they resemble patients with mild Parkinson's disease.

Older subjects are less coordinated when manipulating small objects. They are mildly uncoordinated without frank dysmetria when performing finger-to-nose and heel-to-shin testing. Their movements are slowed compared to younger subjects. Postural and kinetic tremors are increasingly common with advancing age.

Muscle bulk declines with age, especially in the intrinsic muscles of the hands and feet. Power is also reduced. The EMG reveals changes consistent with partial denervation and reinnervation. Paratonia is common in the elderly.

D. Reflexes

Deep tendon reflexes become less brisk as people age, with a distal-to-proximal gradient, although at least 80% of truly normal elderly subjects still have detectable ankle jerks. Babinski signs are rare in normal subjects, regardless of age. All of the so-called primitive reflexes (grasp, snout, root, suck, and palmomental) increase in prevalence with age, but except for the grasp reflex, all of them occur frequently enough in younger normal subjects to limit their clinical value.

E. Sensation

Ability to sense vibration declines with age, again with a distal-to-proximal gradient. Normal subjects who are older than age 70 are commonly unable to detect vibration at the toes. Position, light touch, and pain sensation also deteriorate, but to a lesser degree.

IV. Common Neurologic Complaints in the Elderly

A. Dizziness

In Chapter 14, the distinction between light-headedness, vertigo, and disequilibrium was stressed. This distinction often blurs in older patients because they frequently have several coexisting problems. Arrhythmia, congestive heart failure, and orthostatic hypotension can all contribute to light-headedness, and they are all common in the geriatric population. Many of the medications that are prescribed to older patients can cause either light-headedness or vertigo. The likelihood of ischemic disease in the posterior circulation increases with advancing age. Many age-related changes in sensory function, including visual, auditory, and proprioceptive deterioration, can result in disequilibrium. When an elderly patient is able to give a clear description of a single type of symptom, the evaluation should proceed as it would in a young adult. When the history is more confusing, a careful neurologic examination should be performed with particular attention to the sensory and motor pathways that are important in maintaining balance. In many instances, dizziness is determined to be a result of many different abnormalities, each of which, in isolation, would be too mild to produce significant symptoms.

B. Gait Disturbance

The most common factors in older patients with gait difficulty are cervical stenosis, polyneuropathy, and mechanical problems such as fractures. All of the causes of disequilibrium discussed in the preceding paragraph can also interfere with walking. Other potential causes of gait disturbance that must be considered in elderly patients include parkinsonism, strokes (causing focal weakness, spasticity, or ataxia), cerebellar deterioration (most often from chronic alcohol use), and subdural hematomas (acute or chronic). Normal pressure hydrocephalus is uncommon but should always be considered because of the potential for improvement with treatment. As with dizziness, extensive evaluation of elderly patients with gait problems often reveals a number of potential causes, each of which by itself would produce only minimal symptoms but which combine to cause serious impairment.

C. *Incontinence*

Elderly patients who are incontinent should be evaluated according to the principles presented in Chapter 16. The evaluation can be particularly difficult in demented patients, who often have difficulty providing the historical information necessary to distinguish a spastic from a flaccid bladder. In these patients, diagnosis may depend on associated symptoms, physical examination findings, and results of urodynamic studies. Dementia can result in incontinence because of impairment of the normal cortical inhibition of the micturition reflex, but other causes of incontinence must also be considered. Incontinence may be the only symptom of prostatic hypertrophy or a urinary tract infection in demented patients. Medications frequently contribute to the problem also. Because gait impairment is so common in the elderly, many patients have functional incontinence caused by an inability to reach the bathroom in time. Again, the problem often proves to be a combination of many slight abnormalities, none of them severe enough in isolation to cause significant symptoms. Incontinence could occur in a moderately demented patient with low-grade peripheral neuropathy and mild cervical stenosis, for example. The most important practical objective is to determine whether any of the factors contributing to the incontinence are treatable.

D. *Dementia*

The most common dementing illnesses occur primarily in the elderly population, so the points made in Chapter 7 do not need modification here.

E. *Pain*

The principles of evaluation and management of painful conditions are the same in the elderly as in younger patients, except that older patients are more likely to have more than one painful condition simultaneously. Many chronic painful conditions are incurable, and over time these may combine with accumulated injuries and mechanical stress on the musculoskeletal system to the point where some older patients complain of constant or debilitating pain. Depression may intensify pain and complicate management. Depression is common in the elderly, and chronic pain may itself lead to depression. In addition, older patients have heightened sensitivity to the side effects of drugs, and patients with several chronic conditions are often taking multiple medications. As a result, they can develop confusion or depression, further complicating management.

A few painful conditions occur exclusively or primarily in older patients. Polymyalgia rheumatica (with or without temporal arteritis), post herpetic neuralgia, and trigeminal neuralgia are examples.

V. Discussion of Case Histories

Case 1. Although it is true that Alzheimer's disease can cause incontinence, other possible causes should also be considered, especially in patients whose cognitive impairment is as mild as this patient's. Prostate hypertrophy and urinary tract infections should always be considered. In this case, the examination strongly suggests a spinal cord lesion. There are unambiguous upper motor neuron findings in the lower extremities, indicating a lesion above the lumbar region of the spinal cord. The brisk triceps reflexes further localize the lesion to above the C7 level, whereas the diminished brachioradialis and biceps reflexes indicate that the lesion is not above C5. In short, the reflexes alone localize the lesion to the C5 or C6 level of the spinal cord. The sensory examination cannot be performed in enough detail in this patient to provide precise localizing information, but the suggestion of a sensory level is at least consistent with a spinal cord lesion. Since the patient and his family don't even seem concerned about his gait disturbance, it probably developed gradually, but his urinary symptoms are new, indicating that the spinal cord lesion is getting worse. He needs an MRI scan of the cervical spine as soon as possible. The most likely cause of cervical myelopathy in this age group is compression from herniated disks or osteophytes. Despite his age and dementia, surgery is a realistic option. He appears to be active, productive, and happy; if he were paraplegic, his quality of life would deteriorate markedly and the cost of his maintenance and medical care would rise dramatically.

If the MRI scan shows a mass lesion unrelated to degenerative disease, the imaging characteristics will determine subsequent evaluation and management (including a search for a primary cancer if the mass looks like metastatic disease, and possible steroid treatment and radiation therapy). If no mass lesion is found, nonstructural causes of myelopathy should be considered. These include vitamin B_{12} deficiency, thyroid disease, and neurosyphilis. Motor neuron disease is another consideration, but it would be more likely if there were evidence of lower motor neuron disease at a level below C6. Finally, normal pressure hydrocephalus is always a consideration when the triad of incontinence, gait disturbance, and dementia is present, but this diagnosis is unlikely, given the evidence for myelopathy on examination. Similarly, multi-infarct dementia should be considered in a patient with focal neurologic signs and dementia, but multi-infarct dementia would not explain the reflex gradient or the possible sensory level.

Case 2. This patient's pain is located in her joints, not in her distal extremities, so the cause is much more likely to be degenerative joint disease than peripheral polyneuropathy. The examination findings of absent ankle jerks and decreased distal vibratory sensation are not uncommon in the elderly. Without any other examination findings or symptoms suggestive of peripheral polyneuropathy, no further diagnostic studies are necessary.

Case 3. This patient has many problems that could potentially contribute to disequilibrium. He has impaired vision, presumably due to cataracts. He also has hearing impairment that is probably due to end-organ degeneration, suggesting that his vestibular end-organ might be similarly affected. He has reduced position sense in the lower extremities, probably due to peripheral polyneuropathy in view of the other findings on his examination. All of these sensory deficits can interfere with the ability to determine the position of the body relative to the environment, so they could all be contributing to this patient's gait disturbance.

In addition, this man now has an impaired motor response because of the mechanical limitations imposed by his hip fracture (which may have resulted from a fall caused by his unsteady gait—further questioning would be necessary to determine the cause). A hint of an upper motor neuron lesion exists as well, given the brisk knee jerks, despite evidence for a peripheral polyneuropathy. The most likely cause would be cervical myelopathy from degenerative disease. Finally, psychological factors now seem to be playing a significant role in limiting his gait. He appears to be nervous about walking even though he is not particularly unsteady.

It may prove impossible to identify which of these problems is primarily responsible for the patient's gait impairment. Indeed, each of the problems seems to be fairly mild and in isolation would be unlikely to produce significant disability. All of the problems should be addressed and treated if possible. He should be urged to follow through with the cataract surgery and also to be evaluated for a hearing aid. Although the polyneuropathy is probably due to his diabetes, other potential causes should be explored, especially thyroid disease and vitamin B_{12} deficiency, because these two treatable conditions can cause both polyneuropathy and myelopathy. With no evidence of myelopathy other than the brisk knee reflexes, no surgery would be indicated even if he had significant degenerative disease of the cervical spine, so an MRI scan is not necessary. He should have plain films of the cervical spine, however, to exclude more concerning causes of mild cord compression (e.g., metastatic disease). Finally, the patient should receive additional physical therapy to increase his confidence while walking and to prevent deconditioning. He should be reassured that no evidence of severe ongoing disease exists. Some patients restrict their walking so much because of anxiety that they ultimately develop disuse atrophy that is a more serious limitation than any of their original problems.

Index